QUALITY
IMPROVEMENT
PROJECTS IN
HEALTH CARE

QUALITY IMPROVEMENT PROJECTS IN HEALTH CARE

Problem

Solving

in the

Workplace

Eleanor Gilpatrick

SAGE Publications
International Educational and Professional Publisher
Thousand Oaks   London   New Delhi

For information:

SAGE Publications, Inc.
2455 Teller Road
Thousand Oaks, California 91320
E-mail: order@sagepub.com

SAGE Publications Ltd.
6 Bonhill Street
London EC2A 4PU
United Kingdom

SAGE Publications India Pvt. Ltd.
M-32 Market
Greater Kailash I
New Delhi 110 048 India

Printed in the United States of America

Library of Congress Cataloging-in-Publication Data

Gilpatrick, Eleanor G.
Quality improvement projects in health care: Problem solving in
   the workplace/by Eleanor Gilpatrick.
        p. cm.
Includes bibliographical references and index.
ISBN 0-7619-1166-9 (cloth: acid-free paper)
ISBN 0-7619-1167-7 (pbk.: acid-free paper)
    1. Medical care—Quality control. 2. Medical care—Evaluation.   3. Total
quality management. 4. Medical care—Quality control—Case studies.
5. Medical care—Evaluation—Case studies. 6. Total quality
management—Case studies. I. Title.
RA399.A1   G544   1998
362.1'068'5—ddc21   98-25380

This book is printed on acid-free paper.

99 00 01 02 03 04 05 10 9 8 7 6 5 4 3 2 1

Acquiring Editor: Dan Ruth
Editorial Assistant: Anna Howland
Production Editor: Sanford Robinson/Diana E. Axelsen
Editorial Assistant: Karen Wiley
Designer/Typesetter: Rose Tylak/Marion Warren
Indexer: Trish Wittenstein

Contents

Part II. Cases

List of Tables

List of Figures

Preface

This book is for problem solvers and quality improvers in health services organizations and for students preparing to join them. If you have been working or studying to improve quality as a middle-level manager, service chief, or first-line supervisor, if you have been involved in Continuous Quality Improvement (CQI) or Total Quality Management (TQM) teams, if you are associated with an organization accredited by the Joint Commission on Accreditation of Healthcare Organizations (JCAHO) or another accreditation process, or if you are aware that quality improvement is the next arena for competition in the health field, you may have found that there is a scarcity of detailed guidance on how to actually carry out quality improvement projects not already handled by a department of information management.

If you are a senior administrator, you are increasingly responsible for seeing to it that the departments and service areas of your organization engage in data collection to assure continuous quality improvement, partly in response to regulatory or accreditation requirements, and increasingly in response to consumer-based competitive pressures. Your organization may be engaged in regular collection of a selected number of process or outcome measures, but you need to train staff to carry out intensive research when the measures indicate problems to be solved—or to expand the areas in which your staff engage in quality monitoring.

There is little in the literature about how to design data collection at the departmental and interdepartmental levels to identify the extent of a problem or to determine what is causing it. You may have found that managers jump directly from problem identification to solutions without determining causes empirically, with the result that the problems often remain unsolved.

This book describes the concepts and offers a training manual for health professionals who need to deal with quality issues at the departmental or service level. It deals with data collection design and analysis related to organizational processes and outcomes—except for clinical evaluation of treatments. It acknowledges the framework set by systems such as JCAHO accreditation, fills in some important gaps, and also takes account of issues related to interpersonal communication and organizational culture. It focuses on the collection of data to find or prove the existence and extent of problems or opportunities for improvement, to identify causes, to formulate solutions, to evaluate their success, and to make them operational. The book offers a methodology, a manual, and the experience of applying the method in 14 cases—which were addressed mostly to department-level problems. The book offers guidelines to help bring the department or service area closer to accomplishing its quality objectives.

Although CQI/TQM approaches rely on leadership to disseminate the processes and philosophy of quality improvement throughout an organization, this is not yet a universal accomplishment. This book offers some tools to middle management and supervisors, helping the process to work from the bottom up as well as from the top down, something envisioned by the TQM/CQI philosophy. The book is also one that senior management might want to make available to those members of the organization who will be leading quality improvement efforts at the departmental or service level.

The approach described here was developed while the author was the director of the Master's Program in Allied Health Services Administration at the Hunter College School of Health Sciences, City University of New York. She acted as collaborator, as each student decided on a problem at work that management wanted to have studied, proved whether the problem actually existed and its extent, identified the causes, and recommended feasible solutions.

The students collaborated with coworkers and management to solve organizational problems that usually touched on quality standards formulated by the JCAHO.

In Part I, Chapter 1 offers an introduction that sets the book in the context of the quality improvement literature, accreditation requirements, standards, and indicators. It presents the concepts, terms, and definitions used in and underlying the rest of the book. Chapters 2 to 5 constitute a manual for applying the concepts; they need not be read directly after Chapter 1. They refer to the 14 cases, but it is not necessary to turn to the cases while reading these chapters. The case references are self-contained vignettes to explain the text; the cases are offered separately to illuminate specific problem situations.

Part II contains extended summaries of 14 quality improvement projects selected from the 90 supervised by the author. The summaries describe the key aspects of data collection and the solutions for each case. The emphasis is on the reasoning involved in the design of data collection and the way to choose measures and criteria to prove the existence of problems and verify their causes. The cases can serve as models for managers who have similar problems to solve. Appendix 1 is an outline for the agreement that creates the quality improvement project. Appendix 2 offers examples of detailed tabulations and some practice exercises using data collected for Case 1.

Acknowledgments

The 14 cases reported in this book were carried out by students doing advanced study projects between 1991 and 1994. The students acted as "internal consultants," in each case selecting the projects and carrying out the work. Although continuing to maintain the confidentiality of the organizations involved, I wish to acknowledge the contributions of these students, who worked hard and long to improve their organizations so that they could better serve their patients or clients. The students, in alphabetical order, were Robert M. Debbie, Janet Ghirardi, Jerry Gombo, Alexander S. Kagan, Karen Moskogianis, Tammie Murphy Topel, Gisela Perez, Yvette Robinson, Yvette L. Santana, Errol Seltzer, Linda Q. Stevens, and Anne M. Walsh. Two additional students remain anonymous for reasons of confidentiality.

I would also like to thank the friends and colleagues who read drafts of the manuscript and helped me see where I needed to make improvements. Thanks to Sylvia Feinman, Richard Gottlieb, and Everlena Holmes. Any remaining flaws are my own.

Eleanor Gilpatrick
Hunter College, New York

PART
I

Basic Concepts
and Manual

CHAPTER
ONE

Basic Concepts

Introduction

This book is addressed to the vast army of caring health professionals who, as middle-level managers, supervisors, service chiefs,
quality assurance officers, or quality improvement team members,
combine the search for quality with the need for efficiency; to the senior
managers who are responsible for training staff to carry out continuous
quality improvement; and to the students who will be entering their
ranks.

If you are a middle-level manager in a health service organization
or are involved in quality improvement, you are under constant pressure to solve problems or find opportunities for improvement. You
balance the often conflicting interests of several constituencies, which
management literature calls "stakeholders." You find how best to serve
your particular clients, whether they are called patients, residents, or
consumers or are other departments or professionals who use your
outputs. You consider the needs of your staff, and you may also
interface with the suppliers of the technology that your service or
department uses.

You may be involved with managed care and competitive pressures, expected to keep costs down in the face of prospective payment
systems, managed-care negotiated rates, budget reductions, and
downsizing. You are expected to be fair and to represent the needs of

your staff. You are expected to evaluate new technology while responding to an increasingly critical and articulate consumer population. You are expected to demonstrate improvement of quality as the marketplace brings consumer satisfaction into the arena of competition and because that is among the standards used to evaluate and accredit your organization . . . and you still remember when you chose your career because you wanted to help people.

This book is offered to help *you* with the details involved in evaluating and improving the quality of processes and outcomes in your department or service. It is meant to supplement the guidelines already provided in sources such as the accreditation manuals of the Joint Commission on Accreditation of Healthcare Organizations (JCAHO) and similar quality improvement systems. It adds a level of detail about problem identification and cause verification without which the specifics of data design and collection may be daunting.

Structure of This Book

Part I of this book offers a methodology for research design and data collection to solve operational problems and improve quality. The methodology emerged over a period of 10 years, during which time the author collaborated with 90 health service professionals working in a variety of service delivery organizations. They worked in hospitals, nursing homes, HMOs, municipal health departments, emergency medical services, intermediate care facilities, and home health care agencies and in diverse service areas such as nursing, physical therapy, radiation therapy, pharmacy, medical laboratory, quality assurance, and information services. They also happened to be master's students in health care administration and the author's students.

Each set out to solve a problem or improve quality in the immediate work situation. The problems included excess waiting, errors, omissions, nonperformance, and patient noncompliance. As Deming (1986) indicated, the causes were rarely "people"; they were usually institutional flaws that the organization could change if it had the will to change. As the experiences accumulated, a methodology emerged to carry out the steps needed to run a successful quality improvement project. The first step was always to clarify the problem situation. The second was to prove the existence of the problem and determine its extent through data collection. The third step was to identify the actual causes of the problem through data collection and analysis. The fourth step was to find appropriate and acceptable solutions for the problem. The fifth step was to implement and evaluate the solutions, and the sixth was to make successful solutions operational; in more recent situations, that included recommendations for the ongoing collection of process or outcome indicators.

The best projects were successful because they included rigorous attention to data collection and analytic detail; they were careful to involve staff, who gave input on causes and, particularly, feedback on proposed solutions; they enlisted management in the selection or approval of proofs and predetermined standards or criteria of quality. The projects were generally carried out by middle-level managers. Less senior staff who took the initiative to suggest projects were also able to conduct successful projects, but they were less able to carry them all the way through to implementation.

This methodology is presented within a context in which accreditation agencies such as the JCAHO set standards for systematic quality improvement procedures throughout the organization and expect health care organizations to collect indicator data about some of their key processes and outcomes. To help guide the reader through a complicated set of concepts, Figure 1.1 presents an abbreviated glossary of terms that are used throughout this book. They are more fully developed later in this chapter.

Part I is the conceptual framework for the method and a manual. Chapter 1 provides some background about the concepts involved in Total Quality Management (TQM) and Continuous Quality Improvement (CQI) and about the relationship of those ideas to accreditation requirements. It outlines the steps of data collection design that this book may serve to enrich and presents the relationship of this methodology to JCAHO standards. There follows a presentation of other basic definitions used in the book.

Chapters 2 through 5 are a manual for use in quality improvement projects; the examples draw on experiences from many cases in which the methods were applied. Mention of the cases presented in Part II does not require the reader to turn to the cases; the discussions are self-contained. Works cited in Part I appear at the end of Chapter 5.

Part II presents 14 cases that offer a wide assortment of problem-solving situations and organizations, with explanations of how the methods were applied. The reader can match her or his own situation

Cause: A circumstance, characteristic, or attitude that creates the problem.

Consultant: An individual or group asked to use their expertise to deal with problems in the organization.

Enabling objective (process objective): An event or output(s) that must be produced or accomplished to reach a project objective.

Evaluation: Determining the extent to which objectives are achieved or goals are reached. It involves some measure or success criterion that makes it possible to compare actual results with expected results or standards.

Indicator: A quantitative measure of an aspect of care that represents a level of performance of functions, processes, and outcomes in the organization. Generally a rate, ratio, or percentage that can be compared from one organization to another.

Long-range goal: A desired result related to the problem that is not expected to be accomplished within the time period of the project.

Method: A procedure for achieving a desired result or objective.

Objective: A result that the project is designed to reach, expressed in measurable terms.

Outcome: The result of care from the point of view of the patient; the result of the performance or nonperformance of a function or process.

Problem: Any situation that keeps the organization from meeting its goals, such as a desired level of quality in service or consumer satisfaction. The project is designed to deal with it.

Project objective: A result to be brought about within the period of the project, corresponding to a project question.

Project question: A generic research issue that must be dealt with to understand or deal with the problem. Information that is not yet known. A question that generates major steps to be carried out by the project.

Quality assessment: The evaluation of the care provided by organizations, covering structure, processes, and outcomes.

Quality improvement project (usually referred to as *project*). The specific scope of activities agreed on between the internal consultant and the client to deal with a problem, normally including proving that the problem exists and, if it exists, its extent; identifying and proving causes; finding solutions; implementing and testing solutions; and making the solutions operational. This corresponds to the stage referred to as intensive assessment.

Reference database (performance measurement system): A performance-measuring system tailored to the services and data-gathering resources of the organization, organized to collect comparable data from a network of organizations, thus permitting comparisons of the individual organization's performance on indicators with the group as a whole or with comparable organizations.

Solution: A change that addresses a cause so that the problem is eliminated or reduced.

Standards: Expectations or requirements against which current and future performance is measured. They can refer to structure, process, or outcomes.

Success criterion: A standard with which to measure whether objectives have been accomplished.

Figure 1.1   Brief Definitions of Terms Used in This Book

and perhaps find a model to follow. After the Appendixes, there is a list of sources used by the internal consultants to find ideas about causes and solutions. Appendix 1 is an outline for a project proposal. Appendix 2 presents detailed tabulation models and data from Case 1 and practice exercises for the reader.

Why Another Book About Quality Improvement?

This is not a book about Continuous Quality Improvement or Total Quality Management. It is a book that offers detailed guidelines for the design and data collection aspects of quality improvement projects. There is a vast literature about improving quality in industry in general and in the health services in particular. That literature describes a systems approach that is responsive to customers' needs, promotes interdepartmental cooperation, increases understanding of the functioning of the organization, and encourages employee participation in improvement processes. A good deal of the material flows from the work of W. Edwards Deming (1986), Joseph M. Juran (Juran & Gryna, 1974), and Philip B. Crosby (1979). The systems that have been developed to reflect the work go by many names but are primarily referred to as Continuous Quality Improvement (CQI) and Total Quality Management (TQM), although technically, TQM is a broader concept.

The philosophy underlying these systems is described as having brought about a paradigm shift in the way quality management is viewed because it assumes an ongoing, institutional commitment at every level and a mutual relationship between managers and employees. The approach seeks the causes of problems by looking at *why* rather than *who* and does not assume that errors and omissions are inevitably part of production (Rakich, Longest, & Darr, 1992).

Deming located the source of quality at the point of production rather than in after-the-fact inspection. Quality must be built in. Deming also attributed the bulk of problems to processes rather than to people, so the employee's fear of being blamed is transformed into the desire to find out why things go wrong. Juran enlisted the resources, knowledge, and experience of staff, first-line supervisors, and the managers directly involved in production to identify problems and their solutions. Ishikawa (1990) made the creation of a work environment that elicits employee participation in quality, productivity, and morale a cornerstone of the work. Crosby (1979) insisted that performance standards could and should allow "zero defects."

The TQM/CQI orientation toward the consumer and an institution-wide commitment to quality is reflected in the JCAHO's move from a quality assurance stance, finding flaws, to the 1990s shift to quality improvement and the development of quality output indicators. The JCAHO mandated the application of quality improvement processes in hospitals, and the National Committee for Quality Assurance (NCQA) is attempting to bring a similar consciousness to managed care organizations. In the mid-1990s, the JCAHO embarked on a path intended to include the collection and reporting of outcome indicators, an addition to standards-based evaluation, as a requirement for all accredited health care organizations (Nadzam, Turpin, Hanold, & White, 1993; McGreevey, Nadzam, & Corbin, 1997).

The management philosophy of CQI/TQM has not been universally adopted, nor does it permeate the experience of all health service providers. A given middle-level manager may or may not be in an organization that is committed to CQI or TQM. In a period of mergers, cutbacks, and staff reductions, the spirit of CQI/TQM is hard to maintain. But by virtue of taking part in accreditation processes, the organization is applying some of those concepts. And the pressure is there, if only through market forces, to participate in quality improvement of some sort.

The CQI paradigm assumes that the organization will decide on a clinical area or process to assess and will organize a team to study it whose members are already familiar with the processes and able to understand the ways the processes may break down. The team is expected to identify relevant performance guidelines or standards, find a way to measure adherence to the guidelines or standards, collect data, evaluate the results, select a solution, and evaluate its success, which includes the selection of indicators with which to monitor adherence to the new solution. It is assumed that the team will be able to collect data about the important variables involved, analyze the data, and come up with appropriate improvements.

This book offers guidelines to verify whether a process needs improvement or a problem needs solving; it outlines the steps that can be used to understand the process, including enlistment of employees at crucial stages; it describes how to collect data, especially how to identify and evaluate potential causes, and how to select a solution. It speaks to managers and students who are preparing to enter the field of health services, assuming little background or formal training in administration or statistics.

Health administration literature does not deal with the details of how to design organizational research and data collection to assess problems, how to identify causes, or how to come up with appropriate solutions. For example, the list below is a compilation of tools and techniques from several sources, but rarely are they set into a sequence of logical steps.

1. Events logs record unusual or unwanted occurrences.
2. Control charts show variations in the work process plotted with statistically calculated demarcations of normal upper and lower acceptable limits, such as standard deviations around an average.
3. Flow charts and diagrams explicate production sequences to help the user understand a process.
4. Cause-and-effect Ishikawa (fishbone) diagrams visualize the causes of a central problem (the fishhead) as skeletal branches organized under various broad categories, such as equipment, policies, procedures, methods, and people, and sometimes culture, information, machines, materials, facilities, or the environment.
5. Check sheets are rendered as tables, matrixes, or charts whose columns need only use checkmark entries to verify the presence of items.
6. Pareto diagrams or charts show cumulative percentages and are used to portray the relative contributions to problems of various components in the production process.
7. Frequency distributions show the distribution of variables.
8. Run charts offer time-series data to help the user spot trends.
9. Regression analysis or scatter diagrams show relationships between variables.

The JCAHO (1997a) suggests the use of flow charts, run charts, control charts, and histograms. Some authors do a good job of explaining the tools, such as White and McLaughlin (1992), Amsden (1991), and Johnson and McLaughlin (1994). However, the list does not constitute an integrated methodology. Goonan (1995) suggests the use of "the scientific method and basic diagnostic tools (flow diagrams, simple data collection, cause-and-effect diagnosis, and so on) to uncover the root causes of deficiencies" (p. 141). This involves analysis of performance patterns, identification of below-standard outcomes and processes, formulation of hypotheses about the causes, and testing hypotheses with simple, brief data collection or analysis of existing data; little further explanation about how to do that is included.

The literature sometimes assumes that "someone" is already prepared to design and organize the research and data collection. Orlikoff and Snow (1984) had a facilitator for the quality circle who understood "statistics and basic research design methodology" (p. 9). They acknowledged that "There is little specific training or information available" to aid in verifying causes "other than vague suggestions to review the data collection techniques in the hope that ways to verify the problem's cause will be suggested. It is at this stage that more complicated statistical analysis might benefit the activities" (p. 24). Gitlow and Gitlow (1994) refer to process improvement leaders, Ziegenfuss (1993) calls for the consultation skills of a specialist, and Leebov and Ersoz (1991) have a manager turned *quality manager* (p. 15).

What seems to be missing is material that shows how to design data collection in simple language, that does not presuppose training in advanced statistics, that is process oriented, that covers all the intermediary steps from naming a problem to putting a solution into place, and that can be carried out whether or not a CQI/TQM atmosphere has been established.

This book tries to do that. It offers an experience-based set of guidelines for operational quality improvement and also reports on the experiences of 14 health services professionals who worked as internal consultants to improve the quality of work in their departments. The guidelines are presented as a practical tool for practitioners, regardless of whether their organizations have adopted or maintained the TQM/CQI management philosophy or have assimilated JCAHO or similar standards.

The JCAHO and Quality Improvement

History

By the early 1990s, the health care industry was turning towards quality improvement mechanisms such as TQM and CQI. The Joint Commission's manuals did not insist that health care organizations adopt CQI or TQM systems, but by virtue of the standards, the scoring, and the quality improvement manuals that became part of the accreditation process, CQI/TQM concepts and processes were being incorporated into the functioning of compliant health care organizations. The underlying assumption is that most problems or opportunities for improvement can be traced to weaknesses in processes rather than inadequacies of individuals and that patients and staff need to be consulted about what quality characteristics they consider important; they should also be asked about their satisfaction with outcomes and ideas for improvement.

The JCAHO's accreditation manuals are designed for self-assessment and are the basis for reports by JCAHO surveyors. The JCAHO's (1990) *Accreditation Manual for Hospitals, 1991* aimed to create standards that would address important clinical and managerial functions that are key to quality patient care and to "foster improvement in these areas" (p. iii).

The years 1990 through 1997 marked a transition from standards that indicate capability (structure) to a focus on process performance and outcomes. "Doing the right things and doing them well" is a phrase repeated in each edition of the JCAHO manual. This emphasis reflects a shift in attention to patient care and organizational management. There was also a shift to functional rather than departmental groupings of standards. The functions include assessment of patients; entry to setting or service; nutritional care; treatment; operative and other invasive procedures; education of patients and family; coordination of care; rights of patients; organizational ethics; leadership; management of information; management of human resources; management of the environment of care; the surveillance, prevention, and control of infection; and the improvement of organizational performance. Separate sections present structural standards for organizational governing bodies, management and administration, medical staff, and nursing. The reference to generic functions makes uniform standards across departments and services possible.

Between 1990 and 1997, the number of standards for hospitals was reduced by over 80% (JCAHO, 1997a, p. FW-1). The new standards are expressed as generic performance objectives. Much of the earlier prescriptive detail is shifted to sections dealing with the intent of the standards, implementation examples, appropriate evidence of performance, and scoring guidelines. The organization is given the opportunity to explain to JCAHO its rationales for strategies, so if it can show how it achieves an objective, it can use methods not in the manual and be in compliance.

The manual is seen as a "synthesis of important concepts and methods that health care organizations should utilize as starting points in their pursuit of excellence" (JCAHO, 1993, p. xi). The 1994 issue put the user community on notice that "performance expectations will begin to rise progressively in 1995 and the years that follow" (JCAHO, 1993, p. iii).

The completely revised hospital standards appeared in the 1997 single-volume subscription binder-format manual; it is now updated quarterly, combining standards, examples of implementation, types of evidence, and scoring guidelines in each of the function chapters. Now called the *Comprehensive Accreditation Manual for Hospitals: The Official Handbook* (*CAMH*), the manual's standards are described as being "patient centered, performance focused, and organized around functions common to all hospitals and other health care organizations" (JCAHO, 1997a, p. IN-3). It is the JCAHO's expectation that "any future standards revisions will be made only in response to changes in the health care field or to quality of care issues" (1997a, p. IN-4).

The approach requires organizationwide coordination and integration of quality improvement activities and functions. Individual departments need to look for their standards throughout the *CAMH*. The movement from 1990 to 1997 emphasized the need for "all hospital staff [to] be given the opportunity to view the contents of the manual" (JCAHO, 1997b, p. UM-2). Information management and commitments to ongoing quality improvement are now among the accreditation standards.

By 1997, accreditation standards asked senior management to assure the systematic assessment and improvement of performance, selection of improvement priorities, systematic improvement of the performance of important functions, and assurance of the stability of those functions. Specific standards ask for proof of collaboration among departments, services, and professional groups; coordination of quality improvement activities; assignment of personnel and allocation of time as needed to participate in performance-improvement activities; and staff training in the approaches and methods of performance improvement.

Measurement on a continuing basis is called for—measurement of both processes and outcomes—and assessment of individual competence and performance. This means that data must be collected both for special areas chosen for improvement and as part of a continuing measurement program.

The calendar for accreditation is moving from a survey every 3 years, for which hospitals go into a flurry of activity periodically with interim returns to business as usual, to "continuous accreditation." The hope is that organizations will monitor and improve performance as a regular part of day-to-day operations and be more continually aware of their performance and success in their improvement efforts. They will also be involved in interorganizational comparisons.

In the future, "every accredited hospital will be required to participate in an approved performance measurement system(s). The performance data will be used in the accreditation process" to assist with monitoring between surveys, in planning, and in conducting the on-site survey (JCAHO, 1997a, p. IN-7). An organization will participate in a regional, performance-measuring system (called a *reference database*) organized to collect data from many organizations that can be used to compare performance across organizations. The JCAHO compiles lists of approved reference databases. An individual organization will be able to choose any of the approved measurement systems, one of which is the JCAHO's own IMSystem. There were 60 reference databases listed in the 1997 *CAMH*.

The use of reference databases is expected to "eventually produce feedback loops and correlations to permit the continuous improvement of both standards and performance measures" (JCAHO, 1997a, p. FW-1). Participation in the collection of interorganizational outcome indicators will find many organizations stretching to adapt their organizations well into the 21st century.

The JCAHO Quality Improvement Paradigm

The JCAHO's standards for quality improvement provide a systematic set of procedures that any organization can follow, but they also leave some gaps that this book attempts to fill. The standards ask that the organization adopt a performance measurement system (reference database) and use its indicators to assist in meeting accreditation standards. This assumes that some indicators are in use, but it also includes the possibility that the organization will examine many other processes with indicators created and collected by the individual organization, because the organization is expected to be systematic in its approach to redesigning current processes or acting on opportunities for incremental improvement. The recommended sequence is shown below. Comments in brackets indicate the areas addressed by this book.

1. Management *sets priorities* and selects an area or function for improvement.

2. Management *identifies* specific performance expectations or goals and establishes one or more *performance measures* (indicators) against which the results of improvement interventions can be judged.

3. *Selected indicators* are used to *examine whether there is a problem or an opportunity for improvement*. A comparison is made with past performance and trends in the organization's own data, with indicator rates of comparable organizations, or with recognized standards. If unacceptable or improvable results are found, more *intensive assessment* is considered appropriate. [This is when the guidelines presented in this book are appropriate. The book describes how to carry out such intensive assessment.]

4. An *examination of the process or outcome* is undertaken to provide an understanding of the variables (causes) that may affect or influence the indicator level. The use of "root-cause analysis" is expected to provide detailed information about the process or outcome being studied. [There are no detailed guidelines. This book offers a set of guidelines.]

5. The *specific underlying factors* that may have led to the indicator rate *are identified*. This is expected to result in finding some that are under the organization's control. [This book offers a checklist of possible causes and detailed guidelines for finding and proving causes.]

6. *Selecting and testing an improvement intervention* involves narrowing the list of potential causes and possible solutions to focus on the most relevant factors capable of being influenced or changed. [This is another place where this book has something to offer. Not only are there guidelines for testing *all* possible causes, but a process for selecting solutions is also presented.]

a. *Developing a plan to test an improvement intervention* (solution) includes determining who will be involved in the testing and what education they will require. [This book speaks to that.]
b. Management *involves* relevant individuals, professions, and departments in improvement activities and *identifies* the actions to be taken. [This book speaks to that.]
c. *A plan is developed to test an improvement intervention (solution).* This includes determining who will be involved in the testing and what education they will require. [This book speaks to that.]
d. *A timetable is established for the test* to provide an adequate period for the evaluation. [This book speaks to that.]
e. The intervention and how *it will be tested* is described, as well as what the proof of a successful test will be. A way to ascertain that the test is appropriately and consistently conducted is also described. [This book speaks to that.]

7. *Observing the effects of the intervention* involves continued collection of indicator data as before, to make comparisons possible. The original and new indicator data are compared and related to the success criteria. [This book speaks to that.]

8. *Communicating the results* of the intervention follows. [This book speaks to that.]

9. *Implementing the intervention* (making it operational) follows if the solution is successful. Reversion to the original list of possible causes and redesign of another solution is recommended if the change does not meet the goals set for it. [Returning to the original list and repeating the process is not an efficient option. It can be avoided by the method proposed in this book, which provides a methodology to test *all* possible causes as actual causes.]

10. *Periodic monitoring of the intervention* follows to provide continued assessment and ensure that improved performance is maintained at a desired level over time. This can include *adopting new performance measures* (indicators) if the ones used were created for the project. [This book speaks to that.]

Concepts, Terms, and Definitions

In most disciplines, ordinary words are given technical meanings that precisely express what the speaker or writer wishes to convey. This section provides the basic ideas, terms, and definitions used in the rest of the book. Figure 1.1, presented earlier, is a glossary containing brief definitions of the important terms used in this book. The text below elaborates on their meanings, beginning with terms associated with quality assessment and measurement.

Quality Assessment

Quality can only be measured indirectly. *Quality assessment* is the evaluation of the care provided by an organization. Donabedian (1978, 1980, 1982, 1985) distinguished among three areas that have been used for assessment: structure, process, and outcome. In the health field, quality assessment has been the subject of long, arduous efforts to bring it from indirect structural measures to a closer measurement of the actual quality of the health care provided.

Structural assessment of quality looks at whether the organization is capable of delivering quality care. It refers to the adequacy of plant, equipment, and technology; to the qualifications of staff; to safety and governance; and to policies which, when provided, indicate the potential for the delivery of quality care. Structure has been the easiest to measure and evaluate and marked the earliest approaches to accreditation. In 1996, quality assessment of managed care organizations was criticized for being largely structural in nature (Consumers Union, 1996). But even in 1997, some structural aspects of care were still considered important, such as governance of the institution and medical staff organization, organizational rules, regulations, credentialing requirements, and documented policies.

Process assessment looks at what is done and how well it is done. The focus is on performance. Process is evaluated in terms of standards and protocols established by expert professionals and the degree of compliance with them. The quality level of performance deals with whether what is done is: relevant and appropriate for the patient; done well; made available in a timely manner to patients who need it; effective under usual as well as ideal circumstances; continuous with other care and care providers; and performed in a way that is safe, efficient, caring, and respectful of the patient. These are the *dimensions* of quality performance (JCAHO, 1993, p. 51). Steps prior to the direct provision of care, such as housekeeping, laboratory, and pharmacy activities, can also be evaluated in terms of what is done and how well it is done.

Outcome assessment looks at the results of care from the point of view of the consumer or patient. An *outcome* is the result of the performance or nonperformance of a function or process. It describes the effects on the recipient of the health care. But outcomes are not necessarily the best indicators of quality. Donabedian (1978) noted that "It is not true that outcomes are a more valid measure of quality than is process" (p. 5). To be valid, outcome measures must relate to the antecedent processes of care. "Fundamentally, validity depends on the strength of the relationship between process and outcome, and on our understanding of that relationship" (p. 5).

Outcomes data indicate where the system is falling down from the point of view of the consumer, but it is management's responsibility to find out why. That means another level of measurement, one geared to uncovering the connection between processes, risk factors, and outcomes. Outcome indicators can show whether an organization has a good track record, but it is necessary to know what process standards are needed to achieve good and avoid bad outcomes. Then it is necessary to find out whether the standards are being met and if not, why not. "You need to get underneath the data and find out why something happened" (O'Leary, 1993, p. 490).

Standards

Standards are expectations or requirements against which performance is measured. They can refer to structure, process, or outcomes. JCAHO standards purport to define the structures, functions, and processes needed to achieve good patient outcomes. They not only name the processes or functions but include threshold criteria or limits for what acceptable performance is. The assumption is that "How well an organization performs its primary functions has a large bearing on patient outcomes, the cost of providing effective and appropriate services, and the eventual health status of the population served" (JCAHO, 1997a, p. USI-1).

Indicators

An *indicator* is a quantitative measurement that represents the level of performance of a function, process, or outcome. In the health field, an indicator relates to an aspect of patient care. An indicator might measure patients' length of stay, the number of falls per thousand patient days, the percentage of patients waiting for a procedure beyond an acceptable period, the percentage of newborn deliveries by cesarean section, or the number of deaths within a certain number of days after a surgical procedure. Generally expressed as a rate, ratio, or percentage, an indicator can be compared from one organization to another. When compared with established criteria, an indicator can identify areas that are not doing well and warrant more detailed analysis. Although indicators report on past performance, they can trigger exploration of causes which, when found, can result in system changes that are likely to improve future care.

Outcome indicators can help consumers make decisions about health care providers. Health care organizations can use them as a basis for improving processes and outcomes, for learning what works and what does not, and for evaluating changes; agencies such as the JCAHO use them as a basis for accreditation; and policy makers use them to evaluate the health care system. Thus, outcome indicators are a common interest of consumers and providers. The terms *quality indicator* and *report card* refer to indicators that are expected to help consumers and others decide among health care plans and providers.

Recent concern with health care reform and the public's response to developments in the health care system have focused attention on outcomes. Seemingly the most important, outcome measures have been the most difficult to define, validate, and apply. Outcome indicators measure what has happened to the patient, but what happens sometimes has little to do with the actual quality of the care received. Outcomes are partly determined by the characteristics of the patient, such as risk factors, as well as the contribution of health care professionals to the various stages through which the care progresses. The characteristics of consumers can make them more or less prone to better or worse outcomes. Socioeconomic factors such as race, income, and education are directly related to outcomes, as are psychological factors, attitudes toward health care, the presence of other health conditions, and the extent of insurance coverage.

Factors that are in the hands of providers include whether "the right things are done and whether they are done right." *Process indicators* measure the adequacy of admissions procedures, assessment of the patient's condition, diagnosis, selection of treatment, administering of treatment, management of care, assessment of treatment effectiveness, discharge planning, discharge, and follow-up care. Brook, Kamberg, and McGlynn (1996) consider process indicators to be more sensitive measures of quality because incorrect procedures or omissions of procedures do not always show up as negative outcomes.

In a sense, outcomes, processes, and structures stand in cause-and-effect relationship to one another. The *outcomes* are the end results of the services delivered, such as whether disease has been cured or prevented, whether symptoms have been controlled or ameliorated, whether function has been regained, whether respect for autonomy has been maintained, and whether the patients and/or providers have been kept safe. Inadequate performance of *processes* can be shown to be causes of inadequate outcomes and therefore become correctable problems or opportunities for improvement. The causes of process problems can be related to the design of procedures and/or the presence or absence of essential materials, equipment, plant, or policy. Identifying inadequacies in these areas is the objective of *structural standards*. Structural standards are therefore necessary underpinnings for process, which in turn is necessary for outcomes. None of these levels of quality assessment are direct measures of quality; the relationship of each to the real effects of health care has to be validated for given situations.

Standards and indicators complement each other. Together, they can comprise a comprehensive evaluation system able to predict an organization's future performance (JCAHO, 1997a, pp. USI-1,2). As an example, an *accreditation standard* under patient rights is that the organization "addresses advance directives." The organization must prove that it determines whether patients have or wish to make advance directives and provides assistance to patients who do not have an advance directive but wish to formulate one. A possible *structural standard* to prove compliance is that there are policies and procedures in place that require that patients be told their rights to make advance directives. Proof that staff members are given training in this area would meet a *process standard*. An *outcome indicator* might be the percentage of patients in a specific period of time after admission whose medical records contain advance directives or evidence of a discussion about advance directives. (This standard and its quality indicators was the subject of Case 11, in Part II, in the context of a home health care agency.)

Use of Indicators

Lansky (1993) has suggested that "As the importance of indicator data grows, providers will face a corresponding burden to improve their ability to gather sound data during the course of care, in all practice settings and with the fewest possible intermediaries (for example, transcriptionists, coders, abstractors, entry clerks)" (pp. 549-550).

Solberg, Mosser, and McDonald (1997) warn that the development of indicator data may be confounded if organizations try to satisfy three different and conflicting purposes and collect the same data or use the same methods for all three. The first purpose, *accountability to consumers and regulatory agencies*, usually requires outcome measures that do not in themselves indicate the causes or the solutions to the problems they uncover. The second purpose, *quality improvement*, usually requires process data to identify problems or opportunities for improvement, to obtain baseline measurements of the nature and extent of the problem, and to provide comparison data for the evaluation of changes. (Note that outcome measures for accountability purposes *can* be designed to identify problems or opportunities for improvement. That is one of the objectives of the JCAHO IMSystem.) The third purpose, *clinical research*, usually requires data to test hypotheses about the accuracy of diagnostic procedures, the success of treatments, or the efficacy of other medical innovations or practices.

Accountability data must address desired or undesired outcomes. The definitions and time references must be comparable across institutions so that systemwide, areawide, and nationwide comparisons can be made. *Quality improvement* data must be specific to the institution, detailed, and limited to realistic time periods. The data for identifying a problem and evaluating solutions must be comparable; data to identify causes must be collected if adequate solutions are to be found. *Clinical research* must comply with scientific standards for sample design, requires large numbers of cases, and usually involves a great deal of time and funds. Confusing the standards for evaluation, precision, and sample size for *clinical research* with the less rigorous standards for *quality improvement* can hamper the collection of improvement data because of the view that proper data collection is too expensive and time consuming (Solberg et al., 1997).

Disclosure needs also differ according to purpose. The audience for accountability data includes consumers, payors, and regulatory agencies. Aside from accreditation agencies, there is pressure for disclosure. For example, since 1986, the Health Care Financing Administration has released Medicare mortality reports for hospitals, listing them by name. In contrast, the audience for improvement data is internal to the organization. Solberg et al. (1997) note that the different audiences and objectives for accountability and improvement data may create conflicts. As accountability and clinical research data are of necessity subject to eventual public disclosure, even if not when first collected, there is a built-in bias to "game" the data so that the organization "looks good."

On the other hand, quality improvement data require that the worst practices be uncovered so that they can be changed. The quality improvement approach concentrates on process and not on people; thus the tendency to game because of the fear of being blamed is minimized. "The most powerful improvements usually come from an understanding of processes and from efforts to systematize them, not from . . . exhortation of individuals" (Solberg et al., 1997, p. 138).

Reference databases are in increasing use. As independent performance measurement systems that collect indicator data tailored to the services and data-gathering resources of the member organizations, they are organized to compare data among network members. They make possible comparisons of the individual organization's performance with the group as a whole or with comparable organizations. However, the organization is still faced with the need to collect data about many other processes.

The outcome indicators in the JCAHO's IMSystem and other reference databases are so limited in number and so far down the process pipeline that it will still be necessary for the individual health care organization to collect additional data for its own use, to identify problems at process stages throughout the organization. This is the *intensive assessment* stage. Intensive assessment can mean obtaining detailed data on the extent of a problem and on possible causes so that proper selection and evaluation of solutions can follow. The organization is thereby in a position to try out its own outcome indicators, to trace problems back to process causes, to make improvements, and to then be in good shape to be evaluated in relation to other organizations once comparative data are collected. This is a form of "gaming" the system that could have benefits for all concerned.

Consultant

The terms and concepts that follow deal specifically with the quality improvement projects that are the subject of this book. A *consultant* is usually a specialist asked by an organization to help with a problem it is facing, including how to improve the quality of its outputs. This book uses the term *internal consultant* to mean a single individual, a Quality Improvement Team, a whole department, or any group that identifies quality-related problems, collects data, finds the causes, and shows how to come up with, implement, and operationalize solutions.

Any individual or group asked to engage in such work fills the function of an internal consultant because the work serves the entire organization rather than a particular department or service. An *external consultant* is someone from the outside brought in by top-level management. However, a consultant need not be brought in from the outside. Someone within the organization, an internal consultant, may be asked to deal with problems in the organization.

In either case, the consultant is asked to take a fresh look at a situation, to step back, and to take a wider view. Whole departments may function as internal consultants, helping other departments solve problems. Human Resources and Information Services have consultant functions. A department of Quality Assurance, Quality Management, Quality Improvement, or a related term serves as an internal consultant. CQI/TQM Teams created to deal with specific problems, or individual managers or supervisors who decide to deal with specific problems or improvement opportunities, act as internal consultants.

External consultants have no vested interest in the results; may be able to take a fresh, objective view of the whole situation; and are not affected by past unsuccessful attempts to solve the problem; however, they may not receive access to all the relevant information, may be hindered if staff distrust them, may not have time to get the full picture, may recommend a set of solutions developed for other clients, and do not have to live with the results.

The internal consultant, whether an individual or a team, knows the organization, the staff, and the culture of the organization; expects to be there to live with the consequences of the solutions; and may be able to find solutions that fit the unique characteristics of the organization. Middle-level managers, as internal consultants or as users of internal consultants, can help assure that the work of the consultant is what is desired. The internal consultant can talk with staff so that staff have a chance to learn what will happen and to anticipate change. When people are involved in the process, they are more apt to accept the results.

A senior manager may ask the consultant or team to identify improvement opportunities or problems. Indicator data may have been examined and may show an unacceptable level or trend in performance. The level may be unacceptable compared with absolute standards of performance, such as requiring 100% accuracy in administration of medications; compared with past performance, such as prior near-zero rates of patient falls; compared with other organizations, such as higher rates of voluntary HIV testing among prenatal patients in comparable organizations; or in comparison with standards in the literature, such as smoking cessation rates or national data on vaginal births after a cesarean section. Another spur to initiation of a quality improvement project may be the desire to improve currently acceptable or good performance. A manager or a CQI team may select a process area to improve.

The problem may be an issue such as patients waiting too long for services, patient noncompliance with treatment plans, high rehospitalization rates, improper procedures that produce errors, or something else going wrong or not at optimal levels. The consultant or team is responsible for finding solutions. Solutions require change, and because people generally do not really like or want change, the consultant may also have to help with implementation.

To properly carry out the work, the consultant is required to exercise *leadership*. Leadership is not the same as power, which minimizes the need for leadership. It is the ability to exercise *influence*. It is most required when other people's jobs are not clearly and narrowly defined, when the chain of command is informal, and when the leader has little direct power over the people to be influenced. In most cases, this all applies to the consultant. Whether the consultant is an individual or a team, leadership is exercised through communication and cooperation.

The leader exercises *responsibility* by being able to visualize and be concerned about the consequences of situations for others. To embark on a course leading to change requires the consultant to understand attitudes towards change. When an organization comes into existence, it starts out with a mission to serve its customers, but another purpose quickly comes into being as a motivating force. That is *to survive*. Management and staff can lose track of whom they serve and why, and the organization can function to perpetuate itself. This is especially true for areas such as support services, whose staffs do not see the ultimate population being served. They can be detached from results and feel little stake in quality issues. If they just see the immediate activity, continuing to do what they usually do becomes an end in itself; they lose a sense of responsibility and concern about the people they are serving. If the philosophy of continuous quality improvement has not permeated the organizations as intended by JCAHO standards, the consultant may have to reawaken the sense of responsibility.

The consultant also needs to consider *collaborative planning*, which implies that the planner work with the other people involved as equals. Planning with subordinates or superordinates creates an experience very different from planning with equals, because equals can say "no" and there is no recourse except through leadership. The advantage of collaborative planning is that, if they have been involved as equals, people feel a greater stake in making the plans work. They take responsibility. Collaborative planning can, however, produce dissension if it involves people who are not immediately involved, who are incompetent, or who have strongly negative attitudes.

Ulschak and SnowAntle (1990) divide consultants into those who are process facilitators and those who are technical, task-oriented individuals concerned with problem solving. A process facilitator helps the client carry out the communication processes that make it possible to solve a problem. The task-oriented specialist is more focused on carrying out the research work needed to come up with and implement solutions. This book is geared to the latter function, in which the consultant is involved with the research needed to find and implement solutions. However, to be successfully task oriented, the consultant may also have to use process facilitation skills.

The Quality Improvement Project

The JCAHO uses the term *intensive assessment* to refer to the process of identifying a performance area to improve, finding causes, finding solutions (improvement interventions), implementing and testing them, and making them operational. This book uses the term *quality improvement project*, or simply *project*, in the same way. The quality improvement project refers to the specific scope of activities to deal with a problem agreed on between the internal consultant and the client (management). It normally includes proving that the problem exists and its extent, identifying and proving causes, finding solutions, implementing and testing solutions, and making them operational.

Problems

Quality problems and improvement opportunities will be referred to as *problems*. A *problem* is any situation that keeps the organization from meeting its goals, such as a desired level of performance or consumer satisfaction. It is worth bothering about because it deals with the needs of the people the institution serves or of the staff who perform the services. Examples of problems are patients waiting too long to start physical therapy or postsurgery cancer patients not making appointments for prescribed follow-up visits. The function of quality improvement projects is to solve structural, process, and outcome problems or to act on improvement opportunities.

It is useful to distinguish between quality problems and the research problems addressed by quality improvement projects. To avoid confusion, the term *project questions* is used to mean the generic research issues with which the consultant will deal during the project.

Examples of project questions are: Does the problem actually exist, and what is its extent? What are the causes of the problem? What can be done to solve the problem? and How can the organization implement and test a set of solutions? These generic project questions generate the major steps required to carry out the project.

A *problem statement* says that something is wrong or needs improvement. People sometimes refer to problems in language appropriate for objectives. Long-range goals and objectives are the *results* that are desired, that demonstrate that the problems are solved. For example, "To improve staff attendance at classes" is not a problem; it is a long-range goal. The problem is lack of staff attendance at classes.

It is necessary to prove that a problem exists before trying to solve it. It has been noted that "If it isn't measured, it isn't managed." Proving quantitatively whether the problem exists makes it possible to find the extent of the problem, find where it is occurring, or discover that the problem is really something else. In several of the projects reported here, *proving the problem* uncovered other problems that were not known to exist. Collecting data to prove the problem arms managers with important data with which to argue in support of solutions. It also provides a baseline against which to compare results after solutions are implemented.

The approach to proving the problem is empirical and data based. It assumes that a problem can be expressed quantitatively and studied. Indicators can be created to represent the area of interest. That is, if patients are waiting too long, it is possible to find out how long; if too many charts have missing data, it is possible to find what data are missing and in how many charts; if not enough patients are getting prenatal classes, it is possible to learn what percentage of patients are not attending classes.

Collecting such data is *organizational research*. To carry out the research, the consultant goes to the operations of the department or service where the problem is and collects data over a representative period of time for an appropriate number of units. This depends on what is being examined.

Naming the problem in operational terms means defining how the problem will be measured and the data to be collected, such as average length of wait, percentage of patients waiting above a given length of time, percentage of charts with missing items, or percentage of patients not getting prenatal classes. Management can be enlisted to help decide what average or what percentage would be considered to be a problem in the institution, thus involving them in a key part of the process and preparing them to be convinced by the data. Setting predetermined criteria to evaluate the results is a key aspect of problem identification. The problem is proved after the collection of data in the dimensions or indicators that describe the problem, when the results are compared with the criteria already approved by management.

Causes

A cause is a circumstance, a characteristic of individuals, or an attitude that makes the problem exist. *Objective causes* are work conditions, demographics, and intrinsic qualities. *Subjective causes* are attitudes, opinions, and lack of knowledge. Some causes are preventable by the organization. Staff practices or beliefs, the way the organization functions or organizes work, management policies and standards, and some consumer behaviors are amenable to change. Causes that are intrinsic to the population being served, such as age, sex, diagnosis, or income level, cannot be changed through the efforts of the organization; they are *risk factors* that signal that there are special needs or vulnerabilities to be aware of.

It is necessary to know the causes of problems before suggesting solutions. This avoids suggesting solutions for factors that are not actual causes. Different causes need different solutions. For example, if the problem is that staff are not attending mandated classes, and management decides to develop a program to motivate staff to attend, the truth may be that staff were motivated all along; the cause may be lack of relief staff. Instituting a program to motivate staff would not solve the problem; implementing the false solution would have no effect. As a result, people might think that the problem cannot be solved.

When management or a team decides to address a problem, the tendency may be to say, "This is a problem; let's fix it" and to immediately try to find solutions. But it takes at least two steps before it is possible to talk intelligently about solutions. The first is to determine whether the problem exists and its extent; the second is to identify the causes. The consultant has to understand that it is worth taking the time to do the research.

The first step in finding causes is to decide what all the *possible* causes are. Such a list comes from observing the operations involved or already having some experience with them, consulting the literature of the profession or service involved, and talking with staff, especially those who are doing the work. A generic list of possible causes, presented later, provides the beginning of a checklist. Notice that staff are not asked to *decide* what the causes are, only to name *possible* causes.

The next steps in proving causes are similar to proving that there is a problem. The consultant considers the data needed to show how each possible cause is manifested and can be quantified. There is no elimination of possible causes to investigate; all possible causes that *can* be studied *are* studied. The consultant designs data collection to test whether actual results meet the levels and incidences that would be reached if a possible cause were real.

For subjective causes, it is usually necessary to conduct surveys of staff or consumers about specific attitudes, beliefs, and knowledge. The consultant designs research to find the extent to which subjects associated with the problem answer specific questions differently from subjects associated with an absence of the problem.

The consultant will suggest criteria to prove the causes; that is, levels or thresholds that the data would reach if the possible causes were real. The consultant involves management by asking for approval of the criteria, which can include statistical measures such as coefficients of correlation or t-test results but will usually be simple quantitative measures that make sense. Including management (referred to as *the client*) as part of the process prepares them to understand why some solutions and not others make sense, given the causes proved.

Solutions

A solution is a change or intervention that addresses proved causes so that the problem is eliminated or reduced. Solutions can be changes in how the work is done, in the way supervision is provided, in educational programs, or in how records are kept, among others. A solution should address proved causes and be within management's resource limits.

It is impossible to know the best solution ahead of time, because the actual causes are not yet known. Management may sometimes have a preconceived idea of what the solution should be, but that particular solution may have nothing to do with the actual causes. If alternative causes and solutions have not been investigated, jumping to a solution may cause major difficulties because, without addressing the real causes, the problem will not be solved. It is up to the consultant to convince management to wait for all the results.

Solutions may seem obvious once the actual causes are known, but there is also the literature of the discipline to review, staff to ask, and the consultant's own creativity and experience to draw on. The recommended solutions must be within management's financial and structural limits and must address the greatest number of serious causes in the most efficient way.

Questions of ethics and integrity may arise. If the client has a preconceived notion, such as believing that specific staff are the cause, he or she may not be happy to learn that the causes arise from the way the work is organized. The consultant has to follow where the proof of causes leads. Designing the research to test all the possible causes, enlisting management in setting criteria, and having solid data make it possible to stand up for the more appropriate solutions.

It is tempting to assume that, for any given problem and set of proved causes, there is a set of "correct" solutions. But the correctness of a solution is not a mathematical concept. If there are 10 proved causes, it may be possible to suggest 10 or 20 solutions dealing with individual or groups of causes to alleviate the problem. Even in medicine there is often only a set of options to choose from, each with its own advantages and side effects. Not all solutions can be applied. Some might exceed the limits set for staffing, costs, or restructuring. Some may be rejected by the staff, some by management. The consultant has to consider what is feasible and whose interests will be served by a set of solutions—interests such as those of staff, middle management, executive management, owners, the population served, and the wider community. Some solutions are more efficient in how they deal with resources, some address more causes, and some are easier to implement.

It is important to get the participation and reactions of the people involved beforehand, so they can feel motivated to make the solutions work. The consultant's solutions will not benefit all interests unless there is a conscious effort to find solutions that are optimally accept-able to the different constituencies. If the solutions are not acceptable to management, no implementation will take place. Being successful may mean being concerned with the interests of other constituencies; success implies the need for a strategy to have the relevant people feel from the start that they are included and that they understand what is going on.

Implementing and Evaluating the Solutions

The step after getting approval for a set of solutions is to design an implementation plan. *Implementation* comes prior to and is different from *making a solution operational*. Implementation is the period when a set of solutions is being tried out and evaluated. *Evaluation* is a part of implementation. It is used to determine whether the solutions work. Data are collected to compare the old proof-of-problem data with data collected after the solution has been implemented and is free of bugs. Objective criteria are again needed, such as the amount of improve-ment required for the solution to be judged a success.

Making Solutions Operational

A solution is said to be institutionalized, or made operational, when it becomes a standard operating procedure. This requires the integration of all facets of the solution within the organization, dealing with all the ways in which the new operations interface with other departments and staff, and may require the creation of new data collection forms and manuals, rescheduling, additional purchasing, and a design for training. It may mean collecting indicator data on a regular basis to be sure the solutions continue to be effective. The indicator may be selected for use in a reference database.

Objectives and Evaluation of the Project

Objectives

An objective is a *result* that the project is designed to reach. As an end point, it can be measured in some way or can be said to be present or not. Given the fact that most projects have start and end dates, it is necessary to differentiate between *long-range goals* and *project objectives*.

Long-Range Goals

Long-range goals are desired results that are not expected to be reached in the time period of the project. They are the ultimate aims of the project: the elimination of the problems. However, the goals may not be reached by the time the project period is over. For example, ensuring that all patients receive prenatal education may involve training staff, arranging to schedule patients, designing new curricula, obtaining space, developing new ways of keeping records, tracking no-shows, and, after the program has been operational for a period of time, collecting data to evaluate the results. A project could end before all this has been accomplished.

Project Objectives

Project objectives are the generic results the consultant is committed to bringing about *within* the period of the project. They are the end points related to the generic project questions and are more research oriented than long-range goals. For example, a project question *asking* if the problem actually exists or its extent has, as its counterpart project objective, to *prove* whether the problem exists and its extent.

Each objective includes a *due date*, which is the time at which the consultant promises the objective will be reached; a statement of *what will be accomplished*; and *success criteria* that define what has to be shown to prove that the objective has been accomplished successfully. Long-range goals and project objectives are determined by the problem and the project questions; every problem statement must have a goal or objective that flows from it, and every goal or objective must have as its antecedent a problem statement or project question. A project objective to determine the causes of excessive patient falls must have had a problem question asking what the causes of patient falls are.

Enabling objectives. Enabling objectives, sometimes called process objectives, are prior events and outputs that must be produced to reach a project objective. They are preparatory tasks, and the methods to achieve them are carried out first. For example, the enabling objectives to determine *whether the problem exists and its extent* would include

(a) identifying the basic parameters of the problem and the causes that are to be investigated, (b) designing data collection, (c) getting approval to start data collection, and (d) establishing a set of indicators and criteria to prove the problem. After these enabling objectives, data collection and analysis take place, and the project objective is achieved.

Unlike project objectives, enabling objectives are not ends in themselves. They make it possible to carry out the methods of project objectives, but they are not methods. Enabling objectives are never worded so as to answer the question "How?" They are worded to answer the question "What?" The answer to the question "How?" is a *method*. "Get approval for the project" names an enabling objective that needs its own method, as does "Identify the basic parameters of the problem" and "Design data collection."

Methods

A method is a procedure for achieving a desired result. Methods are the activities carried out to accomplish objectives and meet success criteria. They require an overall strategy or plan. Method is process; it goes on in time. The end point of a method is the completion of an objective. There must be a method for each enabling and project objective. Once a problem and its counterpart objectives are stated, the consultant designs appropriate methods to go from the problems to the objectives. Thus, the project is the set of methods designed to meet the objectives and to solve the problems.

Sequence

Objectives have a logical sequence. Table 1.1 is a model plan of work for a quality improvement project and sets the sequence of objectives. This provides the framework for the chapters and sections in this book. Table 1.1 also presents the evaluation design for the project because it indicates the criteria that must be reached for each project and enabling objective to be considered successful.

In Table 1.1, there are columns for the objectives, due dates, success criteria, and results. The blank columns are filled in later with actual completion dates and results, as the project is carried out. The objectives are shown in order of their due dates, reflecting the logical order

Table 1.1 Project Evaluation Design, Plan of Work, and Progress, in Order by Due Date

Project and Enabling Objectives (1)	Due Date (2)	Date Done (3)	Success Criteria for Each Objective (4)	Actual Results and Comments (5)
Enabling Objectives for Project Objective 1				
Enabling objective 1a: Get approval for the project's plan of work	Date 1		Oral or written approval of proposal from key manager.	
Enabling Objective 1b: Identify project parameters	Date 2		Approval of accuracy by relevant manager(s).	
Enabling Objective 1c: Identify causes to be studied	Date 3		Interview with [how many?] staff and literature review completed. Decision made on final list.	
Enabling Objective 1d: Design detailed data collection for proving the problem and objective causes	Date 4		Approval of data collection forms by relevant manager; successful field test of forms.	
Enabling Objective 1e: Schedule data collection for proof of problem	Date 5		Approval of data collection and schedule obtained.	
Enabling Objective 1f: Identify criteria to prove the problem	Date 6		Criteria approved by key managers.	
PROJECT OBJECTIVE 1: Prove That Problem Exists and Its Extent	Date 7		Data results meet or exceed criteria set in objective 1f. Data checked by ___. Key managers convinced.	
Enabling Objectives for Project Objective 2				
Enabling Objective 2a: Design additional research and data collection on causes	Date 8		Approval of data collection forms by relevant manager; successful field test of forms; survey items understood and/or discriminate between experts and novices.	
Enabling Objective 2b: Schedule data collection on causes	Date 9		Approval of data collection and schedule obtained.	
Enabling Objective 2c: Identify criteria to prove causes	Date 10		Criteria approved by key managers.	

(continued)

Table 1.1 Continued

Project and Enabling Objectives (1)	Due Date (2)	Date Done (3)	Success Criteria for Each Objective (4)	Actual Results and Comments (5)
PROJECT OBJECTIVE 2: Prove the Causes of the Problem	Date 11		Each cause proved meets or exceeds criteria set in objective 2c. Data checked by ___. Key managers convinced.	
Enabling Objectives for Project Objective 3				
Enabling Objective 3a: Identify management's feasibility limits	Date 12		List compiled from interview with key manager approved as accurate.	
Enabling Objective 3b: Get ideas on possible solutions	Date 13		Interviews with [how many?] staff and literature review complete.	
Enabling Objective 3c: Get feedback on selected solutions	Date 14		Of [number of] staff asked for feedback, at least [number] approve.	
PROJECT OBJECTIVE 3: Identify Solutions	Date 15		Solutions reflect proved causes, feasibility limits; approved by key managers.	
Enabling Objectives for Project Objective 4				
Enabling Objective 4a: Design implementation and evaluation plan	Date 16		Content, forms, and success criteria approved by managers.	
Enabling Objective 4b: Schedule implementation and data collection	Date 17		Dates approved by relevant managers.	
Enabling Objective 4c: Determine whether solutions are successful	Date 18		Data meet or exceed success criteria set in objective 4a. Data checked by ___. Key managers are convinced.	
Enabling Objective 4d: Identify steps to make solutions operational	Date 19		Arrangements made to take each required step.	
Enabling Objective 4e: Determine whether new standards or indicators are required to monitor solutions or participate in reference database	Date 20		Approval from key managers on new data collection; collection procedures designed.	

Table 1.1 Continued

Project and Enabling Objectives (1)	Due Date (2)	Date Done (3)	Success Criteria for Each Objective (4)	Actual Results and Comments (5)
PROJECT OBJECTIVE 4: Implement, Evaluate, Make Solutions Operational	Date 21		Implementation complete; criteria for solutions met; new solutions appear in SOP manuals, policy documents, staff orientation, evaluation criteria; new standards or indicators adopted and in use.	
Long-range Goal(s) To eliminate the problem			Time period is beyond that set for the project.	

of events. For Objective 1, *Prove That the Problem Exists and Its Extent*, there are six enabling objectives: (a) Get approval for the project's plan of work, (b) Identify project parameters, (c) Identify causes to be studied, (d) Design detailed data collection for proving the problem and objective causes, (e) Schedule data collection for proof of problem, and (f) Identify criteria to prove the problem.

The due date for Objective 1 follows after the dates of its enabling objectives because they must be completed before Objective 1 can be accomplished. Objectives 2, 3, and 4 have later due dates, all preceded by their respective enabling objectives. In actual use, some objectives may share the same due dates, but each one is presented separately in Table 1.1 for the sake of clarity. As the project is carried out, objectives may be completed before or after their due dates, but the sequence of events largely remains the same.

Evaluation

Evaluation means determining the extent to which the objectives are achieved; it is an integral part of the plan of work in Table 1.1. Standards for judging success are decided before the project is undertaken, and they are applied to the results when the project is completed. Therefore, objectives must be written so that some *measure* is offered for determining whether the objectives have been met. These measures are the *success criteria.*

Success criteria are parameters with which to measure whether objectives have been accomplished, including the dates by which they will be accomplished (columns 2 and 3 in Table 1.1). The measures can be quantitative, statistical, the production of documents, or the occurrence of events, such as approvals. The due dates must be within the time period of the project.

Table 1.1 presents the criteria for each objective. The criteria for Project Objective 1 are that the criteria set in enabling objective 1f (which is the selection of the criteria to prove the problem) are met or exceeded, the data are checked by someone, and key managers are convinced. For Project Objective 2, *Prove the Causes of the Problem,* the success criteria include meeting or exceeding the criteria to prove the causes (set in Objective 2c) and convincing the client.

Enabling objectives also need success criteria—some tangible proof of successful completion as promised. This can be approval from an expert or completed scheduling. The design of a questionnaire has the criterion that the field test be successful.

Success criteria often include getting approval from management or convincing particular people (the clients) of the results. This is important for several reasons. Management people are a source of expertise to draw on; when clients agree to the criteria, they commit to being involved; if clients are involved in setting the criteria, they are more receptive to the results; and, having been convinced of the results, clients are better able to understand the proposed solutions and will be more open to approving and implementing them. (Titles and names of specific individuals should be substituted for the term "key managers" referred to in Table 1.1.)

Organizational Culture and Ethics

In addition to proving whether the problem exists, its extent, and its causes, the consultant is expected to come up with solutions and perhaps help with implementation. The consultant needs to be aware of the organizational climate, understand interpersonal relationships, and needs to be able to communicate effectively by listening as well as giving understandable information. When carrying out the methods for the project, the internal consultant must be aware of how things get done in the organization; must consider what can be expected from an attempt to study and solve a problem; and must know who has to be involved, how, and at what point. The role that trade unions play in the life of the organization must also be understood.

Culture

All this requires a knowledge of the organization's *culture*. Ulschak and SnowAntle (1990) define culture as "a learned pattern of basic assumptions" (p. 175), "a set of assumptions that are learned and expected" (p. 177). *Assumptions*, like beliefs, are given. They are not questioned; therefore they are not proved. People in organizations have assumptions about what staff behaviors are unacceptable, about the proper chain of command, and about what quality of work is acceptable.

Patterns are complex, ordered, repetitive relationships that come into play when problems have to be dealt with, when conflicts arise, when communication is necessary, when the system generates errors, and when new situations emerge. Culture includes relationships whose validity is not questioned and whose design can be so large that no one can see the whole picture. The patterns are *learned*; exposure to the repetitive pattern engenders learning in the participants, whether conscious or not. There is a tendency for peer pressure to move people towards uniformity of belief and behavior. But, if culture can be learned, it can be unlearned and changed.

The culture is said to be *transparent* to its members, who sit within its atmosphere and do not see it. They live within the cultural environment and look out through it. It is *taken for granted*. Cultural patterns tend to be unconscious; they are also implicitly believed to be right. Because the pattern is *expected*, anything other than the pattern will not be accepted easily. People do not take kindly to deviations from the pattern. This has an aspect of coercion. If persons in authority are not questioned, the rebel may be rejected not only by the authorities but by the others sharing the culture. The culture determines whether good work is rewarded and whether the patient as consumer is seen as the ultimate client to be served. This affects the decisions that are made.

The internal consultant needs to determine whether the organizational culture will allow the client or others in the organization to admit the existence of the problem if it is proved and whether a solution will be welcome. The consultant also needs to know if any staff will feel threatened by the project and, when the problem is proved and causes and solutions are found, whether anyone could get hurt by the implementation of the solutions. The consultant needs to know the environment that will be created by data collection, whether the culture supports the flow of valid information, and, if not, how the needed information will be obtained.

The culture of the organization can affect the flow of information through formal and informal channels and what types of information can be shared and with whom. This is important for someone who wants to solve organizational problems. There may be a hierarchical chain of command that determines who gets specific information. The formal norms for behavior may be embodied in organizational rules and documents, but the culture may determine that the informal systems are different and more important. There may be a system of subcultures by department, job title, sex, age, ethnicity, union affiliation, or seniority within which information is shared and beyond which there is resistance to sharing.

Information that cannot be shared is probably considered potentially damaging. What is considered potentially damaging is determined by the culture. Ways of getting around rules, errors, and mistakes and ways of obtaining financial data or long-range plans may be guarded information. If administrators do not consider access to information and criticism to be threatening, information is shared. If criticism is considered to be threatening, access to information will be limited to a small group. An environment that does not share information may be created by an individualistic, distrustful style of leadership; people may try to acquire potentially damaging information about each other to use as leverage. Rather than trying to help the organization serve its consumers, people may try to protect their backs. Where there is an open style, telling the truth is part of the culture, and people tend to cooperate.

In a time-honored analysis of organizational functioning, McGregor's (1960) Theory X corresponds to the assumption that people would like to do as little work as possible, would rather be led, have little ambition, put themselves before the organization, and resist change. This describes the culture of the assembly line, where it makes sense for the worker to do as little as possible while management tries to get workers to produce as much as possible.

McGregor's Theory Y and the philosophy of CQI/TQM correspond to the assumption that, with experience, people can learn to be personally concerned about organizational goals; that management can bring out the part in people that wants to take the initiative and take responsibility; and that management can create situations in which individuals' goals can be met through working for the organization's goals. Neither X nor Y behavior is innate; both can be learned through experience. The more management makes employees feel that their contributions are needed and appreciated or helps employees feel identified with the product, the more Theory Y impulses come into play. The CQI approach may create a Theory Y culture.

In a Theory X organization, data collection on causes could make staff members fear being fired; the client may have to convince staff that no one will be fired as a result of the project and that management is more concerned about *what* is going wrong than in finding out *who* is involved. The consultant might have to show that the very way the data are being collected protects the identity of the staff involved.

The internal consultant is expected to facilitate change. Resistance to change is ubiquitous and will occur in any culture, but organizational cultures do change, even X cultures, because the larger environment is dynamic and evolving. A new service such as a center for women's health or AIDS care may have been instituted; the changing demographics in a community may introduce patients and staff who have different cultural backgrounds; purchasing may become centralized in the institution; government may require wheelchair access to clinic facilities. These will affect and be influenced by the culture of the organization and its day-to-day patterns.

People who resist change may ask the consultant to give up or leave. But there are other choices: Building alliances for reciprocal benefits from the change is one approach; another is finding others who also see the need for change. When people with like-minded views find one another, they build a subculture that can grow and influence the larger culture. The idea that change is impossible is a cultural attitude, but trying everything to help change things is also a cultural attitude.

Culture affects the way solutions are implemented. Management cannot announce that staff initiative is now welcome and expect a great outpouring of ideas; whole patterns need to be changed. Management has to convince employees that it stands behind the transformation to a Y or CQI environment; it must demonstrate this in tangible ways that show up each day as well as in policy statements. This is difficult in a period of retrenchment. If people expect an overnight transformation from the X to the Y culture, they will be disappointed. This then becomes another excuse for not changing; Y is prematurely dismissed as impractical. It takes time to change the cultural environment, and the project and the consultant can be a part of this.

Orienting the organization towards quality improvement is seen by the JCAHO as an opportunity for cultural change. In data collection, the similarities among departments and services become evident, encouraging communication. Common processes used to measure and improve performance encourage staff members to use common process control techniques. When a quality improvement team learns how to use process control procedures, all members learn the "language" specific to their activities. When they share their findings with other staff, additional people come to understand the language and begin using it when dealing with performance improvement. "The development of a common language in turn opens doors to new opportunities for collaboration, creating a stronger sense of shared purpose. And it enables [departments and services] to learn from each other and to adapt resources and systems developed elsewhere in the organization to their own needs rather than 'reinvent the wheel' " (JCAHO, 1993, p. xiii).

Ethics

Ethics deal with principles and rules of right and wrong; they are part of and embedded in cultures. Ethics have to do with good and bad human conduct, and they require value judgments. Ethics, like culture, are not inborn or innate. The ethics of an act can vary with the situation; there is little that is always good or always bad. Personal ethics, organizational ethics, professional ethics, and social ethics all have to do with the degree to which the person or organization can be trusted to behave according to moral standards in situations where choices can affect the welfare of others.

Personal ethics have to do with decisions that arise when the individual can hurt someone else, such as whether the employee will put the organization or the client before personal interests. *Organizational ethics* have to do with whether the product will be misrepresented to the public, whether inferior products will be allowed, whether pricing will take advantage of the consumer's needs, and whether billing will be inflated to enhance reimbursement. *Professional ethics* deal with whether to allow personal feelings to affect the quality of one's work, whether to ignore dangerous behavior in others, whether to observe confidentiality, and whether to administer a prescribed treatment when it is inappropriate. *Social ethics* involve discrimination, treating one group better than another, giving priority to people with better income or with health insurance, deciding whether to ration health care, and deciding whether to support high technology or preventive care.

Ethics for the internal consultant relate to the manner in which the consulting work is done, the accuracy of the data, the confidentiality of what is collected, and the effects of what is determined and/or recommended. The consultant must consider what will happen if the research uncovers abuse of patients, staff, or others, and how the staff and management will deal with proof that such situations exist.

Does the Problem Really Exist?

Roadmap

Chapter 1 presented the basic terms, definitions, and concepts used in this book. Chapters 2 through 5 constitute a manual designed to help the internal consultant carry out a quality improvement project. As these chapters are a manual, the reader is free to skip to the cases or read the chapters as their contents become relevant.

Chapter 2 presents the methods to *Prove Whether the Problem Exists and Its Extent.* Chapter 3 deals with *Verifying the Causes.* Chapter 4 covers *Selecting Solutions,* and Chapter 5 deals with *Implementing and Making Solutions Operational.* The related enabling objectives are discussed in each chapter. Each chapter opens with a list of the major activities to be discussed, taken from Table 1.1.

The descriptions of how to do the work draw on a selection of cases carried out in a variety of service settings. Table 2.1 lists the 14 cases of Part II by number, type of problem, department or service, and the specific problems addressed. In Chapters 2 through 5 the cases are referred to as examples of the procedures or issues being discussed. This does not mean that the reader needs to constantly flip to the cases in Part II; the chapters are self-contained. The references to cases tell the reader where background material on a point can be found for later examination or indicate examples of the matter under discussion.

The cases are meant to be used as examples of research design, to provide ideas on how a wide variety of quality issues were addressed,

Table 2.1 Cases Presented in This Book

Case	Problem Type	Department or Service	Problem
1	Excess waiting	Nursing home physical therapy	New and current residents waited too long to enter a physical therapy program.
2	Excess waiting	Hospital: Radiation therapy	Patients waited too long to receive treatment after arriving at the department office.
3	Excess waiting	Hospital laboratory: Hematology	Physicians waited too long to be informed by the lab of dangerous test results (panic values).
4	Excess hospital stay	Hospital rehabilitation department	Amputee patients remained in Rehabilitation longer than was deemed appropriate.
5	Errors and omissions	HMO offices and central laboratory	Patients referred for lab testing arrived at the HMO's central lab with incomplete referral forms needed for specimens to be taken.
6	Errors	HMO physical therapy	Patients arriving for physical therapy had incorrect fit or incorrect use of canes and crutches provided prior to therapy.
7	Errors and omissions	Hospital laboratory	Blood samples arrived at the lab too hemolyzed for testing; other problems were subsequently discovered.
8	Errors	Hospital pharmacy	Medications arrived at nursing units from the pharmacy with errors.
9	Non-performance	Municipal department	Labor-management committee set up to deal with health and safety issues at the department's sites was not functioning; other problems subsequently discovered.
10	Non-performance	Hospital outpatient department	Nursing staff not attending mandated continuing education classes.
11	Non-performance	Home health care agency; nurses	Nurses not discussing advance directives with incoming clients; when clients had directives, they were not properly documented.
12	Pilot test: patient compliance	Hospital-based physician cancer practice	Postsurgical cancer patients noncompliant with follow-up visits; reminder letter for 6-month postsurgical visit was pilot tested.
13	Pilot test: internal audit	Intermediate care facility	Current internal audit not picking up problems cited later by state audit. New audit for specific problem areas was pilot tested.
14	Finding areas to improve	Emergency medical service	No attempt made to use "unusual occurrence" data to reduce incidents and improve service.

to help in the process of identifying causes and solutions, and to offer practice in data collection concepts. Most of the cases were situations in which the problems were already thought to exist. Case 14 is an example of the search for ways to improve current quality; in this case, the problems were identified once the project began.

PROJECT OBJECTIVE 1: TO PROVE THAT
THE PROBLEM EXISTS AND ITS EXTENT

Get approval for the project plan of work from key manager(s)

Identify the parameters of the project

Identify the causes to be studied

Design detailed research and data collection to prove the problem and identify objective causes

Schedule data collection on proof of the problem

Identify criteria to prove the problem

Carry out data collection and analysis

Getting Started

Initiation of the Quality Improvement Project

Your involvement as an internal consultant may derive from a series of prior CQI steps in which priorities were set regarding activities to be measured, assessed, and improved. Each department may have been asked to collaborate in organizationwide improvement activities. Managers are asked by the JCAHO to provide resources for quality improvement work, including allocation of resources for staff to participate in performance improvement activities, provision of adequate time for participation in performance improvement activities, and staff training. Once a systematic process is used to collect and analyze indicator data, specific conclusions about the need for more intensive assessment may follow.

The decision to conduct intensive assessment may have been the result of comparisons of performance data with pre-established criteria, internal comparisons of the organization's performance over time, comparison with similar process and outcome data from other organizations in reference databases, or consideration of legal or regulatory requirements. When the comparison results in a decision to conduct intensive assessment, the quality improvement project is born.

Your first contact with the project may be as an individual or as part of a team asked to deal with department-level problems that are already the concern of the organization, after management has selected an area for quality improvement. You may be a middle-level manager or part of a team that has identified a problem with a history of inattention in your department, or you may be a staff member with original ideas about a problem.

By the time you or your team are asked (or decide) to embark on a quality improvement project, you will have some idea of the project problem and the project's long-range goal. You may have thought about some of the causes of the problem, and you may know something about the processes involved. However, very little else is fully clear.

This chapter suggests the steps for setting up the project, clarifying the problem situation, and determining whether the problem exists and its extent. The steps follow the order shown in Table 1.1. This stage corresponds to the TQM step called "perception of the problem" (Ziegenfuss, 1993) or establishing the project and verifying that the problem exists (Goonan, 1995). In CQI literature, it is "identify or confirm the existence of actual or potential problems" (Orlikoff & Snow, 1984), or analyze the current situation (Swanson, 1995).

It is helpful to examine the literature of the professional discipline involved in the department or service area to aid you in understanding the problem, finding causes, and coming up with solutions. Although there may be a premium on the amount of time available for this, many people who undertake quality improvement projects will already be reading the journals of their professional discipline or the service area involved.

If you decide to do a literature search, start with journal sources and use a specialized index, searching by subject or key words that describe the problem. *Index Medicus*, the most useful of all the indexes for the health professions, is available in MEDLINE, an international guide to biomedical literature. MEDLINE includes Index Medicus and more. Your organization's library may provide access by way of a separate CD-ROM or through Lexis-Nexis. MEDLINE is also available free of charge on the Worldwide Web, as PubMed.

The Cumulative Index to Nursing & Allied Health Literature (CINAHL) is an index of many nursing and allied health journals and is available on CD-ROM. Other indexes to consider are ERIC (education), PSYCLIT (*Psychological Abstracts*), SOCIOFILE (*Sociological Abstracts*), *Biological and Agricultural Abstracts*, and *Applied Science & Technology Abstracts*.

It is also a good idea to keep a running diary of what is happening, what is being done, responses, and events, much the way scientists keep research journals. This makes it possible to get a perspective and collect material for a progress or a final report, and it helps document problems encountered along the way. Sometimes resistance to the project is an indicator of important organizational problems.

Clarify the Problem

Discuss the problem or improvement opportunity that is to be investigated with the client. This is the time to find out in detail what the client considers the problem to be. The client may confuse the problems to be studied with solutions he or she already expects you to come up with; to guide the discussion, find out what the client thinks is going wrong in the specific delivery of services, what is not functioning appropriately, or what consumers are complaining about.

If you can name what may be going wrong and state or imply what service is being affected, you have identified the basic problem. Examples of problems are presented in Table 2.1. They include patients not receiving treatment soon enough after admission, patients not coming for follow-up visits, incomplete laboratory requisitions, errors in the filling of patients' medication bins in a pharmacy, and staff not attending continuing education classes, among other problems.

If you think that there are additional issues involved in the problem, discuss them with the client and ask for agreement to include the aspects that you think are important. For example, in Case 9, the client said that environmental health and safety problems in the agency's local offices were not being taken to a committee set up to deal with them; the internal consultant believed that, in addition, local office environmental health and safety problems were not being dealt with at all. In Case 3, the client was only concerned about how long physicians waited for critical laboratory results once the results were verified, but the internal consultant wanted to include the entire period during which ordering physicians waited for results from the laboratory.

Identify the Key Organizational Client(s)

Once you have an idea of the problem, be sure that you are dealing with all the proper management people. If the client is a single individual, the consultant has fewer tasks, but the term *client* must include all those who will be asked to approve the criteria to prove the problem, prove the causes, and evaluate the solutions. The client(s) are those who must be convinced of the existence of the problem and the proof of causes, must identify management's feasibility limits regarding a solution, and must approve the implementation of the solutions.

The client may include the person who asked you to assume the role of internal consultant but should also include the manager(s) who need to be convinced that the problem exists and what the causes are—those who will decide whether to implement the proposed solutions. Who has the power to approve changes in process? Who can tell you what management's feasibility limits are? Discover who has the authority to support your position as a consultant or the role of the quality improvement team. Consult the organizational chart, but do not forget the informal system, which will be a useful guide to identifying all those who should be involved. Even if the consultant is a first-line supervisor or senior staff member, a higher level of administration should always be involved, such as the director of medicine or the chief administrative officer.

What About a Collaborator?

If you are the sole person acting as the internal consultant, you may want to enlist the help of a collaborator, someone on the staff who can discuss the project with you, who will check your figures, and who will help you carry out the work. In the 14 cases reported, a college professor was enlisted with the approval of the client. Quality team members can perform this function.

In the absence of a team, consider a colleague, an assistant, or another person who might be willing to help. If management agrees to assign a partner, that is also a good solution, but there may not be funds for another person. At the least, find someone to check your figures.

Is the Management United in Its Interest in the Project?

It is important to discover the extent to which the client in particular, and senior management in general, support the project, because you will need their cooperation. It may help to learn about the history of the problem, attempts made in the past to deal with it, any solutions attempted, and who was involved. Make sure everyone is clear about what is to be accomplished and expresses willingness to invest in a solution as one emerges. For this, your experience with the culture of the organization will help. The advantage of an internal consultant is that, as a member of the organization, you can assess which managers might feel shaky about their leadership and might be reluctant to let the consultant be innovative or come up with answers.

Identify Your Role as Internal Consultant

The role you or your team is assigned in the project will have much to do with how well you succeed in carrying out the work. Determine how much authority you will have to obtain data and how much help to expect in collecting data. To whom will you report? What role will you play in implementation? Will you report on the results of the project to higher levels of management?

Determine whether there will be release time to carry out the work. Sometimes funds are allocated as part of the organization's commitment to JCAHO guidelines for continuous quality improvement. But if, as in the late 1990s, you face tightened budgets and retrenchment, few resources will be available. In the 14 cases reported here, no release time was available, and the consultants integrated the work on the projects into their regular duties and enlisted the help of other staff. The organization *may* be willing to restructure the regular duties of the consultant's job to make room for the work. You need to mutually agree on how your time will be allocated. If some of your duties will be transferred, to whom? What do you return to when the project is over?

When there is already a committee to deal with certain kinds of problems, its members may not be happy to accept a new individual or group, even if the committee has not been actively dealing with the problem. Hostile committees can generate delays in the process by insisting that members not present at meetings must also give approvals to proceed. They may also "take over" without warning and change the project. It is sometimes a good idea to identify a portion of the work or a component of the problem as the province of the consultant to avoid depending on committee approvals. A better alternative is to find the link between the committee's values and the project's and attempt to open up the relationship.

Identify the Specific Approvals, Collaboration, and Cooperation You Will Need

A letter of approval may be needed to give you access to data and staff. If you do need such access, find out whose permission you need, whether permission can be denied, and who needs to sign your letter. Do you need to remember people who, if they are overlooked, could be offended by hearing about the project later? In one case it took a long time to get approval because a supervisor was not brought in early enough and not treated as "important." In the end, higher level managers gave approval and the supervisor had to go along, but the supervisor managed to increase the consultant's workload in nonproject assignments and was otherwise difficult or discouraging. She was finally able to accept the project once she realized that she would share in the praise for its success. In another case, once the consultant explained his study to the trade union representative, the trade union representative encouraged staff to cooperate.

Do you need the help of staff to collect data? Whose permission do you need and how will you enlist cooperation? Will you be asking overworked staff to collect data? Will staff feel involved enough to tell you when the data collection process is beginning to break down? In Case 7, the internal consultant asked staff who drew blood to record the conditions of drawing the blood so she could have data on technique as a possible cause of hemolyzed specimens, but the staff were not asked if they had the time to carry out the record keeping, and the consultant did not check on the data each day. The staff felt too overworked to cooperate; the consultant obtained little data.

When the problem is serious, and if the culture of quality improvement is not fully established, managers may be reluctant to provide data that will prove the problem because they may think it will reflect badly on themselves. It is important to notice the signs of this early. In Case 10, when a manager realized that her staff were not collecting much data on the scheduling of continuing education classes, she refused to supply the data on attendance that she did have. The internal consultant had to go to a different department to obtain collateral attendance data.

Decide on a Preliminary Research Design

Decide on the basic research design for the project in order to prepare the plan of work and estimate the time it will take. The research design for a quality improvement project includes the main objectives of the study, the key variables, such as the problem measures, the proposed subjects (e.g., patients, staff), process measures, outcomes, the study's time period, and the approach to be taken.

The details of the research design are determined during the course of the project. Details may be added when variables are given operational definitions, when crucial additional variables are uncovered, when criteria to test hypotheses are established, and when instruments are designed and field tested. But you need to know in general terms how you will prove that the problem exists, how you will test possible causes, and how you will test any solutions approved. This chapter (in later sections) and Chapters 3 through 5 describe the steps involved. These general comments are an introduction.

To prove that the problem exists and its extent, and to collect data on the objective characteristics of the subjects and processes that may be causes of the problem, you will be engaged in what is referred to as *descriptive research*. This involves data collection about the characteristics of a complete set of subjects, such as patients in a department or service area, or all requisition forms filled during a specific period, or all medication orders filled during specific periods. The relevant characteristics of all the subjects (population) and subgroups are defined and described. You may then compare aspects or parameters of one subgroup with those of another, such as averages, percentages, proportions, and frequencies.

To find the causes of the problem, you will be testing whether a set of hypotheses are false by setting up some likely tests. For quality improvement projects, you will probably be using descriptive data and *associative procedures* to establish whether expected relationships exist among the variables being considered. You may collect data through interviews and questionnaires. Although no causal relationships can be *proved*, if certain events can be predicted and other explanations are ruled out, the results are acceptable for concluding probable causation.

The test of a solution or an intervention may require a research design using *inferential procedures* to make generalizations about an entire population from the data about a sample population. The general term *clinical trial* refers to an experiment that uses controlled conditions to determine the effectiveness of an intervention. The classic study includes a group that receives the intervention and at least one control group, which receives a placebo or an alternative intervention. Individuals are selected and assigned to groups in as random a manner as possible.

A research design should not be judged on whether it is more or less "scientific." Good research design is judged by whether it is appropriate to the questions being asked of it: The design must be a fair test of the hypothesis, and it must be practical.

Consider the Due Dates

Estimate how long the various components of the project will take. You may be able to get extensions, but your reputation as a consultant is affected by how well you meet timetables. The first try at estimating the time needed to do this type of project can be far off the mark. New consultants find that the steps take a good deal longer than they anticipated. Things go wrong; key people whose permission you need to collect data or approve procedures may cancel meetings, go on vacation, get sick, or leave. In checking data, you may discover major errors that require you to redo some work. It will help to visualize what you may have to deal with if you read Chapters 2 through 5 and some of the cases.

Judging by the experience of the consultants whose cases are presented in this book, *proving that the problem exists and its extent* can take 6 to 8 weeks to complete (excluding the time needed to approve the project) if the consultant is also holding down a full-time job without release time. That is because much work on causes is also carried out during this period. *Proving the causes* can take another 4 to 5 weeks, and *finding a solution* can take 2 to 3 weeks. With some release time available to work on the project, time can be reduced considerably. Working with retrospective (past) data eliminates the time needed to collect data in real time.

Examine Your Own Position

Assess how you are viewed by the staff you will be dealing with, their supervisors, any trade unions involved, and how you see yourself, because a major part of the work will depend on interpersonal skills. Examine your own technical and managerial skills. Can you deliver what you are promising? Can you ask for help? Are you willing to be an active agent? Are you enthusiastic about the project? Does it fire your imagination? If all this is agreeable to you, you are ready to go on.

Get Approval for the Project
Plan of Work From Key Manager(s)

Coming to an agreement with the management sponsor (client) about the project is the first enabling objective in Table 1.1. The plan of work for the project is a written or oral agreement between the client and the consultant. It includes the objectives to be reached, due dates, success criteria, ethical considerations, and a delineation of roles and responsibilities. It is best to have the agreement in written form, especially if there is a formal cultural tradition in the organization. An oral agreement may work better in a more loosely run organization. Talk this over with your collaborator and with the client if you feel the need for guidance.

You will want to be sure that all the relevant departments and staff are introduced to the project and what it will entail. If you are asked to make an oral presentation of your plan, your listeners should be able to grasp what your project will be about and what you expect to accomplish. Because you will only have a few minutes, cover the problem and project objectives, mention enabling objectives in passing, make a brief comment on methods, and leave time to deal with ethical issues, answer questions, and negotiate agreements.

Table 1.1 summarizes the project objectives and success criteria; Appendix 1 suggests an outline for the written plan. Select the parts of the outline that suit your project. You may not need to include all the project objectives presented, or you may have variations on the generic model.

The *ethical issues* need to be made explicit (Ulschak & SnowAntle, 1990). You may need to refer to them to reassure staff, and you may need to have a record in case of later disagreements, especially in relation to solutions. The point is to have no one suffer as a result of cooperation with the project. The following are suggested inclusions for the written agreement.

1. Any information that may show a negative impact on patients will be reported to management, with confidentiality of staff identity protected to the maximum degree possible.
2. Any information that may show a negative impact on the organization will be reported to management, with confidentiality of staff identity protected to the maximum degree possible.
3. The identity of individuals who supply information will be kept confidential unless something illegal is involved.
4. The research may not result in the punishment of any individuals or groups outside of appropriate evaluation procedures.
5. Long-term goals will not be sacrificed for short-term gains.
6. If the consultant is unable to fulfill any objectives, this will be promptly revealed to the client.
7. The highest professional standards of skill, competence, and accuracy will be maintained in doing the work.
8. The interests of the client and the population served will come first.
9. No individual involved will be placed at an unfair advantage or disadvantage because of the project.

Ideally, you will now have an approved project agreement and a clear idea of what you will do. In fact, the achievement of a clear

agreement can only come about as the data collection begins to mate-
rialize and those involved find out what the project really involves.

Identify the Specific Parameters of the Project

Once you have an approved plan, it is necessary to know specific
details about the problem so you can design practical data collection.
You may want to collect data about the effect of the problem on the
organization's patients or consumers; you may need to learn the steps
involved in the service you are studying; and you will need to develop
operational definitions if there are important distinctions to be made
among situations, outputs, or people.

Importance

The importance of the problem in terms of effects on outcomes may
have to be established as part of the project. The relationship between
process and outcomes is an ongoing area of interest. In Case 1, which
deals with patients waiting too long to start physical therapy, the
consultant had to establish that starting therapy later than recommended by the literature would have negative effects on treatment
outcomes and patient well-being. In Case 5, studying incomplete
laboratory requisitions sent to a laboratory center, the consultant had
to establish that some types of omissions resulted in unacceptable
delays in the laboratory work.

Relevant Steps

You need to identify the process steps involved in the problem you
are studying because specific steps may be causes of the problem.
While you are collecting data to prove the problem, you need to collect
data about each step. Flow charts can help you find the processes and
contingencies at each step. (A flow chart shows graphically the steps
and contingencies: If this, then A is done; if that, then B is done.) You
may choose to follow a process from the first stage of production to

final consumption, with emphasis on production sequences, or you may find it more appropriate to follow the patient from admission to the department to discharge from it.

In Case 8, the consultant was to find whether patients' medication bins were being filled accurately in the pharmacy. She followed the steps from the receipt of a prescription in the pharmacy to the delivery of the medications to the units, noting errors at each step. Errors might have originated at any point. In Case 2, the patient was followed from arrival at the department to exit from treatment, with all the steps in between, because it was not clear where delays were occurring. In Case 1, each step was identified, from the admission of the patient to the nursing home to the start of physical therapy.

Operational Definitions

Operational definitions are definitions that can be applied unambiguously during data collection, especially if there are important distinctions to be made among patients, situations, or outputs. You need to decide how the problem variables will be measured, such as length of time waiting for a procedure, number of errors in medication bins, or number of negative or positive events, such as discussions of advance directives. Then you decide on indicators, such as the number of patients waiting too long, number of errors in medication bins, or number of new patients with no evidence of advance directive discussions. These should be expressed as a percentage of the total patients, medication orders, or new patients covered during the period of the project—and/or average numbers of the undesirable variables during the period.

Having more than one way of defining the existence of the problem improves the likelihood that the results are valid and reliable and adds information that can lead to finding causes. In Case 2, the average waiting period ("wait") was found to be acceptable, but the percentage of waits above 10 minutes was found to be unacceptable. This meant that some extremely short waits were offsetting an unacceptable number of longer waits.

Bechtel and Wood (1996) explain that "Without a clear, operational definition, two different individuals reviewing the same concept may measure it differently" (p. 22). As an example, in Case 4, the senior physical therapist in a hospital rehabilitation department differentiated between two types of amputee patients: "AP" and "non-AP." AP stood for *anticipated problems*, a set of medical and related conditions that would designate a patient as "sicker" because it was likely that he or she would require more time in rehabilitation. The operational definition of AP was tested to be sure it could be consistently applied using chart information for each patient as he or she entered the study.

Observation Units, Normal Loads,
Quantities, and Time Frame

The population studied in quality improvement projects should be all the subjects of interest for a selected period. The unit of analysis may be an episode of care, such as a patient's stay in a hospital to deal with a specific diagnosis, or a given course of procedures for a specific condition, or a specific product such as a laboratory test. It is important to know how many units, departments, job titles, shifts, and staff there are. A rough idea of the number of "outputs" produced in a normal day, number of patients seen, or number of times the problem situation might arise in a typical period of time affects how long a period of data collection is needed to obtain an adequate and representative set of data.

Generally, the organizational data you collect should cover 100% of the products, services, or problem data produced in the time period selected. You will generally need data for all shifts, hours, days, weeks, and months for services provided around the clock, unless you can be sure that different shifts, hours, days of the week, or months of the year share equally in the problem. Workloads may vary by shift, hour, day of the week, or even by month. To check whether there are patterns, old data can be examined or a quick data-collection pass can be designed to pick up patterns for a specific time period. If you have to choose among periods, it is best to collect data for those that account for more rather than less activity.

If the data you need already exist, a retrospective study will save the time needed to collect new data. Problems for which no data have already been collected will require enough time to design and gather a database. Events that occur infrequently need a longer period of time to collect data than those that occur in large numbers each day.

If the phenomenon being studied is relatively infrequent, such as patient falls, it is best to cover as many departments as possible for each day of the week, and enough weeks to capture data for at least 30 falls. If the project is allowed a short period of time, the data may be very sparse and therefore will not produce conclusive results. If the period is considered to be typical, the data for a few months can be projected and annual rates estimated, but the client and the audience for the report need to be warned about the thinness of the database.

Laboratories usually create enormous amounts of data, as daily tests can be counted in the hundreds or more. One way to reduce the massive amount of data is to select for study typical tests, types of specimens, or special technical procedures. Typical days, days of heavier loads, and specific shifts can be selected.

Solberg et al. (1997) believe that "a high degree of precision" is not necessary for samples of data taken for improvement purposes; the data collection process "needs to be simple and repetitive." Therefore, "small samples, for example 10 to 20 cases per sample" (p. 142), are considered to be appropriate. This seems too small a figure to produce results that can be subjected to meaningful analysis. Bernstein and Hilborne (1993) suggest that sample size should vary to reflect expected differences between groups. (The larger the difference, the greater the significance of the result, and therefore the smaller the sample needed.)

Greater numbers are needed when you plan to study subgroups. Reliance on aggregate data can be misleading. While averages for the total department or institution may be acceptable, some components, such as individual nursing units, may have unacceptable averages, offset in the aggregate by outstanding units (Bechtel & Wood, 1996). In several cases reported in Part II, the aggregate average was acceptable, but problems were found in component units or groupings.

According to Green and Lewis (1986), a conservatively high sample size is 100, because that is needed before you can assume a somewhat normal distribution of the variables you are collecting. The larger the number of component groups, the larger the database needed. If you want to say meaningful things about subsets within the sample, 100 for each subset is a conservative figure (pp. 238-239). (See Chapter 3 for further comments on sampling.)

Identify the Causes to Be Studied

The Original List

It is important to have a list of the causes you will investigate *before* you plan data collection to prove the existence and extent of the problem, because you will need to collect data on some possible causes while you are collecting data to prove the problem. Objective cause data often have to refer to specific observations so that performers and outcomes, or circumstances and outcomes, can be matched. These connections may only be available at the time the performance occurs; frequently, the data cannot be collected later.

CQI/TQM sources often suggest team meetings with people involved in the problem to develop the list of possible causes. The advice is often to "brainstorm" until there is a full list, and then a process is suggested whereby the team decides the order of importance of the causes. Often this results in one cause at a time being investigated. This is not the best approach. As Kibbs and McLaughlin (1994) point out, "any problem is likely to have multiple causes" (p. 323). Ranking causes before they are verified also ignores the interrelatedness of causes and overestimates the judgments that can be made this early in the process. For example, in Case 7, which involved studying the causes of hemolyzed blood samples, it could not be known beforehand that the unit, method of drawing blood, staff titles, and staff training would all be found to be causes, or that they converged on the particular technique of drawing blood in one unit.

The CQI/TQM team approach includes references to finding "root causes" by developing a cause-and-effect diagram and asking "why?" each time a cause is suggested, with the process repeated five or so times until there are no more antecedent causes to uncover (Marszalek-Gaucher & Coffey, 1993). This is an intuitive process at best. The cause-and-effect "fishbone diagram" for finding causes presents the general rubrics of people, methods, machines, materials, and culture (Mears, 1995); people, methods, information, materials, and facilities (Marszalek-Gaucher & Coffey, 1993); or materials, equipment, methods, employees, and environment (Amsden, 1991). The JCAHO (1997a) manual refers to *patient factors*, including psychological, economic, social, and physiological variables; *organizational factors*, including adequate staffing and equipment; *practitioner factors* that influence the type of assessments and treatments a patient may receive and their effectiveness; *environmental factors*, such as payer reimbursement or nursing home availability; and *chance variation*, which includes random variations.

The JCAHO (1997a) "root-cause" analysis looks for the causes of performance variation or a significant negative (sentinel) event by finding "special causes" and then "common causes" in larger systems. *Special causes* are unusual circumstances, difficult to anticipate, such as human error or mechanical malfunction. *Common causes* are found in the processes themselves. A given cause is not inherently special or common; the terms describe relationships of specific causes to specific processes. The focus is on finding common causes because they can be redesigned to eliminate variation or sentinel events. This is a valid point of view but not an explicit method.

The method suggested here starts with a generic list of causes designed to reflect relatively detailed categories experienced in the health field. It neither ranks nor winnows causes before data collection is done, and it requires that all the possible causes be identified before the problem is proved because collection of data on many causes is concurrent with collection of problem data.

The general checklist presented in Figure 2.1 offers groupings that reflect the health services industry. Beside the items are references to other ways of referring to causes. As a start, the consultant can select what applies from the general list, substituting more specific language whenever possible and adding items not covered by the list.

Your list should be exhaustive but include only causes about which you can collect data. For example, collecting data on mental alertness requires access to patients' charts or files; without such access it would be hard to prove mental alertness to be a cause. General causes such as "motivation" are mentioned in the literature but need to be defined operationally as specific attitudes that can be studied with a questionnaire that asks pointed questions related to the problem. For example, in dealing with patient compliance with home exercise, you can ask whether the regimen is painful, whether there is someone able to help carry it out, whether the patient wants to carry it out, and whether the patient thinks it helps. Each of these touches on a separate cause. You cannot ask, "Are you motivated?" because patients could not be expected to answer fully, truthfully, or consistently.

Possible Causes by Major Category	*Other Typology*
Patient/Consumer Risk Factors	Demographic and socioeconomic
Sex	variables, medical condition, and
Age	attitudes not under control of
Diagnosis	organization
Secondary medical condition	
Alertness	
Language used	
Use of English	
Ability to communicate	
Medications	
Mobility level	
Marital status	
Income level	
Type of insurance	
Number of infants, children, individuals in home	
Minority status	
Years of education or highest degree	
Attitude toward problem	
Attitude toward compliance	
Self-care compliance	
Related to Staff	
Specific staff person	Specific
Specific job title	Structure
Years of experience in organization	Structure
Years of experience in profession	Structure
Highest, closest degree	Structure
Attitude toward problem	Subjective
Beliefs about problem/nature of problem	Subjective
Beliefs about consequences of problem	Subjective
Knowledge related to problem	Subjective
Performance skill	Specific
Sense of being overworked	Process/structure
Sense of not feeling accountable	Subjective/structure
Related to Institution	
Specific units	Structure/process
Specific shift	Structure/process
Specific step(s)	Process
Specific procedures	Process
Specific tests or units of procedure	Process
Specific equipment, materials	Specific/structure
No defined policy related to problem	Structure
No standards in administrative manuals	Structure
Way work is organized	Process
Supervisors do not hold staff accountable	Process/administration
Performance on this not part of evaluation	Process/administration
Lack of feedback on problem	Process/administration
Documentation too general	Structure
Documentation poorly designed	Structure
Documentation nonexistent	Structure
Staff do not have authority to do what is needed	Structure/process
Other Causes	
Found through observation, review of literature, interviews with staff or in team/staff meetings	

Figure 2.1 Checklist of Possible Causes and Related Typology

Complete your list and find additional causes by carrying out a literature review and conducting interviews with staff. In some projects, it is useful to interview people doing similar work in other organizations; they may already have faced the problem or may have fresh ideas about causes.

Literature Review and Interviews

The literature review for causes can be part of the review discussed in Chapter 1 under the section on defining the problem. It should draw on the journals associated with the discipline, such as physical therapy or nursing. Textbooks in the field often discuss issues that can suggest possible causes. Look for discussions that deal with similar problems in institutions like yours. Look for indications of what the authors consider the causes to be. (See also the section on "Background Reading Related to the Cases," which follows the Appendixes.)

By far the most important source is the people who are doing the work in your organization; you not only benefit from their knowledge of the situation and its unique features, you are involving staff in the project and providing an atmosphere that creates hope that the problems can be solved.

In a CQI team, the members might be the ones who would be consulted initially. In other situations, select the number of staff to interview, considering how many are involved with the problem and the number you can interview within your time constraints. How many must you interview to avoid having some staff feel left out? If there is a large number of staff, you might select a cross-section by unit, title, or location. On the other hand, if the relevant staff is small, such as eight people, it would be a mistake to ask only six or seven.

In some of the cases reported here, a staff meeting was found to be a useful setting in which to ask for ideas about causes. In others, informal, face-to-face interviews were used. (Be careful about asking management people about causes because they may insist on them later on, despite what you find.)

After selecting the staff to interview about additional causes, use an informal interview approach. Avoid using a questionnaire; you will probably need to do a staff survey later, and you do not want to wear out your welcome. Standardize your questions—that is, present them

The problem being investigated: possible causes and solutions of the problem of long length of stay within rehabilitation for adult amputation patients.

Author number from reference list	Page(s)	Causes Identified	Not New	New	New and Used	Possible Solutions
2	343	Whether there is a permanent home		x	x	Social service should consider community resources, what home support the patient can expect
3	385	Psychological state	x			Psychological help

ID of Interviewee (No Name)	Title and Institution (if different)	Causes Identified	Not New	New	New and Used	Possible Solutions
1	Staff physical therapist	Whether patient has medical complications due to the prosthesis		x	x	Regular in- service classes on topic of prosthetics and care, including developments in the field.
2	Physical therapy super-visor	Prosthesis vendor delivers late, delivers ill-fitting device		x	x	Closely monitor vendors; cancel inadequate vendors; have physical therapists present in clinic when device is delivered
3	Staff occupa-tional therapist	Whether patient has a permanent home	x			Have social service closely involved

Figure 2.2 Model for Causes and Solutions From Literature and Interviews (Excerpts from Case 4)

in the same way each time you ask them. After explaining the problem you are studying, you might ask, "What do you think causes this?" or use similar language.

A useful way to show the results of the literature search and interviews is a table in which you fill in causes and check off your decisions about them. Figure 2.2 is a model excerpted from the literature review and interviews conducted for Case 4, which dealt with the length of stay of amputation patients. The first column identifies each literature source by number or each staff member interviewed by code. For interviews, the job title is in the next column. If you talk with staff in another institution, the name of that institution is entered. The next column lists the causes identified, always using the same language for a particular cause no matter how it is worded by the respondent or the literature. Using the same language makes it possible to recognize how many times the cause is mentioned.

Other columns are labeled "Not New," "New," "New and Used," and "Solutions." If a cause is already on your list, check the column titled "Not New," indicating that you have already identified it. If the cause is not on your list, check the "New" column each time this cause is mentioned. Finally, if a new cause is plausible and you decide to study it, check the "New and Used" column. Any "new and used" cause is evaluated along with the original list. Figure 2.2 shows solutions, but the column is actually left blank until you are ready to find solutions for *proved* causes.

Design Detailed Data Collection to Verify the Problem and Its Extent

The data collection forms are products that you do not need to have ready at the time you define your agreement with the client. All you have to know is the general outline of the research and data collection. This allows you time to refine your approach. Now you are ready to develop ideas and work with your collaborator to design data collection forms. Then, ask for approval from designated managers to field test the instruments. In addition to data collection to prove the existence of the problem and its extent, the work includes the design of instruments for data collection about causes that can be collected at the same time.

Institutional Data

Data to prove the existence of the problem can usually be collected from objective, organizational sources. These include data already collected by the institution in the normal course of work and data collected with instruments designed for the project and collected only during the project.

Objective variables are measures that exist in quantitative form and are not subject to individual judgment or interpretation. They are factual and usually come from operations in the institution or from patient charts. In Case 1, objective variables included the number of days from admission to start of the physical therapy program, as well as patient characteristics such as age, sex, diagnosis, and date of admission. For Case 5, the number of referrals to the HMO laboratory with any of six essential items missing, the number of referrals associated with delays due to missing items, and the number of patients who did not return were all data that could be drawn from existing institutional sources.

If the institution does not generate data that can be used to prove the problem, this may itself be a cause. Any problem worth working on merits regular data collection as a part of normal operations. For example, when the head nurse in a hospital outpatient department studied lack of attendance by staff at mandated classes (Case 10), a major cause was that the department responsible for scheduling had no record of how many classes were held, who was scheduled, or how far in advance staff were notified.

Objective variables created and collected for the project often include information on the start and end times of steps; details on procedures not always collected, such as the blood-drawing technique or type of requisition used; or records of events not previously collected.

If you cannot find records on the start and end times for a step, you need a data collection form on which the people doing the step identify the subjects and list the times the step started and ended. In Case 3, the consultant asked staff to write in on the data sheets produced by the laboratory equipment the time that an important step ended, because no times were collected at that point. In Case 7, data collection instruments had to be filled out by the staff who drew the blood specimens, detailing their techniques, which were linked to patient ID information, because there were no other sources of data on blood-drawing technique. In Case 5, the consultant had to record the type of requisition form used.

Other data collection depends on how the extent of the problem is defined. Identification of the patient, unit, or service provider may be needed. In Case 1, data were collected by patient type, including the presence of a fracture, whether the patient was starting or continuing physical therapy, and whether the patient was a resident of the institution or a new admission coming from a hospital or from home.

The causes being studied determine any additional objective data that need to be collected. So, if you are interested in variables such as equipment used in the process or the way a procedure is carried out, you need to design data collection for this stage, because the data on causes must refer to the same units of observation used to prove the problem; you will not be able to go back to match much of the material later.

Subjective variables, which are sometimes needed to prove the problem but are more closely associated with proving causes, can be produced through interviews and questionnaires. The data are the opinions, attitudes, and knowledge of the specific subjects involved. Subjective variable data have certain limitations. Those answering the questions may not understand them, may not consider their responses carefully, may have faulty memories, may want to please the data collector, may feel intimidated, may not care about accuracy, may be tired, may have a biased outlook, may compare responses with others, or may in some other way respond unreliably. Therefore, the data can be biased and thus unreliable.

Objective variables are preferred when dealing with processes, rates of outcomes, and structural information dealing with the problem. Subjective variables are required when dealing with variables that reflect intangibles such as attitudes, knowledge, beliefs, and opinions.

Questionnaires and interviews can provide important insights, especially if you are sensitive during the field test, are present to answer questions, or ask for opinions. This is the only way to find out how staff view the problem, how patients feel about care, whether staff have the knowledge needed to function properly, and what they think about possible solutions. Questionnaires work best when the items are carefully worded and field tested.

Questionnaires for the 14 cases were tailor-made to identify causes and were sometimes used to collect objective data to prove that the problem existed. In Case 2, a patient-held form was filled out upon arrival at the department and used to record the times of each step, but it also included the patient's opinion on the length of the wait. In Case 9, labor and management representatives filled out questionnaires that led to the identification of health and safety problems and the determination of whether the joint committee was being used to deal with them.

Tables

Design tables to make data collection easy for the data collectors. The title, column headings, and stubs (row titles) should make it clear what the content is, including the units involved. Have columns for all the detail needed later; include columns for the dates. The proportions should be esthetic with respect to the width of columns and the number of rows. A table that fits an 8½" × 11" page is easiest to work with. Provide enough space to include adequate descriptions in the column headings.

Tables have a number, a title, and a horizontal line under the title. Beneath the line are the column headings and another horizontal line. The stubs are in the far left column and show what each row refers to. Beneath the column headings and in the rows are the column/row cells for the data; beneath the data entries is another horizontal line.

Underneath come the footnotes, indicated in the body of the table by symbols or letters (but never numbers, to avoid confusion with data), and sources, unless the data were created for the table. The footnotes in a table provide explanations, such as what abbreviations stand for or how an entry in a column or row differs from others in the column or row in how it was collected or what it refers to. When a table carries over to another page, repeat its title and headings and add the word *continued* after the title, and/or use (for example) "p. 1 of 3" at the top of the page. Tables to be presented in the text of reports are usually numbered in the order presented and appear on the page after they are first mentioned.

To protect the confidentiality of staff and patients, no names ever appear in data tables that anyone may possibly see. The internal consultant creates codesheets that assign project identification numbers to subjects. These tables can include other data, such as demographics, but everyone except the consultant sees them with only ID numbers included. The consultant keeps a set with the names for private reference only.

Code numbers for subjects or units should be assigned in some logical order and should be determined by how you will summarize the data and arrange the original subjects. The subjects might be coded in order as they arrive in the study, by unit, or in some way you will eventually add them as subtotals. Without ordering the subjects, you will not be able to add columns of data easily or find individual items when needed. A logical order also makes it easier to find and correct errors. It is not a good idea to assign project code numbers by the alphabetical order of the subjects' names, because you will never use the names, and the order will never be relevant.

When you design the layout of columns for factual data, such as demographics and other risk factors, it facilitates the calculation of later summary data to use "check sheets," with columns that only need to be checked off. For example, if you want data on marital status, you should not have a column headed "Marital Status" because you will have to write in the status for each subject. Later, you will have to scan the column as many times as there are marital status categories, and there will be no place to show totals and percentages on the same page. You would need an additional table.

The better alternative is to have a column for each subcategory, as shown in the hypothetical model, Table 2.2. All you need to do to record the data is to check the correct column. Totals are easily calculated by adding check marks, and this provides a handy way to check accuracy because the subtotals must add to the grand total. It is also possible to show the percentage share of the grand total by category at the bottom of the same table. The columns need to be wide enough to enter totals and percentages when carrying to one decimal place (e.g., 100.1).

With more complicated variables such as diagnoses, you can designate columns for the most common diagnoses and have a catch-all "other" for more rare diagnoses. Nothing is lost because rare diagnoses do not account for enough instances to be actual causes. The headings in Table 2.2 are abbreviated and explained in footnotes at the bottom of the table.

In Table 2.2 and throughout this text, the data tables are presented single spaced and without lines between rows. For actual data collection, it is easier to work with lines. That calls for more pages but makes

Table 2.2 Demographic Data for Patients in Study

Patient Project ID	Marital Status				Diagnosis[a]				Sex	
	Married	Single	Divorced	Widowed	HD	OA	HT	O	Male	Female
1	x				x				x	
2	x				x				x	
3		x				x				x
4			x					x		x
5				x		x				x
6	x				x				x	
7	x						x			x
8		x					x			x
9			x					x		x
10				x	x				x	
Total 10	4	2	2	2	4	2	2	2	4	6
Percentage of total	40.0	20.0	20.0	20.0	40.0	20.0	20.0	20.0	40.0	60.0

a. HD = heart disease; OA = osteoarthritis; HT = hypertension; O = other.

it easier to be accurate. Having vertical lines between columns is also helpful.

Summary tables are designed to organize the raw data. They contain the information needed to answer research questions such as, "Is the problem proved?" and "Which causes are proved?" Before summarizing the data, be sure that the raw data are accurate. The consultant can check that the data collector has covered what was asked for and has been honest about the figures by spot checking during the actual data collection, by noting whether quantities are plausible, and by asking the collector to describe what he or she is doing.

In Case 3, laboratory technologists were asked to report the time they ended a step. The consultant noticed that some times were impossible because the start of the step, collected elsewhere, showed a later time than the end of the step as recorded by the technologists. This had to be dealt with before she could calculate average time for the steps, so she changed the way some of the data were collected.

The device of using column numbers and showing how columns are combined or acted on to produce other columns tells the reader how calculated columns are derived. In Table 2.3, column 4 is the total of output quality categories derived by adding columns 1, 2, and 3

Table 2.3 Acceptable and Unacceptable Outputs by Unit

Unit ID		*Output Quality*			*Quality as Percentage of Total*		
	OK	*Rejects*	*Salvage*	*Total*	*OK*	*Rejects*	*Salvage*
Columns:	*(1)*	*(2)*	*(3)*	*(1)+(2)+(3)=(4)*	*(1)÷(4)%*	*(2)÷(4)%*	*(3)÷(4)%*
1	230	20	20	270	85.2	7.4	7.4
2	100	30	35	165	60.6	18.2	21.2
3	120	10	12	142	84.5	7.0	8.5
4	140	15	10	165	84.8	9.0	6.1
5	210	18	20	248	84.7	7.3	8.1
6	69	3	5	77	89.6	3.9	6.5
7	70	5	10	85	82.4	5.9	11.8
Total	939	101	112	1152	81.5	8.8	9.7

NOTE: Column 4 is the total of output quality categories derived from adding columns 1, 2, and 3 across. The remaining columns are derived by expressing columns 1, 2, and 3 as a percentage of the total in column 4.

across. The remaining columns are derived by expressing columns 1, 2, and 3 as a percentage of the total in column 4. This gives the distribution by quality category for each of the seven units and the grand total.

A danger with tables is to try to include too much, squeezing many columns onto a page, with headings that are meaningless because of cryptic titles and undecipherable abbreviations. This sacrifices clarity and the reader's ability to understand to what the columns refer. One solution is to use codes or acronyms in the column heads, with footnotes that explain the headings more fully. Another solution is to add more lines to the column heads so that more words can be used in the headings to clarify the meaning (i.e., use several stacked rows in the column heads). Appendix 2 presents a wide variety of column headings used in Case 1.

Getting Approval

Ask the client for approval to field test and use the forms you design to collect data. This gives you a chance to keep the client informed and to make sure there are no issues of data availability, and it gives the client an opportunity to see the logic of the design. When the client sees what you actually want to collect, the project becomes real, but this can lead to the discovery that you do not have access to some data. In one case, the client decided that medical residents could not be asked to provide information on how long their tasks took, even though the project was to study unequal workloads. "Professionals" could not be asked how long they spent on tasks, even though the client wanted to know. (This may have been a trade union issue; residents were in a collective bargaining unit.) The problem was resolved by collecting data on the number of tasks done, information that was available in existing records; management was asked to assign average times to each kind of task. The resulting data were estimates. If the consultant had gone ahead without approval, she would have been in a seriously compromised position, as the client was adamant about not asking the residents directly.

Field Testing

A field test is a tryout of the instruments to be used for data collection in a real application. Objective data are usually collected in tables. All the people who are to collect the data must do the field testing because you want to find out how easily they can use the tables and whether the tables are set up to comfortably record the data. (If you are using questionnaires, field testing is done with a population sample similar to but different from your intended subjects. This is covered in Chapter 3, which is on proving causes.)

Without field testing, you can come to the end of data collection with data missing, with staff ignoring some of the requests, or with data representing staff's own idea of what to collect. Field testing lets you spot and deal with problems before they hurt the project. You might have to consider getting the information another way. Field testing can uncover the fact that data collection will be overwhelming for the staff being asked to do the work.

Important information may be missing from the forms, column headings may mislead staff about what is being called for, or data may not exist in the form being called for. You may discover that the columns are not wide enough for the data, or you may need to add columns for data that are described in more categories than you anticipated. For example, you may have listed three categories for hemolysis—slight, moderate, and gross—and forgotten "none."

The field test is usually conducted during a brief period prior to the start of regular data collection. It might be a few days or a few hours, depending on how many units are seen per time period. Train staff for data collection and field test the instruments with all the staff who will be using the forms. Even if you are the only one who will be collecting the data, the tables need to be field tested. Not doing so may keep you from noticing problems you will then have to face later, when it may be too late to deal with them effectively. Revise any data collection forms as needed after you have evaluated the field test results.

Get Data Collection Dates Into the Calendar

You need to schedule arrangements to start collecting data as planned because it is time consuming and needs to be treated with respect. Arranging for actual data collection may pose new problems, even if you have had a successful field test. Conditions may have changed, the reality of what is involved may have dawned upon the people involved, or you may have neglected to field test some data collection forms. You may discover that your original plans for data collection have been thwarted by unexpected contingencies. Be sure to make all the necessary arrangements to obtain access to data under the control of other staff members, such as medical records or human resources records. This is assumed to have been taken care of when you got approval to do the project; you will have considered who needs to be informed about the data collection and whose permission you need. You need to be sensitive to the structure of the organization so that you do not undermine the authority of those in charge of the people you need to help you collect data. Review arrangements about the original permission they granted with the supervisors of any staff who are to collect data. At this time, be sure you can demonstrate how you will keep the data confidential. In some cases, this means agreeing to work with records in the room in which the data are filed, rather than carrying them away or making copies to work with.

Make sure that each person to collect data for you has been trained in the field test, knows what to do, and still agrees to cooperate. If staff are collecting data about their own work, they may need reassurance about the confidentiality of the data; this may require a meeting to cover how you will protect the identity of the data and how the solutions will deal with everyone and not single out individual staff. You might ask staff what they need in the way of assurances to make them feel safe, and comply with the request. This gives staff a sense that they have some power over the situation.

A supervisor may insist on seeing the data. You might deal with this by making it impossible to obtain data that could identify staff. For example, you could keep the code sheets at home and have only coded data in the office. As an internal consultant, your own reputation for integrity is one of your most important assets; it comes over time through your own actions on a day-to-day basis. The best approach is to already have a stipulation in a written agreement assuring confidentiality.

Staff may be too busy. If staff are too busy to collect data for you, you may have to rethink how you will obtain what you need. In a study about patient falls, the consultant was unable to get the nursing department to agree to collect observation data on falls for the period of the study. He needed to compare incident reports with data from patient charts, and he found three sources for his data without involving nurses. He picked up the incident reports as they came to Quality Assurance; these triggered his review of the patients' charts; on the last day of data collection, he and some coworkers reviewed every chart currently on the patient units to note any falls, which triggered a check for counterpart incident reports. To cover patients who were discharged during the month, he enlisted Medical Records to alert him to charts of patients being discharged that mentioned falls, triggering a check for incident reports.

The data may not exist, may be in archaic form, or may be denied. A consultant who studied rehospitalization rates for an account in a managed care organization found that the account had been handled for only a year. The former manager of the account refused access to computerized records. Only after the consultant had used the one year of data that she had to identify patients who had been rehospitalized in that year was she allowed to see past records for those individuals.

In Case 10, when the consultant studying staff attendance at mandated classes found that the data were not being collected in adequate form to help identify the causes of nonattendance, she was put off from gaining access to the data that *were* in existence; she eventually had to get what limited data there were from another source. To her surprise, however, once she overcame the initial supervisor's fear that the attendance figures would be used against her, the supervisor began to collect data in the way the consultant originally hoped for, without being asked. The supervisor had not been able to visualize how data collection could be helpful until she saw the consultant's data collection forms, which became the model for her own data collection.

The problem may not be what you expected. In a case studying clinic patients' attendance at prenatal classes, the consultant discovered that no classes at all had been given at the main clinic. This affected her decision on what causes to study; those related to patients seemed irrelevant.

The time periods needed may be different. You may find that the original plan did not allocate enough time for data collection or to deal with other difficulties. Your timetable can be affected. You may have to revise your objectives and develop an enabling objective that involves dealing with the difficulties.

Consultants who do well essentially do not take no for an answer about data collection; they assume that they will be able to find a way out of the difficulties and manage to rethink the situation so as to succeed.

What Criteria Will Be Used to Prove the Problem?

The work on criteria to prove the problem's existence should occur while you are collecting data and before you have your results; the criteria must be selected independently from the results. The criteria are the levels of indicator data that would convince management that there is a problem; they are thresholds or limits set or agreed to by management without any recourse to the data being collected. This ensures an objective determination about whether the problem actually exists.

Proof-of-problem criteria are levels of indicators below or above which there would be a problem. They are unacceptable thresholds for rates, proportions, ratios, or percentages in which the problem variables are expressed. The criteria are the points that define *too much* or *too little*, such as the percentage of errors or the percentage of staff who go over the limit. If you are collecting data on waiting time, the criteria would specify the maximum allowable wait and the percentage of patients who could acceptably wait longer than that, and/or a maximum average waiting time. Only the institution's managers, accreditation agencies, and mandated regulations can determine the acceptable levels for the criteria.

Work on your own idea of what the criteria should be and review the literature. Suggest the criteria, and ask for approval from the manager(s) you named in the plan of work agreement. Aside from mandated criteria, which take precedence, be prepared to accept management's views because the managers are the ones who have to be convinced that the problem exists. In Case 1, dealing with waits to start physical therapy, the consultant conducted interviews and did a literature review on the limits for awaiting physical therapy treatment. She found that more than 7 days for patients in general and more than 3 days for fracture patients are the limits beyond which waiting would adversely affect patients. Without management agreement about these limits, the consultant could not establish the proof of the problem. On the other hand, the consultant was free to argue for particular standards.

Table 2.4 is taken from Case 1. It is a model showing the presentation of criteria to prove that the problem exists, its extent, and results. This project established 3 days as the maximum wait allowed for fracture patients and 7 days for other patients. The far left-hand column has the measures (dimensions) to be addressed, and next to it is the threshold above or below which the problem is said to exist. The far right column gives the source(s), usually a summary table from which the data are to come.

The threshold, or cut-off, is set at a level above which management would say there is a problem and below which there would be no problem. In CQI, a level that was once acceptable may now constitute a problem. For Case 1, there were two thresholds. The first was the highest acceptable percentage of patients who have to wait too long and the second was the average wait above which the problem would be said to exist.

The consultant believed that no patient should wait beyond the limit, and suggested a threshold of zero. The client said that some wait over the limit was unavoidable. The consultant said, "OK, is there a

Table 2.4 Criteria for Proof of Problem and Results: Waiting for Physical Therapy (Case 1)

Measure	Point Beyond Which the Problem Exists (Percentage, Rate, etc.)	OKed	Actual Results	Source
Number of days from admission (or from request for physical therapy if already resident)				
Fracture	> 3 days	x		
Nonfracture	> 7 days	x		
Percent of patients with wait longer than limits				Table 1.4
Total patients (74)	> 9%	x	67.6%	Proved
Fracture	> 9%	x	100.0%	Proved
Nonfracture	> 9%	x	60.0%	Proved
Total from hospital	> 9%	x	75.0%	Proved
Starting therapy				
Fracture	> 9%	x	100.0%	Proved
Nonfracture	> 9%	x	60.7%	Proved
Continuing therapy				
Fracture	> 9%	x	100.0%	Proved
Nonfracture	> 9%	x	80.0%	Proved
Total already residents	> 9%	x	50.0%	Proved
Starting therapy				
Fracture	> 9%	x	100.0%	Proved
Nonfracture	> 9%	x	46.2%	Proved
Total from own homes (All starting therapy and nonfracture)	> 9%	x	25.0%	Proved
Average day's wait				Table 1.4
Total patients	> 5 days	x	11.5 days	Proved
Fracture	> 3 days	x	15.1 days	Proved
Nonfracture	> 7 days	x	10.7 days	Proved
From hospital	> 5 days	x	12.2 days	Proved
Already residents	> 5 days	x	10.4 days	Proved
From own home	> 5 days	x	6.8 days	Proved

problem if 2% of patients wait too long? The consultant said, "No," and the consultant worked up. "Is there a problem at 5%? At 10%?" At this point the client said there would be a problem. So the problem was to be proved if more than 9% had to wait too long. (If accreditation standards had been set at 4%, that would have been the limit set.)

The 10% limit applied to the total; to fracture and nonfracture patients; to patients starting therapy or already on it; and to those being admitted from a hospital, from home, or current residents. The second set of criteria specified averages of 3 days for fracture patients, 7 days for nonfracture patients, and 5 days for the total, with anything higher a problem; 5 days were allowed for residents, those coming from hospitals, or from home.

In Table 2.4, the standards for fracture and nonfracture patients are entered at the top, so the reader can see the reference meant when "limit" is mentioned in the criteria. Management accepted the 3 and 7 days. Notice that, because the 3- and 7-day limits were accepted, the same percentage figure for patients above the limit could be used for each category.

The middle column in Table 2.4 has a space to enter an "x" mark when management approves the criteria. Next comes the column to show the actual results. As can be seen, every threshold was exceeded.

With a small number of subjects, the thresholds require special thought. Consider what the percentages mean in terms of people. In Case 12, the internal consultant studied the possible benefit of re-minder letters for women who were due to have follow-up visits. She was to prove the problem with a retrospective study of 100 women and an intervention study of 40 women. Due to the circumstances of the project design, she had a control group of only 20, who received no letter, and 20 in the experimental group, who received a reminder letter. In the study of 100, one patient equaled 1%. The consultant could say that there would be a problem if noncompliance were over 3%; that would be more than 3 subjects. But in a group of 20 subjects, one patient is 5.3%; 3% is .6 of a person and is therefore impossible. In a sample of 15, 1 patient is over 6%. With such small sample numbers, it may be better to choose numerical criteria such as 2 out of 15 or 1 out of 10, because the percentages can be misleading, and the reliability of the conclusions is questionable.

Prove Whether the Problem Exists and Its Extent

Most enabling objectives mentioned so far lead to actual data collection and analysis. After data collection, you need to calculate totals, averages, and percentages as called for by the criteria. You compare the results with the criteria agreed on earlier. You then have your data checked. Finally, you take your results to the key management people you want to convince.

Dealing With Data

When calculating percentages, you will not usually need to take the results to more than one decimal place. Show all the data in a given column to the same number of decimal places; line them up with a fixed decimal position in the column. Never omit the totals when they are called for in tables.

A *percentage change* over time tells the change from a starting point to a later point as a percentage of the original figure. (It is a convention that it is never the change as a percentage of the later figure. The formula is: last minus first, divided by first, times 100.) If there has been a decline, the result has a minus sign. For example, if there were 142 patients in 1990 and 148 in 1992, the percentage change is 148 – 142 (an increase of 6) divided by 142 (the earlier figure), or 4.2%. It would not be 6 divided by 148 (the later figure), which would be 4.1%.

A *rate* is a ratio between two figures, sometimes expressing one as a percentage of the other; for problem indicators, it is negative occurrences as a percentage of the subjects or units being studied. Percentage rates give levels of involvement regardless of absolute size. If, of 120 patients, 40 have TB, then 33.3% have TB. If there were 5 new cases, the rate of new cases is 4.2%. Expressed as new cases per 1000 patients, the rate is 42 new cases per 1000 patients (1000 × .042).

Percentage shares pay attention to proportions, to how large a section of the whole is compared with the whole. For example, one hospital may have a 20% *rate* of TB cases; one out of every 5 patients has TB. However, the total patients in the hospital may be only 2% of the patients in the city's hospitals, a 2% *share*. The hospital would have 2% of all the TB cases in the city if it has a proportionate share of cases. If all hospitals had proportionate shares, each would have the same share of TB cases as its share of patients, and each would have the same rate of TB cases.

Checking Data

Have your collaborator check your figures. A study can be ruined by errors in calculations and conclusions based on them. Always recheck your figures and see whether they make sense to you. Proofread your tables. If you copy data from one page to another, proofread after you do the copying. A good check is to add across as well as down when the data for totals are presented both ways and to check totals from one table to another when the same population is being described. When total observations are tallied for different variables, they should add to the same number of observations.

Comparison With Criteria

When you are sure your data are correct, compare your results with the criteria set earlier, as in Table 2.4, which also tells which tables to consult for each dimension of the problem you are examining. Table 2.4 is completed when you enter the results and make the judgment about whether the particular dimension of the problem is *proved*, *partly proved*, or *not proved*. For Case 1, Table 2.4 shows that each criterion was exceeded, and the problem was proved for each. Not only did the various rates exceed the limits of 3 or 7 days way beyond the 9% allowed, ranging from 25% to 100%, but average days of wait exceeded the limits as well.

Convincing the Client

Take your results to the client who approved the criteria. Because the client helped select the criteria, he or she can be expected to be convinced by the results. You might arrange a meeting and bring Table 2.4 and its source tables; you might send a brief report including copies of the relevant tables. In any case, it is important to have a face-to-face discussion to remind the client of the original criteria and what they mean, to reinforce the significance of the findings, to be sure the client has been convinced, to lay the basis for work on causes, and to ensure that the client does not act precipitously as a result of being convinced.

Sometimes the results are so dramatic, as in Case 1, that the client wants to rush ahead with solutions. In this case the client was shocked at the results, was sure that a particular physician was the cause, and was ready to replace him. The consultant made a point of persuading the client to wait until all the research was completed. This was very important, because unexpected causes were proved, and there was no need to replace the physician.

Progress Assessment: The Progress Report

Once you have proved the problem, you may wish to revise your work plan for the rest of the project. Some remaining due dates may seem unrealistic, some success criteria may need modification, you may have to revise your list of causes to study, the real world experience may have given you a different idea about how to proceed, or you may have found new problems.

You also may have promised to deliver a *progress report*. A progress report is addressed to the client and any other designated audience. Its components are a review of the original project plan of work, a report on what occurred, an assessment of results so far, and suggested revisions for the remaining work. The progress report is an opportunity to make revisions in the plan of work in the context of telling the client what has occurred.

Oral Presentation

If you are to make an oral presentation, you would do well to prepare material to circulate or present as audiovisual aids, provided they are not to be treated as confidential. In your oral presentation, cover what the project is about in the first third of the presentation; explain the main problem or main objectives, and your general approach. In the next third, tell what objectives were due by now and what has happened up to this point. In the last third, tell about your conclusions so far and any revisions you now suggest, plus a summary of what is still to come. Allocate your time so that you have enough left for your last main points. Know what you have proved and how you proved it; don't forget to mention any effects of the project on the organization; and know what you are asking for, such as changes in due dates or modifications of the plan of work. Consider any possible objections and be prepared to answer them.

Practice making a coherent oral presentation. Remember that you are giving the audience a gift. They want to hear your story. To be secure, you need to know your project. Use an outline either on a sheet of paper or cards. (Number the cards in case they fall.) Have the main points you want to make in key phrases and know which specific tables support your points.

When you make your presentation, take a deep breath; feel the audience lean toward you. Relax; you have something to give. Tell what you are about to report on and the purpose of the presentation. Use eye contact for feedback; check to see if you are being understood or need to clarify. This is why it is not a good idea to read; reading can also make the speaker seem boring. Practice delivery and timing with a friend, a tape recorder, or in front of a mirror.

Written Report

The progress report is written with the assumption that the reader knows little about the project. This ensures that all the relevant material will be included and that the report can be circulated to a wider audience if the client decides to do so. The secret of writing such a report is to remember that you are serving the reader and that the objective is to present material that is easy to understand. Writing is a gift to the reader; do not be stingy with explanations or details.

A section called "Review of Project Design" may include the plan of work agreement or a narrative using an updated Table 1.1. Include and refer to a revised plan of work. Table 2.5 shows a revised page from Table 1.1, which is the original evaluation design and plan of work, showing each objective and success criterion in order by due date. Indicate that Table 1.1 has been revised and that it still presents your plan of work and evaluation design, but you have now filled in the columns called *Date Done* and *Actual Results and Comments*. Tell the reader that the table also shows changes in objectives and due dates and that the table is in chronological order by due date. Fill in columns 3 and 5 wherever you have completed objectives. That is what the narrative covers. The due dates remain unchanged in column 2 for all dates already past. However, you may now enter any suggested changes in due dates from the date of the progress report onward.

In the *narrative*, cover the important individual objectives due by name, and give the details. Tell what actually happened as you carried out the work for the enabling objectives and the project objectives they led to, one at a time, in order by due date, with the titles of the objectives as subheadings. Were you successful? Were your success criteria reached? Did you meet your due dates? Tell about unexpected

Table 2.5 Revised Project Evaluation Design, Plan of Work, and Progress, in Order by Due Date (Example; first page only)

Project and Enabling Objectives (1)	Due Date (2)	Date Done (3)	Success Criteria for Each Objective (4)	Actual Results and Comments (5)
Enabling Objectives for Project Objective 1				
Enabling Objective 1a: Get approval for the project's plan of work	Date 1	True Date	Oral or written approval from key manager.	Written approval of proposal from ___.
Enabling Objective 1b: Identify project perameters	Date 2	True Date	Approval of accuracy by relevant manager(s).	Approval of accuracy from ___ and ___.
Enabling Objective 1c: Identify causes to be studied	Date 3	True Date	Interview with [how many?] staff and literature review completed. Decision made on final list.	Interview with___ staff and literature review complete; ___ new causes added to list.
Enabling Objective 1d: Design detailed data collection for proving the problem and objective causes	Date 4	True Date	Approval of data collection forms by relevant manager; successful field test of forms	Approval from ___. Field test results in revision of several tables.
Enabling Objective 1e: Schedule data collection for proof of problem	Date 5	True Date	Approval of data collection and schedule obtained.	Approval obtained from ___and ___. Date set.
Enabling Objective 1f: Identify criteria to prove the problem	Date 6	True Date	Criteria approved by key managers.	Criteria approved by ___ and ___.
PROJECT OBJECTIVE 1: Prove That Problem Exists and Its Extent	Date 7	True Date	Data results meet or exceed criteria set in objective 1f. Data checked by ___. Key managers convinced.	Of ___ criteria to prove the problem, ___ were exceeded. Data checked by ___. ___ and ___ were convinced.
Enabling Objectives for Project Objective 2				
Enabling Objective 2a: Design additional research and data collection on causes	Date 8 Revised		Approval of data collection forms by relevant manager; successful field test of forms; survey items understood and/or discriminate between experts and novices.	In progress.

events or developments and how you handled them. Describe the actual data collection and the tables you used.

Provide your main summary tables and the proof-of-problem table. Tables need to be explained. Identify the tables by number, title, time period, and main purpose. The reader must always know which table you are talking about; this means not jumping from one table to another without telling the reader where you are. Reference to the tables you created should be focused on the parts that bear on the purpose you are addressing, such as totals, rates, and distributions. Show the reader how you arrived at important figures and point the reader to what is important in a given table.

In discussing the results, keep the unit of analysis consistent. If you are talking about percentages, it is inappropriate to switch to totals. For example, to say that 60% of fracture patients waited too long and 18 nonfracture patients waited too long leaves the reader with no basis for comparison. In general, percentages are used for comparison because they express relationships that are independent of the size of the group. If the sample is so small that one case equals 10% or greater, you might give the number as well as the percentage, but this should be done consistently. Similarly, do not switch points of view, such as from attendance to nonattendance rates, in making comparisons.

A *work in progress* section can cover objectives for which you have done work ahead of schedule or in preparation. *Conclusions* are a separate section, in which you draw conclusions about your results. Tell what you learned about the nature of the problem, its extent, unanticipated new problems, or insights about your organization's functioning. *Suggested revisions* are changes you are asking for in the agreement, in your research design, in due dates, or in objectives for the project. Show these in Table 2.5 by crossing out the old language or dates of Table 1.1 and writing in the new ones; discuss them in the report. If approved, the revised plan, objectives, criteria, and due dates will be the ones you are committed to from this point on.

CHAPTER
THREE

Finding and Verifying Causes

**PROJECT OBJECTIVE 2: TO PROVE
THE CAUSES OF THE PROBLEM**

Design additional research and data collection on causes

Schedule data collection on causes

Identify criteria to prove the causes

Carry out data collection and analysis

Design Additional Data Collection on Causes

This chapter covers the work needed to identify and verify the causes of the problem you are investigating. As is the case with other project objectives, the enabling objectives come first.

In this part of the research, the internal consultant is called on to be truly creative, because there are few guidelines in the literature about how to test whether a possible cause is a real cause. Most sources agree that it is not enough to rely on group consensus about the causes of problems. One needs data-based proofs. The collection of data to verify cause-and-effect relationships is "often the most important data collection event in quality improvement" (Swanson, 1995, p. 103). The tests for possible causes are tests of a series of hypotheses.

Data Already Collected

You will have already collected data on the problem variables and a good deal of data on objective causes in connection with proving the problem and its extent, such as demographics and data on the processes, conditions, and other factors involved. Demographic and related data include such variables as age, sex, level of education, diagnosis, and so on. Examples of process data include difficulties with the equipment used, procedures carried out, and length of time for specific steps. Data on conditions might include ratings of the patient's use of English, family size, or degree of alertness. All such data need to be organized in analysis tables, which are created by manipulating already existing data tabulations.

As an example, in Case 2, the problem variable was the waiting period from the time scheduled for the patient's appointment to the actual time the patient was called into the changing room prior to treatment. Each wait was listed in tables by codes for the specific patient visit and patient. There were columns that listed data on possible risk factors or causes such as medical status, mobility status, and whether the patient was an inpatient or not. In Case 4, the unit of analysis was the patient; the problem variable was length of stay; and there were many variables describing the patient, such as age, nutritional status, percentage of cancelled physical therapy appointments, medical condition, and number of persons in the household.

The way to prepare such objective cause data for analysis is to rearrange the data in the tables so that the subjects or units are listed in order, from those with the highest levels of the problem (such as longest waits or length of stay) to the lowest (shortest waits or length of stay). This places the subjects in *rank order* by the severity of the problem. Tables with staff data can be arranged in the same way, by the order of their problem rates and/or proportionate shares of the problem, depending on the project. The same can be done for hospital units, laboratory tests, or any other subject.

Rank 1 is assigned to the subject with the lowest value for the problem variable. Ranks increase in numerical order, 1, 2, 3, and so on, as the variable increases, regardless of the size of the arithmetic distance between two values. For example, if three patients waited 4 minutes, 20 minutes, and 80 minutes, respectively, the ranks would be

1, 2, and 3, respectively. The subject with the highest value of the variable has the highest rank. Subjects with the same value for the variable have the same rank, so there can never be more ranks than subjects, but there can be fewer ranks than subjects.

Once the ranks are assigned, the data in the original tables can be arranged in order by the subjects' ranks. It is then possible to visually examine whether possible causes increase or decrease by rank; it is also easier to identify the characteristics of high- and low-ranked subjects and to calculate totals, subtotals, and percentage shares by subcategories.

For example, in Case 2, there were 132 patient visits. Of these, 19 had excess waits and 113 did not. These are not comparably sized groups, so percentage distributions were needed. Arranging the descriptive variable data such as sex by rank order of the visits permitted the number of visits in each subcategory to be counted and divided between problem and nonproblem visits. The percentage shares by sex could then be calculated for the total (132) visits, the 113 nonproblem visits, and the 19 problem visits. Similar comparisons could be made for variables such as mobility and chemotherapy status.

Additional Objective Cause Data

The new data to be collected will probably fall into four categories: (a) demographic-type data not collected in connection with proving the problem; (b) objective, descriptive data from institutional sources; (c) objective data that can be derived through observation and/or deduction; and (d) subjective cause data that have to do with opinions, attitudes, and knowledge. You decide what data still need to be collected. This section and the next present some guidelines and examples, as do the 14 cases in Part II.

Objective, Demographic-Type
Data Not Already Collected

You may discover that you have forgotten data for some obvious variables; in one case, the consultant forgot to collect data on patients' sex. At this stage it is usually too late to tie problem data to process-related data because the procedures are already completed, but descriptive and demographic data can generally be found in institutional documents such as patient charts, personnel files, and laboratory records. Often the new variables can be inserted into existing tables that were created with wide columns or had space available to add new columns. This also applies to staff data, such as years of experience in the organization and/or in the profession.

Objective, Descriptive Data
From Institutional Sources

Objective, institutional data are needed to investigate causes such as *no defined policy related to the problem, no standards in manuals,* and *performance on this is not covered in staff evaluations.* These are possible institutional causes; they are identified through checking procedural and policy documents or interviewing management. The information is not likely to be disputed because the facts are clear. Data collection is straightforward; results can be tabulated or recorded in notes. In Case 2, for *no standards on waiting times in manuals or policy statements,* the internal consultant examined management-issued manuals and other material available to technologists to see if they said anything about how to handle patient waits.

Objective Data Derived Through
Observation and/or Deduction

Objective data derived through observation are similar to descriptive, institutional data; they must be collected through examination of institutional documents and interviews with management, but they are open to interpretation. Possible causes such as *documentation too general, poorly designed, or nonexistent; staff do not have the authority to do what is needed;* or *the way the work is organized* are given specific detail within the context of the project; the specifics are observed, and conclusions are drawn.

An example is *documentation too general, poorly designed, or nonexistent,* which is really three different causes. Forms being *too general* appeared in a case dealing with patient falls. After examining the forms used to report patient falls, the internal consultant concluded that the form was too vaguely structured and worded to capture the standardized and detailed information needed for an organized quality control program.

A *poorly designed form* was exemplified in Case 5, which dealt with missing laboratory referral data. The official laboratory requisition form did not include a place to indicate whether fasting was required before the specimen was taken for testing, but an unofficial form did. The internal consultant designed data collection so she could compare the rates of patient delays in offices where the official form was used with rates where the unofficial form was used.

No documentation was dealt with in Case 2. The internal consultant examined whether any data were collected on how long patients waited to be seen. In Case 7, the consultant examined whether laboratory reports had a place to indicate whether hemolysis was found in the specimen.

Staff do not have authority to do what is needed was a possible cause in Case 2. The internal consultant investigated whether it was policy for staff to schedule patients in inflexible 15- and 60-minute bookings, because it was possible that such rigidity could result in excess waits.

The way the work is organized requires a description of specific practices that might be causes in the actual project. Interviews and observations establish the facts describing the work, and the connection to the problem comes through deduction and statistical analysis. In Case 2, *the way the work is organized* included, among other things, finding out if inpatients were given priority for visits over outpatients. The consultant interviewed management and examined policy documents to see if the policy existed. The consultant also examined whether "problem visits" were more likely to be among outpatients or inpatients.

Subjective Cause Data: Interviews and Questionnaires

Usually, there are some possible causes that have to do with opinions, attitudes, and knowledge. These call for questionnaires and/or interviews. You may need to develop questionnaires for staff, patients, supervisors, or other relevant "subjects" on possible subjective causes such as *staff attitudes towards the problem; beliefs about the problem, its nature, and consequences; knowledge related to the problem; sense of being overworked; not feeling accountable;* and *lack of feedback about the problem.* These too are general causes that acquire specific detail within the context of the project.

Some subjective cause data can be collected in interviews. An *interview* is a meeting between two or more people designed to obtain or exchange information. An interview need not be face to face. Phone interviews are often successful if they are set up ahead of time. In a *structured interview*, the questions are asked in a standardized manner and order. The resulting data lend themselves to quantification and tabulation. Structured interviews are appropriate when you want respondents to answer a given set of questions and/or choose among a predetermined set of answers, but you also need to adjust the presentation to suit the language skills or experience of the respondents.

An *unstructured interview* is open ended, without preset rules for how the interview will progress. Unstructured interviews should be limited to situations where only a few people are involved because they are time consuming and the results are difficult to quantify. You can use tables to report the results of unstructured interview sessions if the questions lead to answers that can be assigned to predetermined categories or to a set of categories created later to fit the data.

A *questionnaire* or *survey* is a structured set of questions designed to obtain information. You use a questionnaire if it is important that all respondents see or hear the question worded the same way, if the subjects can be assumed to be able to understand the items, and when you have to survey a substantial number of people.

Sample Design

You may need subjective cause data from respondents for whom you already have problem data, such as staff or patients. When you survey such a group of people, the number you survey depends on the situation you are studying, your time, and your resources. If you leave anyone out, you are dealing with a *sample.* If the relevant subjects are all accessible and not too many in number, consider getting data from 100% of the group you have in mind. For example, if you have been collecting data on the bloods drawn by staff, it is best to have questionnaires from all the staff for whom you have data on bloods. If you were studying time spent in rehabilitation by patients, you would want to survey all the patients for whom you have length-of-stay data. If you have the entire group, you are not dealing with sampling, except that any period you select is a sample in time.

If you are dealing with large numbers of people, you might settle for a sample. Sample *size* was discussed in Chapter 2. This section discusses sample *selection*. In sampling, *random selection* means that everyone in the entire group you are interested in has the same chance of being selected for study. You do not impose your own selection criteria. This may be the ideal way to obtain a sample because it gives you the right to make generalizations about the entire group within statistical parameters. But a random sample is often difficult to obtain in the real world of health services organizations.

A good approximation is to use a *systematic sample*. You decide how many out of the total group you will sample, such as 1 out of every 10. You can then select every 10th person, provided you have randomly selected the first subject. The entire group, referred to as the *population* in statistics, is first arrayed by number. If you have 200 in the population, the numbers 1 through 200 are assigned. To give each an equal chance of being included, you might pick a number out of a hat that contains all 200 numbers on slips of paper that have been mixed well, or you might select from a table of random numbers. The number drawn is the number of the first subject to be included in the sample; after that you use every 10th one, coming around to the earlier numbers when you reach the end of the list.

With systematic samples it is important to avoid conditions that can lead to bias. You must be sure that the possible subjects have not been put in order in any way that might bias the results. If the possible subjects have been rank ordered by the attribute you are studying, by alphabetical order, or by self-selected order, the position of the random start can affect the results. You must also avoid having some periodic quality in the list that might correspond to the sampling of "every 10th" that you are using. For example, if the potential subjects were originally assigned to groups of 10 and ranked within those groups, selecting every 10th subject will be biased toward the place in the ranking held by your first subject (Green & Lewis, 1986).

There are instances when you would learn most from *selected nonprobability samples*, especially if you already have problem data. If you were dealing with large numbers of subjects for whom you had problem data, you could arrange them in rank order of their problem variable and select a sample by counting down from the top and up from the bottom until you have a roughly equal number of subjects from both ends of the spectrum. The reason for this design is that you are interested in showing a differential association between problem data and the cause you are studying. A true cause would show a stronger relationship with subjects with more of the problem; it would vary with the extent of the subjects' association with the problem; and the two ends of the problem spectrum would provide more clear-cut contrasts.

If you are *evaluating an intervention*, you might have an experimental group that receives the intervention and a control group that does not receive the intervention, such as in the Case 12 study of the reminder letter. (If there had been another intervention available and in use, it would have been used with the control group instead of no intervention, for ethical reasons.)The subjects were numbered in the order in which their visits were due. The consultant assigned every odd-numbered patient to the experimental group and every even-numbered patient to the control group. This allocated patients to the groups evenhandedly over time and therefore controlled for external events that occurred during the data collection period.

The Questionnaire

Confidentiality is an issue when designing a questionnaire. Asking for staff names might compromise the truthfulness of answers, but you often need to know who answered the questions. You usually need to link the respondents' replies with their performance or association with the problem. If lack of knowledge were a real cause, for example, staff with higher rates of the problem would have more errors on knowledge questions than staff with lower rates, and you would need to match answers to staff.

However, this does not mean that you must ask for names or reveal the identity of the respondents. Use of code numbers and the way you write the introduction to the questionnaire can be helpful. You do not need names if you code the questionnaires or in some other way identify the respondent and then treat the data as strictly confidential. Figure 3.1 presents a variety of opening statements that deal with the question of confidentiality. You need to assure respondents that you

Read to patient:	I am studying the experiences of amputation patients and their adjustments. I would like to ask a few questions. Your name will not be used in my report, so please answer as truthfully as possible. I am interested in whether patients know about the care they need after they leave the hospital. Would you please answer these questions? I will not use your name. Please tell me whether you think things are true, false, or if you don't know.
Write to staff:	Dear colleague: I am trying to find out how well our pharmacy works. Would you please answer the questions below, giving your opinions for each question asked. I would appreciate your help, and thank you for cooperating. My data are confidential, and no names will be used.
	Dear colleague: I am studying the condition of blood specimens that come to the Special Chemistry Department. I would appreciate it if you would answer the following questions as frankly as possible. I am not asking you to write your name, and my results will be based on grouped data. In the questions below, please check the choice that best expresses your opinion, and please answer each question.
Phone or face to face:	I am doing a study on the way we deal with lab test referrals. The information I am collecting is designed to get people's opinions about the referral form information items. The data will be confidential; no names will be used. May I ask you a few questions?

Figure 3.1 Introductions to Questionnaires

are pledged to keeping the data confidential and are not using it against those involved.

Structured questions ask the respondent to choose from a given set of possible answers. The easiest to use are statements of opinion or information relating to the cause that ask the subject to choose *True, False,* or *Don't Know; Agree, Disagree,* or *Don't Know;* or *Important, Not Important,* or *Don't Know.* Trying to get *some* answer is preferable to having an unanswered question, so there must be a place for the respondent to choose *Don't Know.* For knowledge questions, *Don't Know* is important because it can be grouped with the wrong answer choices in later analysis.

Limited choices are preferable if you want to make it easy to carry out subsequent data analysis. Asking the respondent to select among the nuances between *Agree a Little, Agree Somewhat,* and *Agree Very Much* with counterpart degrees of *Disagree* may result in your having few cases within each category, and it may be difficult for the respondents to differentiate among them. As the results will probably be

Which of the following are true or false?	True	False	Don't Know
1. When using a vacutainer, shaking it vigorously can affect whether the sample is hemolyzed.	( )	( )	( )

Please check whether you agree or disagree with the following:	Agree	Disagree	Don't Know
1. I am not always sure that I know the proper way to draw and handle blood.	( )	( )	( )

The following are reasons for not going to the classes. If you have missed any, check how important the explanations below are for you. They can be a main reason, part of the reason (not the main one), or not a reason at all.

Reasons For Not Attending Classes	A Main Reason	Part of the Reason	Not a Reason
1. I would go, but my supervisor says I am needed in the clinic.	( )	( )	( )
9. Other _____	( )	( )	( )

Figure 3.2 Question and Answer Formats

grouped into "agree" and "disagree" categories to prove the causes anyway, fine gradations can be ignored; the point is to have the response be negative or positive rather than neutral.

Open ended questions in which the respondent is asked to fill in requested information are valuable when you cannot anticipate the possible responses beforehand. A useful variation on this is to list all the possible choices you can think of for checking off and also to ask the respondent to fill in anything additional at the end of the list. Figure 3.2 presents some examples of formats for questions and answers. Other examples are presented with many of the 14 cases in Part II.

Validity related to questionnaires has to do with whether or not the instrument is testing what you say it is testing. *Content validity* is about whether the instrument is getting the information you say you want to collect. You need to be sure that the questions ask for the intended information and that the language is appropriate for the educational level and profession of the intended subjects. Nunnally and Durham (1975) suggest that content validity is obtained when the measures are representative of the domain to be studied and if the measures are designed with sensible construction methods. Responses may lack validity because subjects are not willing or able to state directly their true feelings about issues you are interested in. They may be afraid of repercussions, they may want to make a "good" impression, they may think it is none of your business, or they may not know their own opinion.

One of the ways to help assure validity is to frame the questions so that they are most likely to be nonthreatening, free of value implications, acceptably related to the research, and deal with opinions the respondents are likely to be aware of. To do that, the researcher needs to translate causes into neutral, everyday ideas presented from the subject's point of view; this takes experience, which is best gained during field tests of instruments.

To assure professional language and content, select an expert to check work-related questions for professional usage appropriate to the group being surveyed. For example, to interview staff nurses, particularly if *you* are not a nurse, you might go to a higher-level nurse such as the director of nursing and ask her to check for incorrect or awkward language. If you are asking about safety procedures, you might go to the director of infection control.

Whom you select as an expert depends on the kinds of questions you are asking and your intended subjects. Match the expert to the subject matter. The expert could be the client, but it is better to wait for final approval by the client after you have done all the correcting and fine-tuning of the instruments. You then have a better product to show and avoid wasting the client's time on the minutia of creating the instrument.

Field Testing

Once the instruments have been designed, seek the approval of your key management person to field test. Field testing assures the *reliability* of survey data. Reliability allows you to expect that, if the conditions were repeated, the same results would be obtained. Ways to ensure this are to check whether items with similar content get similar results, to standardize the conditions, and to try the instrument on a variety of people and see if you get similar responses from similar people.

You should field test all new data collection forms, but it is most important to field test questionnaires. A question can be hard to understand, it may put the subjects on the defensive, it may be worded too negatively, it may be misunderstood, it may signal the answer you prefer, items may be missing, an item may really be asking two or more different questions, or everyone answering a knowledge question may have gotten it right or wrong.

After the content is approved by the expert, a field test can tell you if the subjects will be able to respond to the questions without bias. The items may actually measure something other than what you intend, such as the ability to read at the grade level of the language or relate to culturally determined experiences not relevant to the information sought.

Field testing with subjects whose backgrounds are similar to the intended group allows you to judge whether your intended subjects will understand the questions and answer what the the questions ask for. You want to know whether you need to make changes. Field testing a questionnaire is done by selecting people *like* the ones you wish to survey. They cannot be the *same* people, because you only get one chance to administer the instrument, and you want to use the final version with your intended subjects. Repeating the use of an instrument contaminates the results because there can be a learning effect.

If your subjects change over time and do not return during the study, such as patients being discharged, your field test group can be patients in the time period just prior to data collection. This makes it possible to include them in your database if it turns out that no revisions of the instrument are necessary. Normally, your intended subjects are a stable group, such as patients undergoing therapy, or staff, and you do not want to contaminate them with trial versions of the instrument. You might field test with staff and/or patients in a similar department, in a unit located far from the one you are studying, or on a shift you will not study. It is best to administer the questionnaire while you are present and encourage the subjects to tell you if anything is unclear. Check the answers at once and ask for explanations of responses that do not seem appropriate for the person responding. Take notes on these exchanges and use them to evaluate how well each item functions in the questionnaire.

Questions on knowledge must be able to discriminate between "experts" who have the information and "novices" who do not. You want to know whether not having the knowledge is associated with the problem. If everyone in the field test answers the same way, you may have worded the question in an obvious way so that even novices get the answers right or in such an obscure way that even experts get the answers wrong. The field test tries out the questions with people whose knowledge you have assessed by other means. They are the experts and novices. An item discriminates if most of your experts get the answer right and most of your novices get the answer wrong. *Most* indicates that there are always exceptions.

During the field test, take note of how how long it takes for respondents to complete the questionnaire or respond to interview questions. That will help you plan your scheduling. Once you have completed the field test, evaluate the results with your collaborator and revise if needed.

Tables for Survey Data

A convenient format for tables with which to present the response data is one in which banks of columns across the top hold a summary of each question at the head of each bank. Below the questions, the columns list the answer choices. This allows the use of check marks to enter the responses from the questionnaires. It is wise to array the responses in a particular order, such as by respondents' rank relevant to the problem, making it easy to add to subtotals and totals. An example is presented in Table 3.1, which is a page from the table used to collect and interpret questionnaire data from staff in Case 7, which deals with the causes of hemolysis in blood samples. The headings are arranged in five banks corresponding to five of the questions, with columns for three possible answers: true, false, and don't know.

As an accuracy check, be sure that the total responses for a question add across to the number of respondents and that the percentage distributions for a question add to 100% for the total and each subset. The comparison of survey results for the highest and lowest ranks allows you to see whether the subjective causes are associated with the problem.

In Table 3.1, 11 respondents are arrayed by rank from 0 to 6, by number of hemolyzed specimens drawn. Rank 0 is none, and rank 6 represents the greatest number. Subtotals cover 10 subjects: ranks 0 and 1 and ranks 3 to 6, with 5 subjects in each group; the rank 2 midpoint is omitted.

Table 3.1 Responses to Questionnaire by Rank Order of Staff (Excerpts from Case 7)

Rank	ID	Title	Q.1 Hemolysis makes a difference.			Q.2 Pulling back on plunger makes a difference.			Q.3 Speed of blood into vacutainer makes a difference.			Q.4 Digging for a vein makes a difference.			Q.5 Shaking the vacutainer makes a difference.		
			True	False	Don't Know	True	False	Don't Know	True	False	Don't Know	True	False	Don't Know	True	False	Don't Know
0	3	PH		x		x			x				x		x		
0	4	PH	x			x			x			x			x		
0	5	RN	x			x				x			x		x		
1	1	PH	x			x			x			x			x		
1	2	PH	x			x			x			x			x		
2	8	RN	x			x			x			x			x		
3	6	RN	x			x			x			x			x		
4	7	RN	x			x				x		x			x		
5	9	RN	x					x			x	x			x		
5	10	HT	x			x			x			x			x		
6	11	HT	x			x				x				x	x		
Total N = 11			10	1	0	10	0	1	7	3	1	8	2	1	11	0	0
Ranks																	
0-1 N = 5			4	1	0	5	0	0	4	1	0	3	2	0	5	0	0
3-6 N = 5			5	0	0	4	0	1	2	2	1	4	0	1	5	0	0
Percentage of Totals																	
Total: 11			90.9	9.1	0.0	90.9	0.0	9.1	63.6	27.3	9.1	72.7	18.2	9.1	100.0	0.0	0.0
Ranks 0-1			80.0	20.0	0.0	100.0	0.0	0.0	80.0	20.0	0.0	60.0	40.0	0.0	100.0	0.0	0.0
Ranks 3-6			100.0	0.0	0.0	80.0	0.0	20.0	40.0	40.0	20.0	80.0	0.0	20.0	100.0	0.0	0.0

NOTE: PH = phlebotomist; RN = registered nurse; HT = hemodialysis technologist.

Schedule Data Collection for Causes
Not Already Dealt With

At this stage, you are likely to need access to institutional documents and interviews with management as well as access to staff so you can administer questionnaires. Make sure to schedule data collection to start by the date to which you are committed by planning ahead. You have already asked supervisors of staff who will be asked to collect data or respond to questionnaires for permission to have them do so; now reconfirm the permission granted earlier. Be sure to train everyone who will collect data and be ready with appointments to administer questionnaires and conduct interviews.

If you administer staff questionnaires at a staff meeting, you can be there to answer questions. For a small number of respondents, administer each one face to face. Sometimes others can administer questionnaires for you at some point in the respondents' day. This may be best if your administrative position might intimidate the respondents should you administer the survey personally. See what makes sense and ensures the most truthful responses.

For busy staff, especially physicians, consider administering the survey by phone. Call first to explain what you would like to do, and then make a telephone appointment if the respondent cannot be interviewed at once. It is important to be able to tell the respondent how long the interview will take. You will have noted this during the field test.

Do not allow questionnaires to be kept overnight by respondents; you do not want them to compare answers. (This happened to a consultant who left questionnaires with staff for several days. All the answers were the same.)

Identify the Criteria to Prove Each Cause

General Approach

You must identify the criteria to prove each cause before data collection is completed because the criteria have to be set without reference to the actual results to ensure that the criteria are not biased.

Unlike proving the problem, institutions rarely conduct research to prove the real causes. Given a problem, there is often a jump to solutions; causes are decided on based on individual experience, conventional wisdom, literature in the field, or what is easy to do and disrupts least. However, years of advanced study projects have shown that things are not always what they appear to be; there have been some real surprises about which possible causes were real causes.

Proof of cause criteria are those combinations of measurements that one would logically expect to obtain if a possible cause were a real cause. You examine all the possible causes to verify or rule out alternative explanations. *Cause* in this context does not imply blame. If a unit or staff member is a cause, you are required to find out what other possible causes are associated.

Work with your collaborator to define what the data must show for each possible cause to be proved to be a real cause, accounting for the kind of data you are collecting. You will have a good deal of leeway in suggesting "proofs," because there are few guidelines in this area. Common sense and basic statistical logic must rule. Consider in what way a real cause would be associated with the problem, and choose threshold values above or below which the cause would be proved. Table 3.2 is an abbreviated model table to show criteria to prove causes and results. It is similar to Table 2.4, which showed criteria to prove the problem. This example is also from Case 1.

The first column on the left gives the cause being studied and includes each cause you originally selected. The next column tells the proof required to prove the cause, followed by a column for "x" marks to show that the client approved the criteria. The last column on the right shows the sources of the data to be consulted, which may include data from interviews as well as from data tables. The next-to-last column on the right is where you enter your results, and the last column also contains your designation of the cause as *proved, partly proved*, or *not proved*.

You may be bewildered by the large number of possible causes you have to find criteria for, but the criteria can be reduced to a manageable set of models. The models can be adapted to similar kinds of possible causes. The section below and the 14 cases in Part II are presented as a guide.

Most *risk factor data* are objective, demographic variables. The underlying reasoning is that a risk factor is proved if it increases or decreases with the degree to which the subjects are associated with the

Table 3.2 Criteria for Proof of Causes and Results: Waiting for PT

Cause and Measure	Proof Required to Prove the Cause	OKed	Actual Results		Source
			Fracture	Nonfracture	
Client Risk Factors					Table 1.4
Whether patient has a fracture	If fracture pts. have a higher % of patients waiting > 3 days than nonfracture patients waiting > 7 days; and if the average wait is longer for fracture patients.	x	Percentage > 3 or 7 — 100.0%; Average wait (days) — 15.1	Percentage > 3 or 7 — 60.0%; Average wait (days) — 10.7	Proved
Whether patient came from Hospital Own home Current resident	If, within fracture and nonfracture groupings, pts. in 1 of the 3 categories has a higher % of pts > limits and if the average wait is longer.	x	Percentage over the Limit — % > 3: Hospital 100.0%, Own home none, Resident 100.0%; Average wait (days): Hospital 12.2, Home 6.8, Resident 10.4	Percentage over the Limit — % > 7: 67.4%, 25.0%, 46.2%	Table 1.4 Proved for Hospital (nonfracture)

problem; subjects with more of the problem have a higher distribution of the risk factor than subjects with less of the problem. Or the problem is proportionately more represented among those with the factor than those without it. The amount of the problem is the subject's rank, amount, rate, or proportion of the problem.

Most risk-factor and process-related causes are either dichotomous or multicategory descriptive variables. A *dichotomous variable* has only two possible conditions, such as sex, whether a subject is an inpatient or an outpatient, or whether a characteristic is present or not. One of the two conditions in a *dichotomous variable* can be said to be a cause if the percentage of subjects with that condition who also have the problem variable is greater than the percentage of subjects with the condition in the entire group or in the nonproblem group, and if subjects with the other condition are a greater proportion of the group without the problem. For example, outpatient status would be a cause of excessive waiting if outpatient status occurred in a greater percentage of patients with excessive waits than with inpatient status (e.g., if outpatients were 70% of the problem group, 30% of the nonproblem group, and 40% of the total) and if inpatient status occurred in a greater percentage of patients without excessive waits (e.g., if inpatients were 30% of the problem group, 70% of the nonproblem group, and 60% of the total).

A *multicategory variable* has more than two possible conditions, such as type of insurance, specific level of mobility, or shift. A subcategory of a multicategory variable can be proved if subjects in the subcategory have higher averages or rates of the problem variable than subjects in the other subcategories, if the subcategory's percentage share of all the problem subjects is more than its percentage share of all the subjects in the study (disproportionate distribution), and sometimes if it accounts for a considerable share of subjects. For example, night shift might be proved to be a cause if its problem rate is at least 10% higher than the other shifts, if its share of the problem is at least 10% higher than its share of clients, and if it accounts for at least a third of all clients.

Special situations, such as having access to equipment or information, can be proved if more than a selected percentage of lower-ranked subjects have or do not have the situation and if this is not true for higher-ranked subjects. The cause must also be tied to the problem logically. Just establishing the situation can prove the problem for causes such as no data being collected about the problem or no policy being in force about the problem. *The way the work is organized* is proved if the situation is verified and shown to be associated with a major share of the problem.

For causes that have to do with *opinions, attitudes, and knowledge*, the criteria are that subjects who give answers that demonstrate the opinion, or attitude, or lack of knowledge must be a large enough percentage of the entire group to make a difference, and that subjects more associated with the problem (higher ranks) give answers that demonstrate the opinion, attitude, or lack of knowledge more than those not associated with the problem (lower ranks). In Case 1, which deals with waits for physical therapy, lack of knowledge was proved if at least 59% of high-ranked physicians gave wrong or don't know answers for relevant knowledge questions and if higher-ranked physicians did worse than lower-ranked physicians.

Staff members, job titles, or *units* are causes if specific members, titles, or units are more associated with the problem. Most of the projects ranked these subjects by *problem rate, disproportionate share of the problem,* and sometimes *share of the work* (i.e., their share of the work was large enough to be able to create the problem). The sum of these separate ranks was used to assign a final rank to the subjects, implying equal weight for each of the ranked variables.

The *rate* of the problem is the number of problem cases of the unit, title, or staff as a percentage of the observations accounted for by the subject. But the rate by itself doesn't tell the whole story. Subjects may all have unacceptably high rates, may all have similar rates, or a subject may account for a tiny share of the total. The *percentage share* of all the observations or all the problem cases pays attention to the extent to which the subject can affect the overall problem. But the percentage share may be high without that particular subject being different from the other subjects. The subject may have a high percentage of problem cases but not a disproportionate share.

A *disproportionate share* of the problem is calculated by subtracting the subject's percentage share of the total observations from the subject's percentage share of the total problem observations. A positive number would mean a disproportionate share of the problem. Zero would mean equal proportions. If each subject has a share of the problem no greater than its share of observations, the problem is distributed proportionately, and no particular subject is a cause. Those with the highest rates tend to have the highest disproportionate shares, but there can be variations. In Case 5, the rate of delay for an office was calculated as *patients with delay*, as a percentage of *patients studied*, but the share of the problem was calculated as the percentage of *days of delay* minus the percentage of *patients*. Proportion of total days of delay was not necessarily the same as proportion of patients with delays.

Once units, titles, or staff are identified as causes, work remains. You want to know *why* these sources are a cause. Is it something about the way the work is done in one unit as compared with others? Is it the training received by one title compared with others? Is it something about the attitudes of some staff? The other cause data help determine this. The criteria require cross referencing with variables such as answers on the questionnaires or years of experience. For example, physicians' knowledge of the consequences of waiting too long for physical therapy was compared with years of experience. Years in the department could be proved a cause if the physicians in higher ranks had a different pattern of experience than those in lower ranks.

In many of the 14 cases, the commonsense criteria described above were used to *screen* for likely causes, and more rigorous *statistical requirements* were then imposed. The statistical tests did not *establish* the causal relationship, because statistics cannot do that; they established the *significance of the results*. Some relatively simple types of statistical analysis can be used to add support to your conclusions—if the consultant has access to a statistical software package and guidance about how to use it. The cases reported in Section II, in which statistical analysis was used, relied on the SPSS®/PC+ package (SPSS Inc.). Norusis (1988) is a very understandable guide.

T tests can be used to determine the statistical significance of differences in problem variable averages based on status in dichotomous (two-condition) cause categories. For example, you might ask, as in Case 4, do female patients have higher average lengths of stay in rehabilitation than males?

Simple correlations measure the extent to which two variables rise and fall together. *Step-wise multiple regression analysis* is helpful when no single variable is sufficient to account for the variations found in the problem (dependent) variable. This method adds variables to the regression equation one at a time so that each one added best explains the remaining variation. Variables can enter the equation at acceptable levels of significance that alone do not correlate highly with the dependent variable.

Significance measures the extent to which a statistical relationship is due to chance. The significance is determined by the probability level of the result. In the cases reported in this book, *t*-test results (the differences between averages of problem data) had to reach the .05 probability level or less, and the coefficient of correlation (*r*) had to be greater than .3 and significant at the .05 probability level or less. Sometimes a variable had to be a significant part of a stepwise regression equation to explain the variations in the problem variable.

With a *control and an experimental group*, the criteria can be that the experimental group must do better than the control group with respect to the problem variable and that statistical tests must be significant. In Case 12, in which the reminder letter was the intervention, the number of patients who received the letter had to comprise a greater percentage of compliant patients than noncompliant patients; among the compliant patients, more than 50% had to indicate that receiving the letter made a positive difference. The coefficient of correlation between compliance and receipt of the letter had to be more than 0.3 and had to be significant at the .05 level or better; the *t* test for comparison of mean differences in compliance between those with and those without the letter had to be significant at the .05 level or better; and receipt of the letter as a variable had to be part of a stepwise regression equation to explain compliance.

In Part II of this book, you will find explicit examples of criteria used to prove causes. They can be a guide for you to develop your own ideas of what the criteria should be. You may also wish to work with someone who understands what you are trying to do, such as your collaborator.

Approvals

When you present your criteria to your client for approval, try to make your reasoning clear; some of the logic may be difficult to understand, so try to present the underlying assumptions. If management has other specific criteria in mind, they take precedence unless they are based on a misunderstanding of what you are doing—because clients are the ones to be convinced. You may want to persist, however, in clarifying your position.

Prove the Causes of the Problem

"Proof" is never all or nothing. Reasonable doubt may persist. Absolute proof of causality is never possible through statistical associations. Proof really means a high probability of finding what you would expect if a factor were a real cause; then you can say that the factor is associated with the problem for the set of data you observed. The larger and more representative the sample, the stronger the association, the more likely that the conclusion will hold for other times and places.

Statistical Analysis

As noted earlier, the criteria that require statistical analysis often involve t tests, correlation analysis, and stepwise regression equations. T test analysis is done with dichotomous variables or variables that are expressed dichotomously as a condition that is present or not. The dependent variable, the problem variable, must usually be a continuous variable, such as length of stay, that is assumed to be normally distributed. The t test is appropriate for most size samples. According to Besag and Besag (1985), the t test is preferable to the Z test for samples below 90, and it is always safer to use, especially because in larger samples the two results converge.

Coefficients of correlation and *multiple regression equations* can be applied to variables that are somewhat normally distributed and can include dichotomous variables, multicategory variables that grade from higher to lower, and continuous variables that take on a variety of graded values from high to low.

The first step for these analyses is to get the data ready for the computer package you will use. In the cases presented here, the data were prepared for use with the SPSS®/PC+ package, which allows the importation of a database on disk. The examples all used the database program dBASE III PLUS. The variables have or are assigned numerical values, starting with the subjects' ID numbers. For dichotomous variables such as sex, assign a value of 1 to one and a value of 2 to the other. The value of 2 can be assigned to having a condition you expect to be associated with the problem variable and 1 for not having it. For graded multicategory variables, such as overweight, normal weight, and underweight, you can assign 3, 2, 1 as values or treat each designation separately as a dichotomous variable. For continuous variables such as age, you can just enter the actual age. When you are ready to work with the statistical package, "import" your database from your disk, including the names you gave the variables. Then you can call them up and select any combination for analysis.

The *t* test is used to test whether the means (averages) of the problem variable for two independent groups (subjects in dichotomous variable categories) are significantly different. For example, to know whether the dependent variable you are studying (e.g., length of stay in rehabilitation) has a significantly higher average among patients with or without anticipated problems (AP), you can assume that the two "groups" of patients are independent of each other; the members are different, unpaired individuals. The *t* test results give the probability that the difference between the two averages was due to chance. The less the probability, the greater the likelihood that the difference was not due to chance. A printed computer report normally presents the number of subjects in each group, the average for the dependent variable (days) for each group, and information about the probability of the differences.

In Case 4, patients with AP had an average length of stay of 76.8 days; those without AP averaged 37.57 days. The two-tail probability indicating whether the difference was due to chance was less than .0005 (.05 is usually the maximum allowed to chance; any lower number, such as .01 or .005, means greater significance). Two-tail probability assumes that the means can differ in either direction. Common sense would predict a higher average for AP patients, so the more appropriate measure was the one-tail probability level, which is half the two-tail probability level. Thus, AP status demonstrated a significant difference at the .00025 level.

The *coefficient of correlation* describes the degree to which two variables rise and fall in a fairly direct relationship. A perfect correlation is one in which there is the same variability in the two. A coefficient of 1.0 is a perfect, positive correlation, and a coefficient of –1.0 is a perfect inverse relationship. The coefficient of correlation is also evaluated for one- or two-tail significance. For AP, there was a positive correlation of .497, with one-tail significance at the .001 level.

A common error is to confuse statistical significance with importance. A coefficient of correlation measures the relationship between the variations in the data collected for two variables. The higher the correlation, the more important the relationship. (The square of the coefficient of correlation tells the percentage of the variations between the two variables accounted for.) A coefficient of correlation of .3 means that about 9% of the variation between the two variables can be explained by the relationship. If a .3 coefficient of correlation between length of stay in rehabilitation and age were significant at the .01 level, this would mean that the correlation is probably not zero and would be due to chance no more than 1 time out of 100, but less than 10% of the variation is *explained* by that relationship. The relationship may be *real*, but it is not *important*. A coefficient of .3 is not very impressive. Even a coefficient of .5 explains only 25% of the variation between two variables.

The difference between the averages in *t* test results can be important if the difference is large, but it may not be significant if the sample is small. A statistical figure such as a *t* test result or a coefficient of correlation "can be statistically significant with a sample size of 100, while the same [measure] . . . would not be significant with a sample size of 50" (Norusis, 1988, p. 232). Large samples increase the significance of the results, but significant results are not necessarily important results. On the other hand, the larger the average difference or the coefficient of correlation, the greater the importance, and the greater the significance. A difference of 30 or an *r* of .3 may not be significant with a sample of 50, but a difference of 40 or an *r* of .4 *may* be significant with the sample of 50.

Sometimes a *group* of variables together account for the variance in the dependent variable. The method of *step-wise regression analysis* adds one variable at a time (within statistical parameters) to best account for the variability. Those that duplicate one another's variability are eliminated, so intercorrelated variables wash out. In Case 4, the variables that best explained days in rehabilitation statistically were medical complications due to the prosthesis, problems specific to the patient, an ill-fitting device, and (in inverse relationship) the number of people in the patient's home. These were in the stepwise regression equation but were not the only variables with explanatory value. Table

C4.2, presented with Case 4 in Part II, is an example of how the important statistical results can be presented.

Comparison With Criteria

Once you have collected and analyzed the data, compare your results with the criteria already set for each cause. Report your results, perhaps as in Table 3.2. When a variable meets all the conditions set as its criteria, it is "proved" for the purposes of the study. When a variable clearly does not meet the criteria, it is "not proved." Sometimes some criteria for a variable are met and others are not. Use your own judgment in deciding whether to call the variable "proved," "partly proved," or "not proved."

Once you have completed your analysis and entered the results in Table 3.2, bring your data to your collaborator and ask to have the data checked. This is a crucial step, because errors can appear in the the most unexpected places.

Convincing the Client

When the data are checked, bring the results to the designated client, whom you will now try to convince. Because the criteria are rather complicated, especially those that involve ranks and statistical computations, you need face-to-face time in which to refresh the client's memory about the criteria, explain the concepts, and convince her or him about the actual causes.

CHAPTER FOUR

Finding Solutions

PROJECT OBJECTIVE 3: IDENTIFY SOLUTIONS

Identify management's feasibility limits

Get ideas on possible solutions

Get feedback on selected solutions

Present solutions for approval

Identify Management's Feasibility Limits

Once you have proved the problem and identified the causes, you are ready to find appropriate solutions. However, it is important to know whether management will place any limits on what you can propose as solutions. Knowing the constraints beforehand and having them in mind when you are trying to come up with solutions is preferable to designing solutions only to have them slapped down as unfeasible. However, it is also important to be prepared to defend really good solutions that may exceed short-term limits but will pay off handsomely in the long run.

Management's constraints are your *feasibility limits*. They may be limits on finances, limits on hiring new staff, prohibitions against increased workloads, or prohibitions against reorganizing the department. A financial limit that is often imposed allows minor one-time outlays but no additions to regular operating costs or major capital costs. Sometimes there are limits set by the nature of the department and its culture. The limits for Case 2, the wait for radiation therapy, included "patient load for department cannot be affected; no new construction or redesign of physical plant; no new staff; no new equipment such as machines or computers."

When you designed your plan of work, you named a management person to interview about the feasibility limits for your solutions, someone who was in a position to know what limitations would be placed on the solutions you might propose. This is probably the client but might be another management person. Undertake an interview and compile a list of the feasibility limits.

The meeting with your management respondent should be face to face, to allow discussion. Clarify that you are talking about the *outer* limits, the point at which a solution would not be acceptable. You might say, "Before I select solutions for these causes, I want to know if there are any conditions that you would place on the solutions we might come up with. Are there any outside limits you would place on a solution?"

Rather than discuss the *specific* solutions you are considering, it is better to discuss *limits on the resources* that might be needed. The reason to avoid being specific about the solutions you are considering is that, at this early stage, you want to avoid prejudicing the client by a weak, premature description or inviting solutions that might be management's pet ideas, with which you do not want to be saddled. You want management's limits before any concrete ideas are presented. You might discuss each limit as the list is compiled; one-time costs might really be acceptable, even if the first response is to allow no financial outlays. Try to have the door left open for a solution that might be costly at first but would save costs in the long run.

Put the feasibility limits in writing and submit them to your interviewee as your understanding of what was agreed to at the meeting. This avoids any later conflict over what was said and gives you something concrete to work with. Show the approved list in the table you will use to present your proved causes and solutions. An example is presented later in this chapter.

Get Ideas on Possible Solutions

Ideas for solutions to the problem come by working with proved causes, using your imagination, interviewing staff, and reviewing the literature.

Your Own Ideas

You can assist the process by first doing your own thinking about the solutions. The way to start is by examining the proved causes. Some of the causes will have been so specific as to make the solutions obvious. For example, the cause "the way the work is organized" can turn out to be as specific as in Case 8, in which the pharmacy technicians were not emptying patients' medication bins before filling them: There was no place to empty the bins, and the staff were constantly interrupted by phone calls. The corresponding solutions were clearly indicated: Redesign the work area to allow emptying the bins; enforce the requirement that the bins be emptied before being filled; and assign, in rotated order, one staff member to answer the phones.

Figure 4.1 contains some generic guidelines. It presents the checklist of possible causes discussed earlier and the kinds of solutions that might deal with them. For more specific ideas, see the cases in Part II; each case includes the causes that were proved and the solutions to deal with them.

If you have proved *specific patients, staff, job titles, shifts, units, service areas, procedures,* and/or *tests* as causes, they probably have something in common. Examine which of the causes cluster together, and the solution may become apparent. The link may be inexperience, inadequate training, working out of title, age or type of equipment, or something else that will become apparent as you look at the results. The solutions will be staff training or education, redesigned staffing patterns, maintenance activity, or some other solution common to the cause areas.

Causes that identify *specific staff* usually also relate to titles or units and are, in turn, linked to the way the work is organized or to inadequate training or supervision. There is rarely anything to be gained from singling out individuals, titles, or units just to draw attention to them. Such pinpointed causes should be dealt with by solutions that cover the department as a whole, such as inservice training or revised manuals. In Case 7, the dialysis unit's method of drawing blood had to be changed. Specific individuals were really not the problem, especially as the evidence indicated that most staff in all areas needed more training. The staff, job title, and unit were clearly linked to the method of drawing blood from an existing line. In Case 1, the steps relating to patients diagnosed with fracture were a cluster of causes that also

Possible Causes by Major Category	Types of Solutions
Patient/Consumer Risk Factors Sex Age Diagnosis Secondary medical condition Alertness Language used Use of English Ability to communicate Medications Mobility level Marital status Income level Type of insurance Number of infants, children, individuals in home Minority status Years of education or highest degree Attitude toward problem Attitude toward compliance Self-care compliance	Highlight proved risk factors and arrange to take special measures to attend to needs so as to avoid the problem. This might be more bedside care, arranging for social service or counseling, providing interpreters, or improved patient education. Indicate risk factor status for the problem in the patient's chart and document compliance with the new procedures.
Related to Staff Specific staff person Specific job title Years of experience in the organization Years of experience in the profession Highest, closest degree[a] Attitude toward problem Beliefs about problem/nature of problem Beliefs about consequences of problem Knowledge related to problem Performance skill Sense of being overworked Sense of not feeling accountable	Avoid public disclosure of specific staff; design and provide for staff education and training in proved subject areas; consider specific support for tuition; consider methods to address attitudes, such as group discussions; consider flexible staffing patterns; demonstration of management's concern with accountability for the problem.
Related to Institution Specific units Specific shift Specific step(s) Specific procedures Specific tests or units of procedure Specific equipment, materials	Use common causes associated with specific steps and procedures to redesign the processes involved. Deal with vendors or maintenance to improve equipment or space.

(continued)

Figure 4.1 Proved Causes and Types of Solutions They Suggest

Possible Causes by Major Category	Types of Solutions
No defined policy related to problem No standards in administrative manuals	Specify policy in documents and provide inservice education.
Way work is organized	Redesign process so steps in process are eliminated or streamlined or provided at a better stage; reassign tasks, provide flexible timing, coordinate steps, etc.
Supervisors do not hold staff accountable Performance on this not part of evaluation Lack of feedback on the problem	Provide for feedback; include in evaluation; collect data.
Documentation too general Documentation poorly designed Documentation nonexistent	Design or redesign appropriate documentation.
Staff do not have authority to do what is needed	Redesign job to include greater authority.
Other Causes Found through observation, review of literature, and interviews with staff or in team/staff meetings.	See cases in Part II for specific solutions.

Figure 4.1 Proved Causes and Types of Solutions They Suggest
a. This includes not only the highest degree attained but any higher degree the subject is close to attaining.

involved physicians, but the solution was to change the way the work was organized to deal with fractures. In each case, the solutions addressed the causes uniting the individuals, titles, or units identified.

If *patient risk factors* are associated with the problem, the patients may need to be dealt with in a special way, such as being given specific attention or support services. Sometimes the identification of previously overlooked risk factors can help avoid a problem. In Case 4, steps to provide preventive attentions were clearly called for.

If *staff knowledge or inexperience* are proved, the solution will probably involve training. In Case 6, it was shown that staff fitting patients with crutches and canes were not trained for the task. If a change in process is suggested, inservice training will be needed to teach the new procedures.

If *institutional factors* are causes, make the solutions specific to the situation. Consider solutions to simplify or reorganize the way tasks are carried out. You may want to suggest ways to restructure jobs, revise documentation procedures, redesign forms, or give staff more authority to make efficient decisions. Think of what can be done to make supervisors and staff feel responsible and accountable if corresponding causes have been proved. Consider how evaluating performance in the problem area can be used as a positive incentive; suggest how the solutions or new standards can be represented in manuals; think of what data need to be collected to provide staff with feedback on their performance and how it should be presented.

Interviews and Literature Review

The staff and literature review are important resources to draw upon. The best people to ask about possible solutions are the staff you interviewed about possible causes. They will already be familiar with the project, will understand what you are doing, and will appreciate being involved. Getting ideas from staff not only increases the possibility of finding good ideas, it is also a way of providing staff who will ultimately be affected by the solutions with a sense of participation and identification with the success of the solutions you finally propose. This objective helps develop allies.

Ask for ideas on solutions in much the same way you asked for ideas about causes, but first make sure to present the *proved* causes, because you want to avoid getting solutions for nonexistent causes. Face-to-face informal interviews are best because they allow discussion to clarify ideas, but an open session for staff may also be productive. In either case, it is a good idea to take notes. You may also want to examine the same literature you used in looking for causes, add additional sources, and consult with institutions that faced similar problems.

Do not ask managers for suggestions at this point, especially not the client, because if someone in higher management gives you a solution, he or she will probably expect you to accept it, and you do not want to take on a needless battle if you come up with better solutions.

Once you have completed your analysis, the interviews, and the literature review, you can record the results in a table such as Figure 2.2, which you originally used to report causes in connection with your interviews and literature search. You now fill in the last right-hand column, Solutions, with proposed solutions to correspond to causes, but you fill in solutions only for the proved causes.

Examine the possible solutions, including your own. Decide on the best possible solutions by considering the problem, the proved causes, and the feasibility limits. The solutions you choose should address the largest number of important causes at the least cost. Some causes may be interlinked; one solution may deal with several causes. Usually, every cause proved or partly proved should be dealt with except for trivial causes that affect a relatively small aspect of the problem.

Get Feedback on Selected Solutions

If the organization has staff who are union members, consider having informal discussions with union representatives to make sure you are not creating a labor relations problem. If you are considering solutions that the union might like, you will have an ally when the time comes to implement them. It is important to be clear during these talks so that you are not misunderstood by either union people or management.

When you have come up with what you think are the best solutions, make sure each one is within the feasibility limits, can be financed within existing limitations, or can be justified as cost effective in the long run.

Ask for feedback from staff. It is easiest and best to go back to the staff you have talked with about causes and solutions. You will again want face-to-face meetings or a group meeting in which staff feel free to speak. If you are part of a team, a group discussion is expected. Staff can often spot technical flaws in proposed solutions and can help in fine-tuning suggestions or pointing out potential implementation problems. Involving staff will help assure that they will be allies during the implementation period. The principle that nothing that management does should be a surprise applies here.

Table 4.1 Causes, Constraints, and Solutions: Waiting for PT (Example
From Case 1)

Feasibility Limits: 1. No increase in nonmedical professional staff.
                    2. Additional documentation by MDs to be limited.
                    3. Additional costs not to exceed $1,000.

Causes Proved	*Solutions*
Fracture patients	
PT, X ray, and orthopedic consult orders not automatic at admission	Set policy: New admissions or current residents with fracture must receive orders for X rays, orthopedic consult, and physical therapy consult upon admission or injury.
Response to X-ray order and order for orthopedist consult	X rays and orthopedist orders and consults shall be answered promptly

NOTE: PT = physical therapy.

Make changes in your solutions to reflect useful feedback on your ideas. When considering the solutions, consider what indicators would be needed to measure the success of the solutions and monitor compliance. These might be the indicators used to prove the problem, but you might need to design data collection to make sure new steps are being carried out or that documentation requirements are being fulfilled. The design of such indicators is discussed in more detail in Chapter 5.

Presenting the Solutions

Table 4.1 is an abbreviated model for a table with which to present the proved causes, the feasibility limits, and the solutions you propose. It is excerpted from a longer table prepared for Case 1. There is a place to list the feasibility limits at the top. On the left are some of the proved causes, grouped by relationship to a particular issue: in this case, fractures. On the right is the related set of solutions. In the example, two suggested solutions cover three causes.

After identifying the causes, after getting input from others and from the literature, after coming up with reasonable ideas and examining them to check that they are feasible, and after getting feedback from staff and making any last-minute changes, take your solutions to your client, the management person who can implement them.

At this point, you will reap the benefits of how you have been relating to the client. If the client has been involved at every step of the way, the solutions will not be a shock, because the client will have been convinced about the problem's existence and extent, will have been convinced about the causes, and will have presented you with the feasibility limits. Now you can show how you propose to deal with each proved cause. Because you know the feasibility limits, it is unlikely that you will offer a solution that can be rejected out of hand. Also, because you have asked staff to respond, you are reasonably sure of a positive reception from staff.

If you have waited until now to bring the proof of problem and proof of cause data to the client's attention, perhaps because the client was too busy to really be involved, you now have to walk the client through all the thinking involved; this may require more than one meeting. You may need to be aware of tactical issues in setting up the meeting to get approval. For example, if there has been any competitiveness with your immediate supervisor, you may want to arrange to make your presentation to your supervisor and the client at the same time, so that everyone is present at the same meeting and no distortions can result from secondhand information.

In all likelihood, there will be a series of meetings. In the first, you will present your solutions to the client. If institutional factors are causes, you will need to use your consulting skills to help him or her see the need to remedy the situations. You may be asked to present an oral or written report to a decision-making body such as a board of directors. The main thing you want to get from your initial meeting with the client is a positive response to your suggestions and a mutual agreement on the next steps.

The Executive Summary

Before or after your meeting with the client, you will probably be asked to prepare an oral and/or written report, even if the project is scheduled to continue through to implementation and making solutions operational. In either case, you will need to introduce the report with an executive summary.

An executive summary is a concise statement of the main points you wish the reader to know. It is undertaken because decision makers feel inundated by paper. They prefer to have a summary of the major points they are being asked to grasp. They generally read only what they need to to make decisions, to run things, or to protect themselves. They respond more favorably if the material they need to know is predigested for them and is brief.

The executive summary is written to suit the needs of the specific readers you want to reach, such as the client, higher-level managers, a group of professionals, a department, or the public. It should be no more than two pages in length and may have appended the latest update of your plan of work. This will give your audience or reader some idea of what your project has been about and will make it easier to write no more than two pages.

Tell the reader the key facts about what you have been doing and your results so far. What the reader is most interested in finding out from you must be clear in the summary. *Say the most important thing you have to say precisely, so it can be quoted.* Include as much background information as needed for the information to be understandable. Try to incorporate it within the material you expect to be quoted. Include anything else you want the reader to know, and say it clearly, including any needed background. Below is an outline you may wish to follow.

1. Scope of the project and role of consultant.
2. Problems addressed: why undertaken and what was done to prove they exist.
3. Causes proved and what was done to arrive at conclusions.
4. Solutions proposed and why proposed.

The Oral Presentation

You may have to describe your project in an oral presentation. First, find out *how much time* you will have. Second, learn *who* will be there and how much they already know about the project. Third, find out *why* you are presenting. Is it to say what you have found or accomplished, or are you also being asked to suggest a course of action, solutions, and implementation? This tells you what to concentrate on and how much detail to present.

For a successful oral presentation, you have to know and understand your own project in detail. You will be asked questions; your credibility hinges on your knowing what everything you present means and how you arrived at it. Also, realize that the audience needs you to either teach or interest them. You are in a giving position, and if your main aim is to give what you know to them as a gift, you will feel less defensive.

You may be able to distribute the executive summary before the oral presentation. That will put the audience on familiar ground when you present. In any case, consider what you can hand out or present visually to help you avoid throwing numbers at the audience that they will have a hard time holding in their heads. What you distribute or show depends on the degree of confidentiality of the data. Generally, you would show your key proof of problem, proof of causes, and solutions tables and explain them. You might also show the summary tables they are based on, but not if that will be overwhelming.

You can arrange for some ground rules with your client. For example, you might arrange to have questions held until you finish your presentation, except for those asking for clarification. You might ask to have the handouts returned at the end. Talk these issues over with your client.

Do not plan to read your report; it is boring, and reading will involve you in too rigid a structure to sense or adjust to what the audience needs. If you speak from an outline, you can react to audience feedback. An outline on a sheet of paper allows you to see the overall structure of your report and makes it easier to change. Some people like index cards with individual points on them. If you use them, be sure they are numbered, because they can fall.

Practice beforehand to see how long things take to explain and to get used to the feeling of the delivery. Ask someone whom you trust to listen and give you feedback. Choose someone who knows nothing about the project and ask the person to tell you where you are confusing or what is unclear. You will then know where you need more introductory information or detail. The next best thing is to tape the presentation and listen to how you sound.

When you begin your presentation, take a few deep breaths. Feel the audience lean toward you. You have something they want to hear. Start by saying what you are reporting on and what you are going to do. Then say how the project came into being, the main problems you were addressing, and your main methods. Then tell what you accomplished. Lead the audience through your displays. Always explain how a table is set up and what to look for.

Remember that you have had approvals and enlisted staff all along the way. Give credit and thanks to all the people who helped. If you feel nervous, stop and take a deep breath. The audience is there because they want to hear what you did. If you had to prove the problem exists, explain what the indicators and proofs were. If you proved causes, show or tell the types of causes you studied and general criteria for those causes; concentrate on the ones you proved. Have a list of proved and disproved causes ready for the question period.

When presenting solutions, tell what constraints and criteria you took account of. You may say what alternatives you considered and why you rejected them. Offer your proposals and give your reasons. If the proposals could be controversial, consider the best arguments you can think of *against* them and prepare answers. Allow plenty of time for questions. Be open to suggestions or expressions of concern from your audience.

The Final Written Report of the Project

The final report of your project is addressed to the person(s) for whom you have been a consultant. It tells why the project came about (introduction), what it addressed (problems), what it set out to accomplish (objectives), and what you accomplished (methods/evaluation).

The report will likely be disseminated to other managers. It is introduced by an executive summary and probably need not include details on most enabling objectives unless the client is interested in the details. It may cover implementation, but the outline presented below assumes that the project has ended with the recommendation of solutions.

Pay attention to the appearance of the report. Use a consistent heading style. Do not allow your word processor or printer to leave a heading alone at the bottom of a page and its text without a heading on the next page. It is very important to proofread your report, even if you use a spellchecker program. Extraordinary mistakes, loss of key words, and duplication of paragraphs plague all writers who do not check. A suggested outline follows.

▷ Title of the project.
▷ Executive summary.
▷ Introduction: The introduction may be similar to that in the progress report. Present the background of the project, the client, and you as the consultant.
▷ Problems and objectives: Present long-range goals and project objectives, with some mention of enabling objectives covering the establishment of criteria and feasibility limits. If you list the causes you were to study, include the *final* list with the causes you added as a result of your search.
▷ Method(s) (Evaluation): Describe the research design you selected: what was to be done, period of time, numbers involved, indicators, and who did the collecting. Mention and give thanks to the people whose approvals you received and who participated in data collection. In reporting what happened for project objectives, describe data collection and the tables you used; tell the reader what they show. Describe important tables by number, name, and what each was designed to do. Discuss the extent to which criteria were met. Discuss the causes you *proved* by presenting them in related groups.
▷ Conclusions/Recommendations: Tell what conclusions you reached and your recommendations on solutions. Refer to the feasibility limits, the causes you proved, and your proposed solutions. Summarize what you have demonstrated, what you have learned about the institution, and anything else that might be helpful to your client. Are there any ethical issues that have to be raised? Tell about any possible impacts of the project on the institution, staff, patients, or the public. You might have learned about how the institution functions, something needed for improved patient care, or what to do in a future situation. The final section should tell what you suggest should happen next.
▷ References: List any published works or other documentation you cited in the report.
▷ Appendixes (supporting materials and tables).
▷ Bibliography: Cite any literature that helped you with the project or that relates to project issues. The bibliography contains all the sources in the reference list plus any others you might wish to recommend as supplementary or background reading. It is not essential for the report.

Implementing Solutions and Making Them Operational

PROJECT OBJECTIVE 4: IMPLEMENT, EVALUATE, AND MAKE SOLUTIONS OPERATIONAL

Design implementation and evaluation plan

Schedule implementation and data collection

Determine whether solutions are successful

Identify steps to make solutions operational

Determine whether new standards or indicators are required to monitor solutions or participate in a reference base

---

Introduction

Once a solution has been accepted, it has to be put into place. The early stage of putting the solution into place is called *implementation*. It has its own set of steps, including planning and evaluation.

Implementing solutions means change. The first stage in the change process, according to Kurt Lewin (1935), is *unfreezing the current conditions*. Staff may question a current situation; negative consequences may make staff aware that there is a problem. Openness to change can also come with the arrival and report of an accreditation team, when staff become aware of a quality improvement project, when a quality team is set up, or when the internal consultant proves

121

the problem. Having staff aware that the problem was proved empirically helps keep the attitudes unfrozen while work goes on to find causes. By the time you are ready to implement solutions, staff should expect some changes.

Even though change may already be anticipated, and no matter how much change was desired, implementation will feel like an imposition and a burden to people who really never expected that *their* daily experiences would have to accommodate the solutions. A CQI philosophy can eliminate the sense that change is imposed by an authority. In other situations, understanding how to work with people will be key, as will systematic identification of all the steps needed to install the solutions. Planning for implementation includes taking account of resistance and can ease the process.

Staff may be excited about the change, but they will be resistant if things go wrong in the installation process or if cherished ways of doing things are brushed aside. Setbacks can make the whole idea seem misguided. However, if it is a good solution, at some point the bugs will be worked out and people will begin to habitually practice the new ways. They may begin to see results; there will be a glimmer of insight that the changes will work. Then they will become more optimistic and accepting.

Implementation and Evaluation Plans

Planning

Planning is crucial to successful implementation. You need to plan for any new documentation or procedures, transferring and/or training staff, purchasing, and reorganizing departmental communications. A flow chart can help you map sequences and identify how one step depends on another. But implementation will involve people; knowledge of the organizational culture, respect for ethics, and your skills as an internal consultant will surely be needed. For each solution, the consultant needs to be prepared to suggest (a) how to prepare staff to deal with the changes, (b) what the resistances will probably be about, (c) what can go wrong, and (d) how to handle it.

Consider all the people and departments that need to be involved in applying the solution(s), including any changes in the way staff interface with other departments. The interface is those points of contact between independently functioning units, such as admissions with service departments, service departments with purchasing, and nursing with rehabilitation. First, be sure *approval to implement* has been given and that all staff people involved have been notified about the changes. Supervisors and professionals should be involved in identifying how the changes will affect their operations and should be asked to suggest how they can assist. This may mean a series of meetings introduced by brief written material.

Decide on the *sequence* in which the new solutions should be carried out. Some solutions are more important than others; some can be instituted at once; others need more time. You need to put the solutions in order of importance and in order by functional time sequence. Lay out a work plan and chart to show the due dates of steps and the people involved, including the sequence for what gets done, who is involved, and the time required.

Then identify *what will be different*. If new documentation or record keeping forms need to be designed, the new designs must be produced and approved, and printing must be ordered. Staff must be taught how to use the forms and which practices to discontinue. If new procedures need to be installed, this means delineating the procedures, deciding who does what, which staff should be trained, who will design the training, who will do the training, and when the training will take place. Staff need to see the advantages conferred by the different way the work will be done. If any staff need to be transferred, they should be involved in the decision. Arrangements must be made to incorporate changes in the staff scheduling process. If the solutions require education of staff, the training has to be designed, the educator selected, and classes scheduled.

The planning process must pay attention to providing the proper interface with other departments and existing operations in the organization. This involves considering how the old procedures impinged on other departments and noting what changes have to be made in the way the departments communicate.

Evaluation Design

A period of time must go by before the new system is *evaluated*. Time is needed to get rid of the bugs and overcome the persistence of old ways. How much time to wait is a function of how many changes are needed, how easily they are adopted by the organization, and how soon they are all in use and working as planned. In Case 1, which deals with physical therapy at the nursing home, once the physicians were convinced of the existence of the problem, little time was lost before the new procedures became routine. But three months were allowed for the solutions to take hold.

If solutions are put into place in a piecemeal way, you have the option of conducting several evaluations or waiting a considerable time before you do an overall assessment. Some solutions are so obvious that management may decide not to measure the results in any special way. Normal operations themselves are the test. But there must be data to follow the progress of the solutions.

Part of planning for evaluation is to design the data collection forms to show whether the new solution has reduced the problem. Ideally, the same kind of data collection forms used to demonstrate the problem can be used to compare the old data that proved the problem with the results from using the solutions. In some cases, a new set of baseline data is needed. In a case where the consultant proved that few staff were receiving mandated inoculations against Hepatitis B, the consultant could not use the data she had originally collected to prove the problem because she could not know how many staff were inoculated between the time she proved the problem and the time she was to start implementing her solutions. She had to have a baseline accurate as of the day before the solutions were implemented. Only proper planning can produce that kind of fine-tuned timing of data collection.

Another type of data collection for evaluation is questionnaires for staff or patients dealing with satisfaction or morale. Do people like the changes? If the changes are objectively successful but people are feeling rebellious about them, you might want to know that. On the other hand, if people feel good about the changes, that lends support for making them operational.

Work again with colleagues to develop the data collection instruments needed to evaluate the solution. This might include the design of indicators to show whether the solution is being applied or to show the effect on problem indicators. Get approval to field test any new instruments. Field test, and then revise the instruments based on the results of the field test.

Criteria to Evaluate the Solutions

You need to have some idea of how much of a change in the problem can be realistically expected from the solution. Your solutions might not be able to totally eliminate some problems; it may be enough to reduce them to some agreed-on percentage. For example, the reminder letter in Case 12, which deals with patient noncompliance with follow-up visits, was not expected to produce total compliance; noncompliance has many causes and is notoriously resistant to solutions. Among the criteria to assess whether the follow-up letter was a good solution was a drop in the experimental group's noncompliance rate by at least 20 percentage points more than the control group's rate. To judge the success of a solution in terms of patient or staff satisfaction, you need to decide on the percentage of your respondents who would have to indicate acceptance or a positive response to the changes.

Below is a checklist for the implementation stage of problem solving that summarizes what this section has described.

1. What changes in operations are being proposed?
2. For each change, state the staff who will be involved.
3. Which administrators have to be involved?
4. Will anyone have resistance to the changes? Why? What will you do about it?
5. Is there anything to be newly designed?
6. If so, who will design it, and who must approve?
7. In what order should the changes be introduced?
8. Describe what will now be different for each staff member involved.
9. What meetings will be needed? When?
10. Will any staff training be needed? If so, who will design it? Give it? To whom? When?
11. Will the changes affect the interface with any other departments? How? How will the interface change be introduced?
12. For each change, what could go wrong? How would you handle it if it did?
13. How long a period should elapse before the solution is evaluated?
14. What data need to be collected to evaluate the solutions?
15. What should the success criteria be for evaluating the solutions?

16. Who will approve the criteria to evaluate the change(s) and judge whether the solution is a success?
17. What indicators would you recommend be adopted to monitor the solutions?

Schedule Implementation and Data Collection

After an implementation plan is designed, the timing for its installation must be approved by all the relevant supervisors and, perhaps, the staff. You will also have to arrange for any needed baseline and evaluation data to be collected.

Determine Whether the
Solutions Are Successful

At some point comes the moment of truth, when the evaluation data are examined to see whether the new solutions have met the criteria to prove their success. You compare the pre- and postsolution data with the criteria that have been selected. Again, ask your collaborator to check your data results, then take your results to the client.

The cases in Part II do not all deal with solutions that were evaluated. Not all of the consultants went on to implementation and evaluation. Some went directly from solutions to operational changes, and still others were ignored or stalled due to reorganization and financial crises. The best examples of the implementation phase are Cases 1, 13, and 14.

Identify the Steps to Make
the Solutions Operational

Once the solution has been demonstrated to be worthwhile, it enters into a period when it is made part of normal procedures; it becomes operational. That is the third of Lewin's (1935) stages, *refreezing the changes*. Making the solutions operational is a more permanent activity than implementation. Having the solutions written in manuals, policy documents, staff orientation curricula, staff evaluation protocols, printed standard operational procedures, and even job descriptions shows the final commitment of management to the solutions. It may be the task of the consultant to identify and monitor the steps needed to formally make the successful solutions operational.

The internal consultant's role may also include making sure that the implementation steps are completed or shepherding the solutions through to final acceptance. The internal consultant makes sure that the institutional decision makers have carried out the steps needed to incorporate the accepted solutions in all the ways appropriate to the nature of the solutions. Executive summaries, oral reports, and final written reports may be needed as well. They have already been discussed.

Consider Adopting New Indicators to Monitor the Solutions

When the quality improvement project has been successful, another step may include the determination of whether a new indicator and new standards should be adopted by the organization to monitor the solutions newly put in place. The JCAHO includes a standard asking that the improvements be maintained through measurement and assessment activities, and this may be an activity with which the internal consultant will become involved.

You may decide to suggest continued collection of data that were important in proving the problem; your organization might be interested in establishing an indicator for use internally or as part of its participation in a reference database. The development of indicators for reference databases is a complicated, time-consuming task, with new material appearing all the time. See, for example, Kane (1997). The following section provides some summarized, rule-of-thumb concepts and ideas.

Background

The JCAHO's reference database, the Indicator Measurement System (IMSystem), is a national comparative measurement system composed of indicators that have been developed by expert clinicians, rigorously tested for relevance, reliability, and validity, and risk adjusted using patient characteristics. [It] . . . was designed to help health care organizations measure and improve their performance, assist the Joint Commission in evaluating health care organizations, and meet the national mandate for sound measures of patient outcomes (Koss, Nadzam, & Loeb, 1995, p. 99).

The IMSystem began to accept data in 1994. By the spring of 1997, it had data on almost a million cases from over 80 hospitals (McGreevey et al., 1997). The reporting unit is the *patient episode of care*, a particular stay in the hospital by a specific (though not identified) patient. In 1997, the IMSystem's 42 indicators dealt with perioperative, obstetrical, trauma, and cardiovascular care, oncology, use of medication, and infection control. There were plans for indicators for home care, long-term care, behavioral health care, and ambulatory care (JCAHO, 1997b).

The IMSystem allows choices in software for data collection and submission; organizations can develop their own or may purchase a commercially available system, but computer-based data in an electronic, machine-readable format, such as modem transfer, disk, or tape, is required. In 1997, at least 10 vendor products had successfully been used to submit data, with that many more in the pipeline for approval. McGreevey et al. (1997) report that 10% of those who selected the IMSystem have in-house software solutions.

In 1995, the Joint Commission decided to serve as an evaluator of other performance measurement systems. It was anticipated that hospitals and long-term care organizations would select a JCAHO-approved measurement system and, by 1997, choose several indicators relevant to a portion of their consumer population that would be relatively important from the point of view of the public's confidence in health care (Berman, 1996).

The JCAHO (1997a) asks that the organization use and contribute to collections of performance data from multiple institutions. These may include multihospital system databases, disease- or diagnosis-specific databases, procedure-specific databases, management databases, investigational databases, proprietary databases, quality improvement databases, purchaser or payer databases, and state agency databases. Rosen, Schroeder, Hagan, Acord-Szczesny, and

Garavaglia (1996) suggest, as indicator sources, retrospective ICD-9-CM diagnosis and procedure codes and Medicare diagnosis-related groups (DRGs) assigned at the time of discharge.

The database selected should provide feedback reports and should have known specifications adhered to by all participants, such as mechanisms to screen and filter out bad data and uniform and consistent data definitions, codes, and classifications. The feedback data should be useful for comparison purposes and decision making, should have been subjected to risk adjustments and validity and reliability testing, and should include an adequate number of participants in similar organizations (JCAHO, 1997a).

In 1996, the National Committee for Quality Assurance (NCQA), which accredits managed care plans, required that plans measure patient satisfaction, but it did not require that they reach any minimum level of satisfaction. Although it is generally understood that healthy people tend to be more satisfied with their health plans than sick people, few plans study only ill clients.

The NCQA database is the Health Plan Employer Data and Information Set (HEDIS). HEDIS data collection began in 1993. In 1996, Consumers Union found inconsistencies in what and how measurements were done, some inadequate data collection systems, and insufficient information to judge the way plans serve their members. For example, a plan that appears to be twice as good as another on making cholesterol screening available by providing a free examination each year, compared with a plan that provides this only every second year, might not be twice as good at making sure that the members actually come in to have the tests done (such as with use of reminder letters) and may not achieve a high percentage of patients who are actually tested. They may also not be as successful in persuading patients to change behaviors in order to lower their cholesterol levels (outcome), but it is possible to develop useful measures.

Developing Indicators

The indicators in current databases may be too far downstream (close to clinical outcomes) to reflect the processes in your particular department. In that case, you may be involved in developing more department-specific indicators. Each indicator is always defined in terms of the component or aspect of care involved. The upper portion of the indicator rate or proportion (numerator) and the lower portion of the rate or proportion (denominator) should be specified. For example, a current IMSystem indicator for obstetrical care is *rate of cesarean delivery*. Its numerator is the number of patients delivered by cesarian section during a specified time period, such as the past quarter; its denominator is all deliveries during the same period. An example that is further upstream (less close to clinical outcomes) might be the rate of correct medications sent by the pharmacy as a percentage of all the medications sent by the pharmacy (Case 8).

Bloomberg et al. (1993) suggest that, for managed care, the indicator be pertinent to an important clinical area, represent an outcome or process that can be improved upon if needed, be specific enough to be measured in a variety of treatment settings and in different payment structures, be relatively easy to measure, be able to be measured in a short period of time, and be applicable across a variety of managed care plans. The operational definition would specify who is involved in the count, the specific population or age group, the length of time in the plan or in a previous plan, the principal diagnosis, the form of insurance coverage, and the data source.

For primary care and managed care organizations, the following are examples of the kinds of indicators that might be developed:

1. Percentage of patients diagnosed with diabetes who had blood levels checked a specified number of times within a specified period.
2. Percentage of patients diagnosed with diabetes who had retinal examinations within a specified period.
3. Percentage of patients over a specified age who had flu shots within a specified period.
4. Percentage of children within a specific age group who had specific immunizations by a specific age.
5. Percentage of women between specific ages who received mammographic examinations within a specified period.
6. Percentage of women between specific ages who received cervical cancer screening within a specified period.
7. Percentage of women who were pregnant for a given duration greater than three months who received prenatal care during the first trimester of pregnancy.
8. Rate at which calls coming into the central switchboard are completed.

In developing indicators, in addition to *reliability* (the ability to obtain the same results over time and across observers), *validity* must be established. *Content validity* is the extent to which the measure describes the intended process or outcome. *Predictive validity* is the ability to forecast future events or performance, such as future negative outcomes if procedures are not up to standard, or good outcomes if the threshold standard is met or exceeded. *Concurrent validity* measures the strength of the relationship between the chosen indicator and other measures of the same content.

When designing an indicator, you may need to present it in a computer-ready format. The numerator and denominator are expressed as data elements. McGreevey et al. (1997, p. 592) present a sample format for a data element from the IMSystem dictionary. In general terms, it asks for the following:

1. The *name of the data element*
2. The *indicator numbers* that use the data element
3. The *definition* of the data element
4. A *short name* (which will be used in edit statements)
5. The *format*, such as length (number of digits), type (numeric), value if the element occurs in the data sources (such as patient records), with 1 meaning it is present
   a. An edit message number to signal an invalid value
   b. An edit message number to signal that the data must be numeric
6. *Allowable values* (for the aggregate data), such as 1 through n
7. A *data entry prompt*, such as the data element name and spaces for the designated length so that the figure can be entered into the field
8. *Data entry edits*, which is an if/then statement (example):
   a. *If:*   short name for a condition that makes this element relevant is more than zero (> 0),
   Then: short name of the data element must be more than zero (> 0)
   b. An edit message number to signal a logical inconsistency
9. *Presubmission entry edits*, which consist of if/then statements (example):
   a. *If:*   no diagnosis or other data element that make this element relevant appears in a location (< 1),
   Then: short name of the data element is not needed.
   b. An edit message number to signal a logical inconsistency
10. *Segment position* in the system

This format includes feedback to make sure that the data are "clean" by way of editing commands and messages. The reporting system identifies all the indicators that use a given data element, so all using the same element would be consistently served by the same information.

Final Comments

If the descriptions in these five chapters have whetted your appetite for more details, please go on to the 14 cases presented in Part II. They are offered as examples to help you understand the processes involved. Some may serve to generate ideas about your own problem situation or as models you can use to carry out your own quality-improvement project. Appendix 2 presents detailed examples of data collection forms and tables based on Case 1.

References

Amsden, D. M. (1991). *SPC simplified for services: Practical tools for continuous quality improvement*. White Plains, NY: Quality Resources.

Bechtel, G. A., & Wood, D. (1996, March). Improving the accuracy of total quality management instruments. *Health Care Supervisor, 14,* 21-26.

Berman, S. (1996, July). Putting it (performance measures) together: An interview with Jerold Loeb. *Joint Commission Journal on Quality Improvement, 22,* 518-526.

Bernstein, S. J., & Hilborne, L. (1993, November). Clinical indicators: The road to quality care? *Joint Commission Journal on Quality Improvement, 19,* 501-509.

Besag, F. P., & Besag, P. L. (1985). *Statistics for the helping professions*. Thousand Oaks, CA: Sage.

Bloomberg, M. A., Jordan, H. S., Angel, K. O., Bailit, M. H., Goonan, K. J., & Straus, J. S. (1993, December). Development of clinical indicators for performance measurement and improvement: An HMO/purchaser collaborative effort. *Joint Commission Journal on Quality Improvement, 19,* 586-595.

Brook, R. H., Kamberg, C. J., & McGlynn, E. A. (1996, August 14). Health system reform and quality. *Journal of the American Medical Association, 276,* 476-480.

Consumers Union. (1996, August). How good is your health plan? *Consumer Reports, 61,* 28-42.

Crosby, P. B. (1979). *Quality is free*. New York: McGraw-Hill.

Deming, W. E. (1986). *Out of the crisis*. Boston: Massachusetts Institute of Technology.

Donabedian, A. (1978). *Needed research in the assessment and monitoring of the quality of medical care* (DHEW Publication No. [PHS] 78-3219). Hyattsville, MD: NCHSR Office of Scientific and Technical Information.

Donabedian, A. (1980). *The definition of quality and approaches to its assessment*. Ann Arbor, MI: Health Administration.

Donabedian, A. (1982). *The criteria and standards of quality*. Ann Arbor, MI: Health Administration.

Donabedian, A. (1985). *The methods and findings of quality assessment and monitoring*. Ann Arbor, MI: Health Administration.

Gitlow, H. S., & Gitlow, S. J. (1994). *Total quality management in action*. Englewood Cliffs, NJ: PTR Prentice Hall.

Goonan, K. J. (1995). *The Juran prescription: Clinical quality management*. San Francisco: Jossey-Bass.

Green, L. W., & Lewis, F. M. (1986). *Measurement and evaluation in health education and health promotion*. Palo Alto, CA: Mayfield.

Ishikawa, K. (1990). *Introduction to quality control*. Tokyo: 3A Corporation.

Johnson, S. P., & McLaughlin, C. P. (1994). Measurement and statistical analysis in CQI. In C. P. McLaughlin & A. D. Kaluzny (Eds.), *Continuous quality improvement in health care: Theory, implementation and applications* (pp. 70-101). Gaithersburg MD: Aspen.

Joint Commission on Accreditation of Healthcare Organizations. (1990). *Accreditation manual for hospitals, 1991. Vol. I: Standards*. Oakbrook Terrace, IL: Author.

Joint Commission on Accreditation of Healthcare Organizations. (1993). *1994 accreditation manual for hospitals. Vol. I: Standards*. Oakbrook Terrace, IL: Author.

Joint Commission on Accreditation of Healthcare Organizations. (1997a). *Comprehensive accreditation manual for hospitals: The official handbook*. Oakbrook Terrace, IL: Author.

Joint Commission on Accreditation of Healthcare Organizations. (1997b). *Comprehensive accreditation manual for hospitals: The official handbook* (Update 1). Oakbrook Terrace, IL: Author.

Juran, J. M., & Gryna, F. M. (Eds.). (1974). *Juran's quality control handbook* (3rd ed.). New York: McGraw-Hill.

Kane, R. L. (1997). *Understanding health care outcomes research*. Gaithersburg, MD: Aspen.

Kibbs, D. C., & McLaughlin, C. P. (1994). The family practice center. In C. P. McLaughlin & A. D. Kaluzny (Eds.), *Continuous quality improvement in health care: Theory, implementation and applications* (pp. 317-334). Gaithersburg, MD: Aspen.

Koss, R., Nadzam, D., & Loeb, J. M. (1995, January 11). From the Joint Commission on Accreditation of Healthcare Organizations. *Journal of the American Medical Association, 273*, 99.

Lansky, D. (1993, December). The new responsibility: Measuring and reporting quality. *Joint Commission Journal on Quality Improvement, 19*, 545-551.

Leebov, W., & Ersoz, C. J. (1991). *The health care manager's guide to continuous quality improvement*. American Hospital Association: American Hospital.

Lewin, K. (1935). *A dynamic theory of personality*. New York: McGraw-Hill.

Marszalek-Gaucher, E. J., & Coffey, R. J. (1993). *Total quality in healthcare: From theory to practice*. San Francisco: Jossey-Bass.

McGreevey, C., Nadzam, D., & Corbin, L. (1997, March/April). The Joint Commission on Accreditation of Healthcare Organizations' Indicator Measurement System: Health care outcomes database. *Computers in Nursing, 15*(Supp.), S87-S95.

McGregor, D. T. (1960). *The human side of enterprise*. New York: McGraw-Hill.

Mears, P. (1995). *Quality improvement tools and techniques*. New York: McGraw-Hill.

Nadzam, D. M., Turpin, R., Hanold, L. S., & White, R. E. (1993, November). Data-driven performance improvement in health care: The Joint Commission's indicator measurement system (IMSystem). *Joint Commission Journal on Quality Improvement, 19*, 492-500.

Norusis, M. J. (1988). *The SPSS guide to data analysis for SPSS/PC+*. Chicago: SPSS, Inc.

Nunnally, J. C., & Durham, R. C. (1975). Validity, reliability, and special problems of measurement in evaluation research. In E. L. Streuming & M. Guttentag (Eds.), *Handbook of evaluation research* (pp. 289-352). Thousand Oaks, CA: Sage.

O'Leary, D. S. (1993, November). The measurement mandate: Report card day is coming. *Joint Commission Journal on Quality Improvement, 19*, 487-491.

Orlikoff, J. E., & Snow, A. (1984). *Assessing quality circles in health care settings: A guide for management*. Chicago: American Hospital.

Rakich, J. S., Longest, B. B., & Darr, K. (1992). *Managing health services organizations* (3rd ed.). Baltimore, MD: Health Professions.

Rosen, L. S., Schroeder, K., Hagan, M., Acord-Szczesny, J., & Garavaglia, M. (1996, July). Adapting a statewide patient database for comparative analysis and quality improvement. *Joint Commission Journal on Quality Improvement, 22*, 468-481.

Solberg, L. I., Mosser, G., & McDonald, S. (1997, March). The three faces of performance measurement: Improvement, accountability, and research. *Joint Commission Journal on Quality Improvement, 23*, 135-147.

Swanson, R. C. (1995). *The quality improvement handbook: Team guide to tools and techniques.* Delray Beach, FL: St. Lucie.

Ulschak, F. L., & SnowAntle, S. M. (1990). *Consultation skills for health care professionals.* San Francisco: Jossey-Bass.

White, J., & McLaughlin, S. S. (1992). Measurement and standards in continuous quality improvement. In J. D. Dieneman (Ed.), *Continuous quality improvement in nursing* (pp. 75-93). Washington, DC: American Nursing Association.

Ziegenfuss, J. T. (1993). *The organizational path to health care quality.* Ann Arbor MI: Health Administration.

Additional Reading

Al-Assaf, A. F. (1993). Data management for total quality. In A. F. Al-Assaf & J. A. Schmele (Eds.), *The textbook of total quality in healthcare* (pp. 123-156). Delray Beach, FL: St. Lucie.

Bateman, T. S., & Ferris, G. R. (1984). *Method and analysis in organizational research.* Reston, VA: Reston/Prentice-Hall.

Carefoote, R. (1995). The TQM—reengineering link. In S. S. Blancett (Ed.), *Reengineering nursing and health care: The handbook for organizational transformation* (pp. 50-60). Gaithersburg, MD: Aspen.

Gift, R. G., & Mosel, D. (1994). *Benchmarking in health care: A collaborative approach.* American Hospital Association: American Hospital.

Graham, N. O. (1995). *Quality in health care.* Gaithersburg, MD: Aspen.

Griffith, J. R., Sahney, V. K., & Mohr, R. A. (1995). *Reengineering health care: Building on CQI.* Ann Arbor, MI: Health Administration.

Hradesky, J. L. (1995). *Total quality management handbook.* New York: McGraw-Hill.

Jaeger, B. J., Kaluzny, A. D., & Roth, A. (Eds.). (1993). *Management of continuous quality improvement: Case studies in health administration. Vol. 9: Case studies in health administration.* Chicago: Foundation of the American College of Healthcare Executives.

Kaluzny, A. D., & Veney, J. E. (1980). *Health service organizations: A guide to research and assessment.* Berkeley, CA: McCutchan.

Keys, P. (1998, July). The betrayal of the total quality movement in Western management: Managed health care and provider stress. *Family & Community Health, 21*, 1-19.

Schroeder, P. (Ed.). (1994). *Improving quality and performance: Concepts, programs, and techniques.* St. Louis, MO: Mosby—Year Book.

Stratten, A. D. (1991). *An approach to quality improvement that works.* Milwaukee, WI: ASQC Quality.

PART II

CASES

Getting Nursing Home Residents
Into Physical Therapy in a Timely Fashion [1]

Timeliness of performance is one of the dimensions of quality care. This case demonstrated that excessive waiting for care can adversely affect patient outcomes. The case is the most complete of the series, going from proof of the existence of the problem to making the solutions operational.

Proving the Problem

The Problem

Anna was the director of physical therapy at a 320-bed nursing home. She believed that residents were waiting too long to begin physical therapy, and she chose to take the initiative and investigate. Current hospital and long-term care accreditation standards include initial assessment and screening within 24 hours of admission, but there is no standard for the commencement of physical therapy.

The Client

The client was the nursing home administrator, who was very interested in the project. However, both he and Anna considered the

Please note that fictitious names have been used throughout the case presentations.

medical director to be an important decision maker, and he was involved. Anna usually met first with the administrator, who then set up a joint meeting with the medical director.

Importance

As the director of physical therapy, Anna saw patients become discouraged, frustrated, physically weaker, or even injured while waiting for their physical therapy programs to begin. Some anxious patients attempted to do things on their own, and this caused some accidents. Other patients finally began their programs feeling disappointed in or angry with the institution and the therapists because they had had to wait so long.

Anna knew that she could not influence the situation unless, in addition to showing how long residents were actually waiting, she established a link between waiting too long to start or continue physical therapy and outcomes. She had to determine the amount of time patients could wait for physical therapy before experiencing detrimental effects and whether this varied according to patients' diagnoses or whether they were beginning or continuing physical therapy. She undertook a survey of the literature as well as interviews with physiatrists and physical therapists in nursing homes and hospitals.

Anna's review indicated that most physical therapy patients can wait no longer than 7 days before starting physical therapy; patients with fractures can wait no longer than 3 days. Although fractures, amputations, recent strokes, or other neurological damage make patients likely candidates for physical therapy, no diagnosis other than fracture was consistently considered a basis for differentiating the length of time patients can wait. Whether a patient was starting or continuing physical therapy did not appear to affect the limits.

Anna found that some of the consequences of over-long waits for fracture patients are higher risks of injury, accidents, swelling, blisters, skin breakdown, and medical complications such as pneumonia or phlebothrombosis. She found that waiting more than 7 days can result in decreased joint mobility and contractures, decreased muscle strength, increased osteoporosis, higher risk of deep venous thrombosis, urinary tract disease, respiratory problems, skin breakdown, and infection. Anna also found that the harmful effects could delay progress for 3 to 4 months and that there could be permanent damage such as joint contractures—even fatalities if medical complications were serious.

Relevant Steps

All quality improvement projects that deal with waits must identify each of the steps and must collect data on the elapsed time from the first to the last step and for individual steps. However, the complexity of the actual situation can make it difficult to sort out the individual steps; the familiar can be overlooked, and the sequence of events can be confused by contingencies. Anna found that when residents were first admitted, all were treated the same, regardless of whether they came from home or from a hospital, whether a physical therapy program had been underway or not, or whether it was a current resident who became a candidate for physical therapy. For anyone to be able to receive physical therapy, various consultation (consult) orders were required, but these *consult orders* could be delayed and might not be ordered on the day of admission or when physical therapy was first suggested.

No physical therapy could begin without a request for a physical therapy consult with the physiotherapist. The *PT Consult Order* form had to be signed by a patient's general physician (one of the eight general medical physicians, including the physiatrist, who also served as a general physician). For fracture patients, a request for radiography (X rays) and, usually, for an orthopedic consult, also had to be made by a general physician. Only the physiatrist could order physical therapy, but this had to await the PT consult order, which in turn would await the results of X rays, the orthopedist's consult, or other consults such as for cardiology or neurology.

Physical therapy was notified of a new resident's arrival by a card from the admissions office, which would generally arrive late in the day, Monday to Friday, after admissions occurred. As a result, Anna would see the card the next morning. She was expected to evaluate (screen) whether the new resident was a candidate for physical therapy the day she received the card; she was also asked to screen when a current resident was thought to need physical therapy. If, upon screening, Anna thought the patient would benefit from receiving physical therapy, and if a PT consult had not been ordered, Anna would ask the physician for the PT consult order by writing in a *communication book* located at the nursing station. There were eight books, one for each floor, corresponding to the eight general physicians. For fracture patients, Anna might also request orders for radiography and an orthopedic consult.

The communication books were reviewed by physicians about twice each week. When Anna's requests were noted, physicians would write the consult orders. Once Anna had written her requests, she would prepare a list of patients on Fridays to alert the physiatrist, who did his physical therapy consultations on Saturdays. She included on her list all the patients she had identified that week, even if the PT consult orders were still pending.

On Saturdays, the physiatrist would evaluate the patients who had PT consult orders. Patients without PT consult orders had to wait until the following Saturday to be evaluated, assuming the orders were in by then. When the physiatrist was away or on vacation, no one took his place. Once the physiatrist ordered physical therapy, the treatment program would generally begin on the next working day.

Based on this information, Anna identified the steps from the point of view of a patient, starting with admission to the nursing home, through to the start of physical therapy. There were eight steps, as shown below. Steps 3, 5, and 6 were generally required only for fracture patients. Steps 1, 2, and 3 have admission as the starting point; these and other steps could be concurrent as well as sequential.

1. From admission to notice to physical therapy for screening
2. From admission to the physical therapy consult order
3. From admission to orders for radiography/orthopedist consult or orders for other special consults
4. From physical therapy consult order to physical therapy's request for the physiatrist
5. From the X-ray order to completion of the X rays
6. From orthopedist or other consult orders to the consults
7. From the request for the physiatrist to the physiatrist's physical therapy order
8. From the physical therapy order to the starting date of physical therapy

Observation Units, Normal Loads,
Quantities, and Operational Definition

Because not all residents required physical therapy, Anna had to know how long a period she needed in which to collect a reasonable sample of cases from chart and current data. Upon examining past data, she calculated that an average of eight new patients per month entered physical therapy. Anna decided that she would study a 100% sample over a 9-month period, including every resident who was screened as positive for physical therapy. She expected to cover about 75 patients; she actually had data for 74 new patients and residents.

Anna needed an operational equivalent of the admission date for current residents who required physical therapy. She chose the date of the in-house initial request for physical therapy, which could be the date of injury.

Final List of Possible Causes

Anna identified a list of 16 possible causes, culled from interviews with staff, her collaborator, a literature review, and her own knowledge.

Patient Risk Factors

1. Whether the patient had a fracture
2. Whether the patient came from a hospital, own home, or was a resident
3. Whether the patient was starting or continuing physical therapy
4. The patient's diagnosis
5. Whether X rays and consults were needed

Related To Staff

6. Specific general physicians
7. The physician's knowledge that there are consequences with delays beyond the 3- and 7-day limits
8. Whether the physician was unconcerned about the problem
9. Whether physicians were aware of the problem of delays for therapy

Related to the Institution

10. Specific steps
11. No defined policy on how long a wait is allowed or when steps should occur
12. The way the work was organized (also applies to items 13, 14, and 15)
13. Too many steps for patients to pass through
14. No coverage for the physiatrist when away
15. Physical therapy did not have timely access to admission information
16. Lack of communication about what the steps are

Research Design

The research design to prove the problem and gather objective cause data involved current and past chart data for 74 patients. Anna had access to all the records she needed. To prove the problem, Anna collected data on the start and end dates for each of the steps. She then calculated data for the total wait, average wait, excess waits, and excess wait rates by risk factor category.

Data Collection Instruments

Anna designed two codesheets, one for physicians and one for residents, to provide ID numbers so that names could be kept confidential. The patient codesheet listed the 74 residents by code numbers 1 through 74. There were columns to check whether the patient came from a hospital, from home, or was a current resident; whether the patient was starting or continuing physical therapy; the patient's diagnosis, including fracture; and whether tests or consults had been ordered.

This provided data on causes as well as for grouping the proof-of-problem data. (See Appendix 2 for the layouts of the tables and data.) The physician codesheet listed physicians and their floors by the same numbers, from 2 through 9 (Code 1 was assigned to the medical director, who was not a general physician); no patients were on floor 1.

The key variable was the total days wait from admission to the start of physical therapy. After Anna calculated the wait, she rearranged patient data in ascending order of wait and ranked them, with rank defined by the number of days of wait. Ranks went from 1 (4 days) to 20 (27 days). The same number of days received the same rank. Related patient data included the code for the general physician; whether there was a PT consult at intake; and dates for intake, the X-ray and orthopedist consult orders for fracture patients; the physical therapy request for a consult order, when (if) a nurse was enlisted to ask the physician for the PT consult, the PT consult order, when X rays were taken, the orthopedist consult and other consults ordered, when they were completed, the physical therapy request for the physiatrist, when the physical therapy order was received from the physiatrist, and the order to start physical therapy. Also included was the number of days the physiatrist was away during a given patient's wait.

A summary table showed the total wait, the wait over 3 days for fracture patients, and the wait over 7 days for nonfracture patients. Anna calculated totals, average days of wait (days divided by patients), and the percentage over the limit for every patient category of interest.

Criteria to Prove the Problem

The client and medical director accepted Anna's recommendation that a 3-day wait for fracture patients and a 7-day wait for all other patients be the limits for acceptable waits. The table used to show the criteria to prove the problem was presented in Chapter 2 as Table 2.4. It shows the criteria Anna and the client agreed on. The far-left column shows the 18 indicator measures, which cover totals and patient risk factor categories. The indicators are stated as percentage of patients above the limits and as average days of wait for each category.

In the next column are the thresholds above which the problem would be said to exist. The client overrode Anna's more stringent suggestions of zero tolerance and decided that there would be a problem if more than 9% in any category had to wait too long and if average waits exceeded 3 days for fracture patients, 7 days for other patients, and 5 days for the combined total. The column with "X" marks shows the client's approval of these criteria. The far right column gives the source of the data, Table 1.4 in Anna's project.

Results

Table 2.4 also presents the results. All categories exceeded the 9% limit. Twenty-five percent was the lowest rate (for nonfracture patients coming from home and starting physical therapy). The highest rate was 100% for fracture patients, whether starting, continuing, coming from the hospital, or already residents (no fracture patients came from home). Average days of wait ranged from 6.8 for patients coming from home to 15.1 days for fracture patients, with an overall average of 11.5 days. Patients without fractures had an average wait of 10.7 days.

The 6.8 average for patients coming from home exceeded the 5-day limit, but, as it turned out that there were no fracture patients who came from home, this limit probably should have been 7 days. Patients coming from home may have done best because they had no fractures or because they had the benefit of involved family members to spur the process, but it is just as likely that, with only four patients in the group, the figures were not reliable.

The meeting at which Anna presented her results included the client, who was shocked by the results, and the medical director. The client indicated that he had never realized the extent of the problem, and he was ready to start suggesting changes at once. Anna persuaded him to wait for the proof-of-cause results.

Identifying Causes

Research Design

The design to prove the causes used raw data on elapsed days for the steps, other objective cause data collected earlier, responses to a physician questionnaire, and interviews with management on documented policies.

Objective Cause Data

Objective cause data had been collected for seven possible causes: (a) whether the patient had a fracture; (b) whether the patient came from a hospital, his or her own home, or was a current resident; (c) whether the patient was starting or continuing physical therapy; (d) the patient's diagnosis; (e) whether X rays and consults were needed; (f) the patient's general physician; and (g) the time taken for specific steps.

Anna calculated elapsed time for each step from data she had already collected, which she arrayed separately for fracture and non-fracture patients and in rank order. She determined for each step a suggested maximum number of days a patient could ideally be expected to wait for the step to occur. These maxima were set to be realistic as well as ideal but were more stringent for fracture patients than nonfracture patients. The total days had to make it possible for fracture patients to wait no more than 3 days and nonfracture patients to wait no more than 7 days. As an example, for fracture patients, the elapsed days from the admit date to the admit notice and screening date was set at zero, to occur on the same day, but one day was allowed for nonfracture patients.

In tabulations for each step, Anna showed (a) the actual number of days of wait, (b) whether this was within the ideal limit, or (c) if it was over the limit, the number of days over the limit. Anna also calculated which step had the longest wait and its percentage of the individual patient's total wait. Some totals were calculated excluding specific consultations or days the physiatrist was away.

Anna evaluated each physician as a possible cause, using work-sheets that used data already collected but which she now aggregated for each physician's own patients among the 74. She worked with data on the steps involving the general physicians: days from admission to orders for X ray, to the orthopedic consult, and to the PT consult. These data were used to calculate overall ranks for physicians in relation to the waits.

Anna calculated for a given physician's patients: (a) total days from admission to the physical therapy consult order corresponding to the same patients and (b) the corresponding total days over the limit for the step (which totalled 328 days for the 74 patients and 8 physicians). The *excess wait rate* for each physician was excess days wait as a percentage of total days wait for a physician's patients: (b) as a percentage of (a). This excess wait rate was then ranked. The lowest rate was assigned rank 1. The highest was rank 8. Each physician's percentage share of the 74 patients was (c), and was ranked. The physician's percentage share of the 328 days over the limit was calculated as (d) and ranked. To find *disproportionate shares of the excess waits*, Anna subtracted the physician's share of total patients (c) from the physician's share of excess days (d). A positive number meant a disproportionate share of excess waits. The difference, (d) – (c), was also ranked.

Thus, there were ranks for rate of excess days, proportion of patients seen, proportion of excess days, and disproportionate share of excess days of wait. A similar analysis was done for days between admission and the order for X rays or other consults, covering 14 X-ray consults and three other consults, for a total of 17. Anna then calculated the sum of the ranks for the two sets of scores and ranked the final combined scores. A physician's final rank was a composite measure of responsibility for the results.

New Objective Cause Data Related to the Institution

There were four objective causes for which Anna set out to collect data. Anna was to verify whether there was (a) *no defined policy on how long a wait is allowed and when steps should occur* in an interview with the client during which she asked for evidence for a policy on when orders were due for the PT consult and for X rays, on how soon the physiatrist was supposed to respond to a PT consult order, and on limits for the allowable wait for physical therapy. For (b) *the way the work was organized*, Anna asked management for evidence of whether any action was required prior to admission for a patient coming from a hospital, whether X-ray orders were required automatically on the admission of fracture patients, whether the physiatrist was supposed to act on PT consult orders only on Saturdays, and (c) *whether physical therapy had timely access to admissions information*. She also had to verify that she waited until Fridays to compile requests for physical therapy and that there was (d) *no coverage for the physiatrist when away.*

Subjective Cause Data: Interviews and Questionnaires

Anna collected data for 3 subjective causes: (a) *physician's knowledge that there are consequences with delays beyond the 3 and 7 day limits,*

(b) *whether the physician had an unconcerned attitude towards the problem,* and (c) *whether the physician was aware of the problem of delays in patients starting physical therapy.* She created a questionnaire for the physicians (see Figure C1.1). The field test demonstrated that the knowledge questions could discriminate experts from novices; it also helped Anna eliminate two vague questions and focus the instrument. The questionnaire explained Anna's interest in the patients' wait to begin physical therapy and asked the respondents to select *agree, disagree,* or *don't know* as answers to its 10 brief questions.

Questions 1, 2, and 7 tested whether physicians knew that there are consequences from a delay in physical therapy beyond the 3- and 7-day limits. For Question 1, either a or b was accepted as correct. Though 3 days is the correct answer, a more rigorous answer was allowed. The right answer for Question 2 was c, but a and b were also accepted. For Question 7, the right answer was a. Questions 4 and 10 tested whether the physicians were concerned with the problem. Whether physicians were aware of the problem was tested with Question 3. Question 5 partly tested the physicians' knowledge of whether there was a defined policy on how long a wait was allowed and when steps should occur. Question 8 tested lack of communication about the steps. Questions 6 and 9 asked about possible solutions, to see if there would be support from the physicians for their ordering a PT consult ahead of admission when a patient on physical therapy was to be admitted from a hospital or for providing the PT department with computerized admissions data on patients.

As the director of physical therapy, Anna had good connections and support among the physicians. She was able to make appointments to personally administer each of the questionnaires and sat there while each of the eight was filled out, to ensure their completion. There was no particular emphasis given to confidentiality, although it was assured; Anna correctly assumed that physicians do not get intimidated by questionnaires.

Anna arranged the responses in order by physician rank, with the ID codes in the stub and a bank of possible answers under each summarized question across the top. The responses were added for all eight and for ranks 1 through 4 (those who had the fewest problems) and ranks 5 through 8 (those with the most problems). Below the totals for each question were the percentage distributions.

Dear Physician:

I am examining the wait of physical therapy patients from the time it is decided they need physical therapy (PT) services to when they start. Would you please check the answers below that best express your opinion.

	Agree	Disagree	Don't Know
1. Fracture patients need to begin PT:			
a. The next day	( )	( )	( )
b. Within 3 days	( )	( )	( )
c. By 7 days	( )	( )	( )
d. By 14 days	( )	( )	( )
2. Nonfracture patients (such as CVA, amputee) need to begin PT:			
a. The next day	( )	( )	( )
b. Within 3 days	( )	( )	( )
c. By 7 days	( )	( )	( )
d. By 14 days	( )	( )	( )
3. At this nursing home, residents do not wait too long for PT to begin.	( )	( )	( )
4. It is a usual concern of mine to see that residents start PT early.	( )	( )	( )
5. There is no nursing home policy on how soon PT consults should be done.	( )	( )	( )
6. It would be a good idea to order a PT consult ahead of admission when a patient on PT is to be admitted from a hospital.	( )	( )	( )
7. Fracture patients need to have X rays ordered:			
a. Upon admission	( )	( )	( )
b. Within 3 days	( )	( )	( )
c. By 7 days	( )	( )	( )
8. I feel well informed about the steps leading to and following from a PT consult order.	( )	( )	( )
9. If it helps speed things up, I would be in favor of providing the PT department with computerized admission data on patients.	( )	( )	( )
10. How long residents wait to begin PT is not something I am concerned about because it is not a problem.	( )	( )	( )

Figure C1.1 Physician Questionnaire

Criteria to Prove the Causes

To prove that a *fracture* was a risk factor, the percentage of fracture patients waiting more than 3 days had to be higher than the percentage of nonfracture patients waiting more than 7 days, and the average wait had to be longer. A similar criterion was required to prove whether *coming from a hospital, coming from home*, or *being a current resident* was a risk factor within fracture and nonfracture categories; this also applied to proving whether *starting or continuing physical therapy* was a risk factor.

A given *diagnosis* would be a risk factor if its proportion among patients ranked 10 to 20 was more than 10% above its proportion among patients ranked 1 to 4 and if the diagnosis accounted for at least 15% of the 74 patients. The *need for consults* (X-ray, orthopedic, neurologic, or cardiologic) would be risk factors if the number of days from the times consults were ordered until the times they were carried out exceeded, respectively, 15% of the total number of days of wait over the limits (428 days).

Specific general physicians would be judged to be causes if they ranked high in three out of four criteria: (a) rate of excess days, (b) disproportionate share of excess days of wait for the admission to PT consult step, (c) disproportionate share of excess days of wait for the special consult steps, and (d) if one to three of the physicians showed markedly higher scores. The *physicians' lack of knowledge that there are consequences with delays beyond the 3- and 7-day limits* would be a cause if answers to questions 1, 2, and 7 were incorrect for 60% or more of physicians and if those in ranks 5 to 8 did worse than those in ranks 1 to 4. Similar requirements would determine if *physicians had an unconcerned attitude towards the problem*, based on answers to questions 4 and 10. *Whether the physicians were aware of the problem* of delays in patients starting physical therapy was to be proved in similar fashion from answers to question 3.

Among factors related to the institution, any of the 8 *steps* would be a cause if its excess wait rate was more than 20% over its limit and accounted for more than 15% of the total of all days over the limit (428 days). Only data for fracture patients were used for steps 2, 3, and 4. *No defined policy on how long a wait is allowed and when steps should occur* would be proved if Anna found that there was no policy on when to write the PT consult order, when to order X rays, when the physiatrist must respond to the consult order, and the maximum allowable wait for physical therapy, or if at least 60% of physicians responded to question 5 by saying that there was no such policy or that they did not know. *Lack of communication with physicians about what the steps are* was to be proved if answers to question 8 showed that 60% or more of physicians did not know the steps and if those in ranks 5 to 8 did worse than those in ranks 1 to 4. *The way the work was organized* involved four issues that would be proved if, upon interviewing management, Anna found:

1. No action was required prior to admission even if the patient were coming from a hospital and if the admit to PT consult order step was proved.
2. The PT/X-ray/orthopedic consult orders were not automatic at admission and if these steps were proved to be causes.
3. The physiatrist acted once per week and this was proved to be a cause.
4. Physical therapy waited for the physiatrist's day to do consults before issuing requests and this step was proved to be a cause.

Too many steps for patients to pass through was also related to the way the work was organized. It would be proved if more than two steps averaged more than two days over the limits for more than 10% of the patients or if any patients had no steps more than two days over the limit but had excess waits anyway. *No coverage for the physiatrist when away*, related to the way the work was organized, would be proved if calculation of waits excluding days the physiatrist was away could reduce the average wait by at least one day. *The physical therapy department not having timely access to admission information*, also related to the way the work was organized, would be proved if, upon interviewing management, Anna found that there was no policy on providing early access and if more than 10% of residents waited more than one day for the step from admission to the screening date.

Results

Of the 16 possible causes, Anna was able to prove 11, partly prove 1, and disprove 4. Four proved risk factors were *having a fracture, coming from a hospital, having a diagnosis of fracture*, and *needing an orthopedic consult*.

Fracture was proved as a risk factor and as a diagnosis. Fracture patients were 100% over the 3-day limit and had a longer average wait than nonfracture patients. Their wait was prolonged by X *ray and orthopedist consults,* but the orthopedist consult was the greater problem. The diagnosis of cardiovascular accident was most prominent among the total of 74 physical therapy patients, but it appeared almost equally as a percentage of the highest- and lowest-ranking residents (43% and 46%); by contrast, the *fracture diagnosis,* although only 8% of ranks 1 through 4, was 29% of ranks 10 through 20. Fractures were 19% of total patients; thus this diagnosis was proved, echoing its role as a risk factor already proved by other criteria.

Fracture patients coming from a hospital and current residents with fractures had equally high over-the-limit rates, both at 100%, but *coming from a hospital* had a higher over-the-limit rate for nonfracture patients and longer average waits than nonfracture patients coming from home or residents.

Proved *staff* factors were *three specific physicians* and *physicians not being aware of the problem.* Physicians 2, 3, and 9 had disproportionate shares of excess waits and high excess wait rates. Anna was surprised to find that 100% of the physicians were unaware of the problem and that most had knowledge of the consequences; she was glad to find that most were concerned.

The bulk of the causes were *institutional.* Three *steps* played a major role in the delays: the step *from admission to the physical therapy consult order* had an excess wait rate of 90% and an 85% share of days over the limit. The step *from the physical therapy consult order to the request for physical therapy* had a 77% excess wait rate and a 33% share of days over the limit. This was because physical therapy waited until Friday, anticipating the physiatrist's arrival on Saturdays. The third step, *from the request for physical therapy to the order to start physical therapy,* had a 44% excess wait rate and a 23% share of days over the limit, reflecting the fact that the physiatrist came only once per week.

Five *ways in which the work was organized* were proved: (a) there was no action prior to admission even if the patient came from a hospital; (b) the PT consult, the orthopedist consult, and X-ray orders were not automatic for fracture patients on admission; (c) the physiatrist acted once per week on PT consult orders; (d) physical therapy waited for the day the physiatrist came to issue requests; and (e) there were too many steps. Three additional institutional causes were proved: *lack of communication about the steps, no defined policy on how long a wait is allowed and when steps should occur,* and *physical therapy not having timely access to admission information.*

Whether the patient was starting or continuing physical therapy made no difference and was not proved. Lack of knowledge about consequences was not a proved cause, but the worst-ranked MDs tended to know less about waits for fractures. Not being concerned about the problem was not proved; not having coverage while the physiatrist was away was also not proved to be a cause.

The administrator and the medical director were convinced of the causes. The medical director seemed impressed by the large number of contributing causes and pleased that his staff were not being blamed. Anna again had to ask that the administrator hold off on solutions, and probably saved a physician his job at the nursing home.

Solutions

Feasibility Limits

Anna met with the administrator and medical director to find out what constraints would be put on any solutions she might suggest. The limits were no increase in nonmedical professional staff; only limited additional documentation, especially by physicians; and no additional costs exceeding $1,000.

Choice of Solutions

Anna met with staff members and physical therapists from other nursing homes and hospitals, reviewed the literature, noted the responses to questions 6 and 9 on the physician questionnaire, and came up with a series of solutions that were enthusiastically supported by the staff members she asked to review them.

To deal with no defined policy on the allowable wait for physical therapy and on when steps should occur, Anna suggested having a documented policy for each step and a maximum total wait: Physical therapy would have to begin within 3 days of admission or injury for fracture patients and within 7 days for nonfracture patients. For the cause that physical therapy did not have timely admissions data, Anna's solution was to have the admissions office notify physical therapy early on the day of admission via an admission card. Anna also asked for access to any newly computerized admissions data that would be designed as part of the expansion planning currently underway.

For the cluster of causes related to fracture patients, Anna suggested a new policy. First, for new or current residents with fractures, there would be orders for X rays, orthopedic consults, and physical therapy consults on admission or injury. Orders for X rays and orthopedist consults were to be answered promptly.

To deal with patients coming from the hospital and the step covering the PT consult order, Anna's solution was also a new policy. All new admissions and readmissions receiving physical therapy prior to admission were to receive a PT consult order upon admission. All new admissions and readmissions with recent diagnoses of fracture, CVA, amputation, and dementia were to receive a physical therapy consult order upon admission (as they would be likely candidates for physical therapy).

For the physiatrist step and the fact that the physiatrist acted only once per week, the solutions were that the physiatrist would be on call for acute fractures, would visit such a resident at once, and would answer other PT consult orders 3 times per week (Saturday, as he already did, plus Tuesday and Thursday). In addition, the physiatrist would be asked to prescribe "weight-bearing status" for a fracture and place the resident on a physical therapy program while awaiting the orthopedist consult.

The step covering physical therapy's request for the physiatrist was also dealt with by a new policy. Physical therapy would screen the patient within one day of admission, would notify the physiatrist of a PT consult order the same day as the screening, and could reach the physiatrist at once for fracture patients because he would be on call. The physical therapy program was to start the day after the physical therapy order.

The cause that there were too many steps for the residents to pass through was addressed by the other solutions; the steps were reduced from eight to six:

Step 1. Upon admission: PT, X-ray, and orthopedist consult orders auto-matic for fractures and PT candidates as appropriate. Notice of admission to physical therapy: same day.

Step 2. From admission notice to PT screening and request for physiatrist: within one day.

Step 3. From X-ray order to completion of X ray for fracture patients: ASAP.

Step 4. From request for physiatrist to physiatrist evaluation and order for PT program: at once for fracture, others within 3 days.

Step 5. From orthopedist consult request to consult: ASAP.

Step 6. From order for PT program to start of PT program: next day.

The cause that specific physicians were a problem was handled as part of the solutions for physicians not being aware of the problem and lack of communication about the steps. Each physician was to receive a copy of the new policies and was asked to attend a facility medical board meeting at which the report of the project and the new policies would be presented.

The client was pleased with the solutions and appreciated having waited for all the results. The solutions he had expected to implement would have involved personnel changes and additions, would have been more expensive, and would not have been as much to the point. The medical director subsequently accepted the solutions and pre-sented them at a medical board meeting, where Anna was credited for the study and the solutions were accepted. The medical director appeared to be pleased with the results, particularly because the medi-cal staff was not unduly affected. For her part, Anna learned that the administration and the physicians really did care about the patients receiving timely physical therapy, and all parties involved came out of the experience with increased respect for one another.

Implementing Solutions and Making Them Operational

The administrator decided to start implementation at once. He and Anna had drafted the new policies together and presented them to the medical director together. Prior to the meeting of the facility medical board, there was a meeting with the physiatrist to assure his approval.

The physiatrist readily agreed to being on call for fractures and agreed to prescribe weight-bearing status for patients while waiting for the orthopedist consultation. He saw no problem with handling physical therapy requests 3 days each week.

The new policies were distributed as part of the facility's *Manual of Administrative Policy and Procedures*, thus making them operational; each physician received a copy of the new policies, and a copy was placed in the physicians' communication books as an added reminder.

The solution to computerize the facility's admissions data and provide access to physical therapy needed approval from the owner of the facility. A doubling of the physical therapy department was already planned, so the client saw no problem in suggesting the computer system. Permission was granted; however, progress was slow, and a year later, the expansion had taken place, but the installation of the computer system was just starting.

Among the major changes, the admissions clerk now places a copy of the patient's admission card in the physical therapy mailbox immediately upon the patient's admission to the facility. As an additional safety check, the clerk places a copy of the admissions list for the day and the anticipated admissions for the following day in the physical therapy mailbox. The general physicians now follow the policy on issuing orders for physical therapy consults, orthopedist consults, and X rays on the day of a patient's arrival.

The physiatrist experienced the greatest change, because he is now on call for fracture patients. However, because the physiatrist was affiliated with two nearby hospitals, this was not a problem. The 3-day schedule for PT consults was even less a problem: Saturday was already scheduled, and Tuesday and Thursday were days he normally came to see the patients on his assigned floor, where he served as a general physician. A side effect of the change was that the physiatrist, who is now assessing more patients, has increased reimbursement matching his increased work load.

Evaluation Design

The plan to evaluate the solutions allowed 3 months to phase them in, with a 3-month quality assurance audit to follow, based on patient waiting times and comparable to the initial data. Three months after implementation, Anna collected 3 months of data on the time between admission and the start of physical therapy. This covered 38 patients, of whom 9 were fracture patients and 29 were nonfracture patients, and included 3 in-house residents. The criteria were 0% over the limits of 3 days of wait for fracture patients, 7 days for nonfracture patients, and average days of wait no longer than 3 days for fracture and 7 days for nonfracture patients.

Results

None of the 38 patients had a wait over the limit; the longest wait was 3 days. The average wait over the 3-month evaluation period was 2.0 days for fracture and nonfracture patients as well as for the total, which meant that the solutions were a complete success on all criteria. Management adopted as policy the periodic review of patient waits for physical therapy, seeing it as a useful indicator of patient care.

Additional benefits came about because receiving restorative physical therapy, which applies to most patients on program (i.e., those receiving physical therapy), qualified a patient for Medicare Part A. The more timely placement on program speeds up the process whereby patients qualify for Part A, and the facility receives reimbursement. There are more PT evaluations now, so there is increased reimbursement, because the facility is reimbursed for an evaluation even if a patient is not placed on program. Management is enthusiastic about the success of the project and considers it a resounding success.

Even in 1997, JCAHO standards did not mention the timeliness of admission to rehabilitation care after assessment. What was accomplished at Anna's organization anticipated a needed change. The percentage of patients receiving timely physical therapy could serve as a useful indicator in a reference database.

Note

1. Yvette L. Santana was the internal consultant for this project. Appendix 2 contains detailed tables and practice exercises related to this case.

Case 2

Patients Waiting for Radiation Therapy
During Scheduled Visits[1]

In this case, patients who came to receive radiation therapy were waiting to be seen. The case was an example of the variety of methods that can be used to identify real causes.

Proving the Problem

The Problem

Bob was a senior radiation therapy technologist in a 6-technologist radiation therapy department of a county hospital. The technologists had been concerned about the length of time patients seemed to be waiting for treatment after they arrived at the department for their scheduled visits; when the issue of quality improvement arose, they suggested this problem for study. Bob asked to function as the internal consultant.

The Client and Importance

The clients were the chief physician and the administrator of radiation therapy.

Most "patients' bills of rights" require that patients have specified appointment times and either punctual treatment or prior notice of delay. No further substantiation of the importance of the problem was needed. The clients gave oral approval to the project and granted access to patient information. The project was presented to the entire staff of the department and was generally welcomed by everyone.

Relevant Steps

When patients, whether inpatients or outpatients, arrived at the radiation therapy department, they normally waited to be called to the dressing room prior to receiving treatment; they could also go to see the nurse or go to the laboratory to have blood drawn while they were waiting.

Observation Units, Normal Loads, Quantities, and Time Frame

The department saw about 65 to 70 patients each day. They were cared for in three rooms, one for each type of machine: a LINAC machine, a cobalt machine, and a simulator. The simulator was used to plan the setup for a new treatment phase so as to provide optimal coverage with minimal exposure to healthy tissue. Each room was assigned a permanent team of two radiation therapy technologists. All the technologists scheduled their own patients. The unit of data collection was the individual visit, identified by visit ID, patient ID, date, time of appointment; one of three team/machine/room assignments; type of treatment, and phase or reason for the visit. There were six treatment types: (a) simulation, (b) whole field, (c) off cord, (d) first cone down, (e) second cone down, and (f) whole body. Patients could go from one type of treatment phase to another. Three reasons (phases) for the visit were *P1*, the setup for a new phase (not always with the simulator); *T1*, the first treatment of a new phase; and *RT*, a regular treatment.

Operational Definitions

The wait for radiation therapy was defined as the number of minutes from the time of the appointment to entry into the dressing room, because a patient's perception of being seen usually starts with his or her entry into the dressing room. The appointment rather than the arrival time was named to avoid too-early or too-late arrivals. Because there could be intervening steps, such as going to the laboratory or seeing the nurse, the actual variable was the *net wait*: from the appointment time to entry into the dressing room, minus time spent going to the nurse and/or to the laboratory if these came after the time the patient arrived at the receptionist's desk. Bob also decided to record data on the length of time spent in the dressing room and in treatment, as these might prove of interest later.

The clients determined at the start of the study that the net wait should not exceed 10 minutes, that time in the dressing room should not exceed 5 minutes, and that treatments in the LINAC and cobalt rooms should not exceed 15 minutes, with 60 minutes as the maximum for the simulation room. Technologists scheduled patients for 15- and 60-minute slots, respectively.

Final List of Possible Causes

Bob came up with 40 possible causes by examining the literature; by interviewing staff, who were very responsive; and by drawing on his own knowledge.

Patient/visit risk factors

1. Specific patients with chronic excess waits
2. Age
3. Sex
4. Whether the patient is a member of a minority group
5. Education (high school and less or more than high school)
6. Use of English (good or not good)
7. Type of insurance (Medicaid, Medicare, or private insurance)
8. Health status (excellent, good, fair, poor)
9. Mobility (able to walk, using a wheelchair, or on a stretcher)
10. Whether an in- or outpatient
11. Mobility combined with in- or outpatient status
12. Disability status on the 10-point Karnofsky Performance Scale (major disability at 4 and normal at 10)
13. Whether having chemotherapy
14. Whether the treatment was palliative or curative (a stand-in for prognosis)
15. Tumor size: 1 cm, 2 cm, 3 cm, 4 cm, 5 cm and greater
16. Number of visits during the study period

17. Whether patient had a prior visit on the same day
18. Whether the patient knew the correct time for the appointment
19. Whether the patient came early
20. Whether the patient came late

Staff factors

21. Years in the department
22. Educational level attained
23. Taking patients out of turn
24. Whether technologists consider scheduling routine
25. Whether technologists feel accountable for waits

Institutional factors

26. Specific machine (LINAC, cobalt, simulator), room, and team
27. Reason (phase) of treatment (setup for new phase, setup and first treatment of new phase, or regular treatment)
28. Type of treatment (simulation, whole field, off cord, first cone down, second cone down, and whole body)
29. Whether the patient went to the nurse after arrival
30. Whether the patient went to the laboratory after arrival
31. Lack of adequate wheelchair access for outpatients
32. Whether prior treatment ran more than 5 minutes beyond next appointment
33. Whether waiting time is a high priority for management
34. No standards on waiting time in manuals or policy statements
35. Whether performance on patient waits is a part of staff evaluation

The way the work is organized

36. Whether inpatients are given priority over outpatients
37. Whether the amounts of time for treatments reflect patients' needs
38. Whether staff have authority to schedule patients based on needs
39. Whether records of appointments are poorly designed
40. Whether there is documentation of patient waits

Research Design

The research design called for equal representation of patients for each treatment type. Bob was to collect data on each patient who arrived for a new phase until there were 27 representatives for each treatment type or until the last day planned for data collection was reached. As the result of another concurrent study Bob was conducting about patient knowledge, he required that the visit be the first one for a new phase. This limited the visits that could be included in the database and adversely affected sample size.

The patients were the primary data collectors. A survey form was designed and was given to the patient on arrival at the receptionist's desk. The name of the patient was put on the back by the receptionist, and a code number was assigned by Bob after he referred to the appropriate scheduling data and codesheets; the name was then erased.

Patients were asked to write in the time they got the survey form and the time of their appointment. Objective data on the appointment time was also available from departmental data. Patients were asked to fill in or have someone else fill in the times they reached the dressing room, therapy room, and when therapy was over. There were also places to write in the times of arrival and departure to see the nurse and/or to have blood drawn. One question asked whether the patient thought the wait for treatment that day was too long. (Other questions were designed to elicit patients' knowledge about their treatment for the concurrent study.) After treatment, the patient put the survey form into a collection box supplied for each treatment room. The technologists were asked to check that the surveys were filled out completely and not carried away.

The survey form was approved and successfully field tested with 18 patients in the nuclear medicine department, as radiation therapy patients were all potential participants in the study. Project data were collected over 6 days, covering 100% of new phase appointments for each treatment type, until a sample of 27 was complete for each type or until data collection had to stop and analysis of data begin.

Data Collection Instruments

Bob assigned code numbers to each technologist and collected data on years in the department, level of education, and patients seen by the technologist. Bob organized the data taken from the technologists' scheduling sheets, each machine's daily logs, and the survey forms. A visit was given an ID number as it entered the database. At the end of the data collection period, there were 27 visits for four treatment types but only 17 visits for the relatively rare second cone down and 7 for the rarer whole-body treatment. There was data for 132 visits, representing 68 patients, listed by visit and patient code, by machine/room/team, by appointment date and time, by treatment reason (phase), and by type. Times were recorded in European style, from 7:45 hours to 16:45 hours.

Data included start and end times for the nurse, the laboratory, the dressing room, and the treatment. Bob derived data for elapsed times from the appointment to entry into the dressing room, time with the nurse, time in the laboratory, time in the dressing room, time in treatment, net waiting time, and total time from appointment to exit. Early and late arrivals were flagged. Maximum allowable times for steps were subtracted from the data on elapsed times to show any excess waiting according to the standards set by management. Other data associated with specific visits included the patients' responses to Question 12 on the survey, "Do you think you waited too long for treatment today?" Total visits, net waits, average net waits, excess wait in minutes, number of visits, and average waits above 10 min were shown for the six treatment types and the total. Finally, the rate at which patients thought the wait was too long was summarized.

Criteria to Prove the Problem

Management set a net wait of more than 10 minutes as unacceptable. As Table C2.1 indicates, the problem indicators, for the total and by treatment type, were the percentage of visits with net waits over 10 minutes, average waits, and patients' opinions about the wait. The clients agreed that the problem would be proved if more than 5% of visits for any treatment type or the total had waits beyond 10 minutes, if any average net wait was over 10 minutes, and if more than 5% of patients in the survey judged that they had waited too long. This came to 21 criteria.

Results

Table C2.1 indicates that 13 of 21 threshold criteria to prove the problem were exceeded. Over 14% of visits had net waits to enter the dressing room longer than 10 minutes. There were variations by treatment type, from 42.9% for whole-body to none for whole-field treatments. Average wait was not proved to be a problem for any treatment type

Table C2.1 Criteria for Proof of Problem and Results (Radiation Visits)

Measure	Point Beyond Which the Problem Exists (Percentage, Rate, etc.)[a]	OKed	Actual Results		Source
Percentage of Visits Over 10 Minutes Wait					Table 1.6
Simulations	> 5.0%	x	14.8%	Proved	
Whole field	> 5.0%	x	0.0%	Not Proved	
Off cord	> 5.0%	x	14.8%	Proved	
Cone down 1	> 5.0%	x	22.2%	Proved	
Cone down 2	> 5.0%	x	11.8%	Proved	
Whole body	> 5.0%	x	42.9%	Proved	
Total	> 5.0%	x	14.4%	Proved	
Average Wait Per Visit					
Simulations	> 10 min	x	6.9 min	Not proved	
Whole field	> 10 min	x	2.4 min	Not proved	
Off cord	> 10 min	x	5.0 min	Not proved	
Cone down 1	> 10 min	x	8.0 min	Not proved	
Cone down 2	> 10 min	x	5.9 min	Not proved	
Whole body	> 10 min	x	14.7 min	Proved	
Total	> 10 min	x	6.1 min	Not proved	
Percentage of Questionnaires by Patients Stating That They Waited Too Long (N = 132)					Table 1.6
Simulations	> 5.0%	x	18.5%	Proved	
Whole field	> 5.0%	x	0.0%	Not proved	
Off cord	> 5.0%	x	18.5%	Proved	
Cone down 1	> 5.0%	x	18.5%	Proved	
Cone down 2	> 5.0%	x	11.8%	Proved	
Whole body	> 5.0%	x	42.9%	Proved	
Total	> 5.0%	x	15.2%	Proved	

a. Limit on wait in minutes, after time of appointment, to be called to dressing room: > 10 minutes. N = 132 visits, 68 patients.

except whole body, which had an average wait of 14.7 minutes. With 62% of the criteria met, the clients agreed that the problem was proved, but they noted that 19 problem visits was a relatively small number.

Identifying Causes

Research Design: Objective Cause Data and Criteria

Bob rearranged data on visits in order of net waiting times and ranked them. Those with the same net wait had the same rank. There were 132 visits in 25 ranks: 113 visits in rank 1 had no wait; ranks 2 to 11 had waits from 1 to 10 minutes. These were the acceptable waits. Ranks 12 to 25 included 19 visits, from 1 excess minute (rank 12) to 27 excess minutes (rank 25).

The 40 possible causes were to be proved with a smaller group of model criteria because similar criteria could be applied to similar causes. Thirteen *dichotomous variables* included patient's sex, whether the patient was a member of a minority group, education (high school and less or more than high school), use of English (good/not good), in- or outpatient status, whether having chemotherapy, whether the treatment was palliative or curative (a stand-in for prognosis), whether there was a prior visit on the same day, whether the patient knew the correct time for the appointment, came early or not, came late or not, and whether the patient went to the nurse or had blood drawn in the laboratory after arrival. The first-step criterion for dichotomous variables was that the share of visits in one of the two subcategories must be more than 15% higher among ranks 12 to 25 than in ranks 1 to 11. Once this was established, more precise statistical tests were applied.

A group of 11 possible causes had multiple categories. These were type of insurance (as a stand-in for socioeconomic status), health status, mobility (able to walk, using a wheelchair, or on a stretcher), status on the 10-point Karnofsky Performance Scale, tumor size in centimeters (cm), number of visits during the study period, the specific machine/room/team, the reason (phase) for the treatment, the type of treatment, and the three types of mobility combined with in- or outpatient status. To test the multicategory variables, the first-step criterion was that the average wait for visits in one of the subcategories must be over 10 minutes, and its percentage share of the visits over 10 minutes must be more than 10% higher than its percentage share of all visits. Once this was established, the more precise statistical tests were applied.

Three types of statistical analysis were used. First, *t* tests were run to measure the significance of differences of waiting time averages for dichotomous cause categories or those that could be characterized as having or not having a characteristic, such as having whole-body treatment or not. With only 19 cases in the group with excess waits, it would not be easy to reach significant results. The second analysis was simple correlations with cause variables that had graded values. The dependent variable was the actual values for net wait, except that

1 minute was added to each wait to avoid zeros. The minimum acceptable coefficient of correlation (*r*) was .4; the 1-tail significance level had to reach .05 or better (an *r* of .432 was usually significant). The third method was stepwise multiple regression analysis, with significance at the .05 level or better.

Of eight miscellaneous variables, *specific patients* would be proved if patients with more than one problem visit accounted for at least 50% of the problem group or if all their visits were in the problem group. *Age* would be proved if the average age for visits in ranks 1 to 11 was at least 5 years different from the average age for ranks 12 to 25; a second stage was the coefficient of correlation as described above. *Lack of adequate wheelchair access for outpatients* required that wheelchair use combined with outpatient status be proved and that there be agreement by management that wheelchair access from the new parking lot was inadequate. *Staff years in the department* and *educational level* would be proved if staff for a room and machine that ranked highest in excess waits had a pattern different from the others.

There were three possible causes that depended on data on visits paired with data on the previous visit in the same room. *Taking patients out of turn* would be proved if more than 25% of visits in ranks 12 to 25 showed that they were taken out of turn later than scheduled and if this was a higher percentage than for ranks 1 to 11. *Prior treatment running more than 5 minutes beyond the next appointment time* was to be proved in a similar way: if more than 25% of visits in ranks 12 to 25 showed that a prior treatment had run over the patient's appointment time, and if this was a higher percentage than for ranks 1 to 11. *Amount of time for treatments did not reflect patients' needs* would be proved if more than 25% of visits in ranks 12 to 25 showed prior treatments that ran longer than 15 (or 60) minutes and if this was a higher percentage than for ranks 1 to 11.

Bob created a table to show paired visits for which there were data on the immediately preceding visit in the study in the same room on the same day. There was a lack of data on this, caused by the nightmare of so many data gatherers. The original surveys were thrown away before data on prior visits were recorded; consequently there were data for only 47 such pairs. Of these, 42 pairs were in ranks 1 to 11 and 5 were in ranks 12 to 25; this was 37% and 26%, respectively, of the two groups.

Analysis of the paired data uncovered the fact that patient 20, whose appointment was at 13:30, was seen out of turn at 14:04, following patient 21's 13:45 appointment and patient 22's 14:00 appointment. Patient 20 had come late and was taken out of turn, after a long wait. It was strange that patient 22, with the 14:00 appointment, was listed as being taken into treatment at 14:03, a minute earlier than patient 20, so the two were listed as being treated simultaneously in the same room.

Upon further investigation, it appeared that there were 10 pairs out of the 47 that showed evidence of overlap between the end of the prior visit and the start of the next treatment. Nine of the 10 were in ranks 1 to 11. This suggested that the data collection was flawed and/or that it underestimated waiting times, because *actual* overlap in the rooms was a physical impossibility.

Research Design: Interviews, Subjective Causes and Criteria

Ten possible causes required additional data collection. To collect data on staff attitudes, Bob conducted an informal face-to-face survey of five technologists, including himself. All were asked, "When you schedule, is it pretty routine, or do you think each one out?" This was a stand-in question for not considering scheduling important. The other question was, "Do you think your supervisor cares about how long your patients wait to be seen?" This dealt with not feeling accountable for waiting time.

For *waiting time not being a high priority* and *lack of adequate wheelchair access for outpatients*, Bob interviewed the clients and made observations. Bob also had to note whether wheelchair and outpatient status was proved as a combined risk factor. *No standards on waiting time in manuals or policy statements* required an examination of documents such as manuals or other material available to technologists to see if anything was said about how to handle waits. *Performance on patient waits not being part of staff evaluation* required an examination of evaluation protocols to see if anything was included about waiting time.

The way the work was organized included *inpatients being given priority over outpatients*. This called for a search to see if there were a policy statement to that effect and a check on whether outpatient status proved to be a risk factor. *Staff do not have authority to schedule patients based on needs* required that Bob examine whether average treatment time for a treatment type proved to be a cause was longer than the appointment time allowed for it; whether staff were expected to always follow fixed booking periods; and whether staff had no authority to schedule patients based on needs.

For *documentation of appointments poorly designed,* Bob examined scheduling forms to see if they could be used for flexible scheduling. For *no documentation of patient waits,* Bob investigated whether there was any evidence that data were normally collected on how long patients waited to be seen.

Results

Of the 40 possible causes studied, 12 were proved and 5 were partly proved, as listed below. Twenty-three were not proved.

1. Using a wheelchair (partly proved)
2. Being an outpatient (partly proved)
3. Being an outpatient with a wheelchair
4. Not knowing the correct time for the appointment (partly proved)
5. Not coming early
6. Coming late
7. Staff consider scheduling routine (partly proved)

The bulk of the proved and partly proved factors were *institutional:*

8. Whole-body and first cone down treatment types
9. Going to the laboratory after arrival (partly proved)
10. Inadequate wheelchair access for outpatients
11. The prior treatment ran more than 5 minutes beyond the next appointment
12. Waiting time is not a high priority
13. No standards on waiting time in manuals or policy statements
14. Performance on patient waits not a part of staff evaluation
15. Inpatients given priority over outpatients
16. Staff do not have authority to schedule time for whole-body patients based on needs
17. No documentation of patient waits

The proved and partly proved causes seemed to fall into four main clusters. The first was *patient behavior*: coming late and not knowing the correct appointment time. The second cluster suggested a *rigid way of scheduling patients* into 15- or 60-minute time slots regardless of individual needs. The third cluster combined *inadequate attention to access for outpatients in wheelchairs* with *a higher priority given to inpatients*. The fourth cluster was a *lack of policy or documentation* to support concern about patient waits and technologists not being able to administer visits more fairly.

Examination of the 19 visits with excess waits indicated that the most prevalent cause was the outpatient status of all but one of the patients involved. The combination of wheelchair and outpatient status accounted for 10 of the visits; coming late accounted for 7 visits. Two of the excess waits were not associated with any risk factors beyond outpatient status.

The combination of variables that best predicted excess waits through stepwise regression was *coming late, being an outpatient with a wheelchair,* and *having whole body or first cone down treatment* ($r = .6$, significant).

These causes were reinforced by *administrative policy* that required staff to book standard times regardless of patient need, technicians having no materials on handling patient waits, no standards in manuals, no records being kept on waiting time, inadequate wheelchair access for outpatients, and staff not being evaluated for their patients' waits. It seemed that management cared about waiting time but did not have the procedures in place to back up its concern. The clients were pleased to see that no single, glaring cause accounted for the bulk of the excess waits, and they tended to regard the proved causes as danger signs. They expressed interest in the solutions Bob would next address.

Solutions

Feasibility Limits

Bob interviewed the two clients to learn the feasibility limits for any solutions. These were *patient load for the department cannot be affected; no new construction or redesign of the physical plant; no new staff; and no new equipment such as machines or computers.*

Choice of Solutions

To select solutions, Bob reviewed the literature and interviewed the staff who had been involved earlier in suggesting possible causes. Staff were enthusiastic participants. After selecting the best solutions, Bob returned to them for further feedback and received helpful suggestions about wording and details. He then presented his solutions to the clients. The most significant changes called for new departmental policies assuming that reducing patient waits was to be given greater priority. The solutions are summarized as follows:

1. A review and revision of priorities on patient waits by management
2. A review of procedures for whole-body and first cone down treatments combined with a trial period of "flex scheduling" to allow technologists to book patients for more or less than the 15- or 60-minute periods, as the cases demanded; this would be accompanied by a request to technologists to plan their scheduling to avoid excess waits rather than doing it routinely
3. Guidelines to deal with waits to be developed, including no priority given to any class of patient except patients in apparent distress
4. Spot checks on waiting time to be made periodically
5. New policies to be reflected in material to be distributed to the technologists in manuals and used in staff evaluation
6. The administrator would contact plant management to hasten the provision of wheelchair access to outpatients from the new parking lot and to have an assessment made of internal pathways to and within the department. (Bob did not think that this would violate the no new construction or design limits set out in the feasibility limits.)
7. Patients not to be sent to or kept in the laboratory while they were waiting, if this could run into treatment appointment times
8. Further work to be done to find out why patients come late. Patients would be given written appointment cards; technologists would not use loss of turn unduly to punish patients who came late, especially if they were late due to lack of wheelchair access.

Implementing Solutions and Making Them Operational

The clients treated the results of the project as a consultant's report and acted on the suggested solutions without involving Bob further.

Bob was not a participant in implementation planning but continued to be treated with respect in the department. He has been acting more or less as an associate administrator since that time.

The suggested solution that work be done to see if there were preventable reasons for patients coming late was implemented by a request to technologists to interview patients with chronic patterns of coming late. This resulted in the discovery that specific appointment slots assigned for a patient's whole series of treatments were sometimes difficult for individual patients to come to on time. Management then declared the policy that technologists could switch patients' regular appointments with other patients, provided that each patient in such a switch agreed. Since then, technologists have not had to use loss of turn as a punishment for lateness.

The suggested solution to review the processes in whole body and first cone down to see if the procedures could be streamlined coincided with a clinical reconsideration that resulted in more fractionated whole-body treatments. This meant more visits but shorter treatments, and it eliminated a major portion of the treatments that ran too long. In addition, although the feasibility limits excluded any new equipment, the cobalt machine was replaced. It had been the machine most associated with longer waits. Shortly after the study was completed, a prior request for a new linear accelerator was approved; the cobalt machine was retired; and the newer machine did indeed streamline operations and shorten treatment time.

"Flex scheduling" on an experimental basis was not adopted, but technologists were allowed to schedule patients in more than one continuous block of time, such as for 30-, 45-, 60-, or 75-minute periods, according to individual needs and without requiring permission. No alteration was made in the booking slots or scheduling forms, but the effect was the same because, as a result, technologists could group 15-minute periods, were encouraged to think through their scheduling, and were given authority to do what was needed.

Lack of wheelchair access for outpatients was handled in two ways. First, plant management agreed to provide smooth pavement for the access route from the new parking lot to the department; second, in addition to the ramps, the closest parking spaces were reserved for patients with impaired mobility.

Policy changes resulted in the requirement that, if treatments were running 15 minutes late, the technologist would announce this in the waiting room and post a sign. This helped patients decide whether to go to the laboratory while they were waiting. There is still no ongoing collection of data on waiting times, but patients now sign in and a time of arrival is recorded by the receptionist for use in case of disputes. No formal evaluation was carried out, but Bob, the staff, nurses, and patients seem to be aware of much better experiences in the department and a major reduction in the problem.

The 1991 JCAHO standards for hospital-sponsored ambulatory care services required that services be accessible to patients, that appropriate procedures for appointments and scheduling be in place, and that waiting times be appropriate to the type of care to be provided. Standards specified the elimination of physical barriers for the physically, visually, hearing, or speech impaired and required that the hospital gather, evaluate, and take appropriate action on information relating to patient satisfaction with all aspects of care. These standards disappeared into the more generic standards subsequently adopted by the JCAHO, but the intent, examples, and scoring of patient care standards attend to timeliness and attention to the needs of patients. The data collection carried out by Bob and the organizational changes induced by the project improved the quality of care.

Note

1. The internal consultant for this project wishes to remain anonymous.

Late Notification of Critical Values
by a Hospital Laboratory[1]

W hen critical limits of specified test results are exceeded, medical laboratories are expected to provide immediate notification to the physicians responsible for the care of the patients. In this case, physicians may have been waiting too long for results.

Proving the Problem

The Problem, Importance, and the Client

Physicians in a voluntary hospital complained that the hematology laboratory was not providing them with timely notification by phone of first-time *critical values*. Critical values, also called *panic values*, are test results that vary from established norms to such an extent that they represent a life-threatening condition. Knowing the results at once allows the physician to react appropriately and rapidly.

Clara, who was a laboratory technologist in the clinical hematology department, offered to investigate. The client was the laboratory manager. She wanted data on whether first-time criticals were being called in within 60 minutes after verification of the results, as mandated, but Clara and her collaborator considered prior periods important too.

Normal Loads, Quantities, and Time Frame

The laboratory operated on a three-shift, 24-hour, 7-day basis. The client was not willing to allow staff to help Clara collect data during the night shift. Clara determined that the day and evening shifts accounted for about 93% of critical values during a representative week, and she agreed to the restriction. Clara further suggested that, to minimize the data collection time each day, the study be confined to two tests conducted simultaneously: hemoglobin (Hgb) and hematocrit (Hct). Critical values for these can indicate that the patient is bleeding internally; they were performed in large enough numbers to keep data collection on first-time criticals to a workable period.

Relevant Steps

When specimens arrived, ID data were entered into the computer, the samples were inspected for clots, they were then placed in tubes on racks that held up to 12 samples, and the tests were run. The laboratory technologists identified a first-time critical value by noting test results in the critical range and examining the computerized patient record. If critical results were inconsistent with a previous history and/or prior notation, and if retesting and reporting to the ordering physician had not yet been done, the results were called *initial [first-time] critical results*. There was no concern about when specimens arrived or were tested, so the first item Clara was concerned with was the time the test was run; this was shown in a computer printout that also gave the test results.

The technologists decided when to examine the results, which was done on the computer screen; comments and entries could be made through keyboard access. The time that the technologist examined the results and decided whether there was a first-time critical was not recorded during usual operations. Clara had to enlist staff to record this. As Table C3.1 indicates, Clara referred to the time from the test run to the time the technologist examined the results as *Step 1*.

The operative standard at the hospital was that the technologist must verify (rerun) critical results. The technologists also decided whether to rerun a critical at once or to go on checking other results and do the reruns in a batch. Sometimes instruments were tied up; there was an observed tendency to accumulate retests. The retests were

Table C3.1 Case 3 Steps and Associated Staff Members

Step Number	From/To	Staff Member
1	Time test is run to time technologist examines results	Technologist
2	Time technologist examines results to time of rerun	Technologist
3	Time of rerun to time results placed in slot	Technologist
4	Time results placed in slot to time of call as shown in the computer	Clerk
5	Time results placed in slot to time of call as shown in the logbook	Clerk

run manually, on a different part of the same instrument or on a backup instrument. A record of the time of the rerun was generated automatically. Table C3.1 shows this as the end of *Step 2*. From the point of view of an ordering physician, Steps 1 and 2 were important parts of the wait, but waits for these two steps had no time standards, although they could compromise the larger objective of prompt reporting of criticals.

If the critical value was verified, the ordering physician had to be notified by telephone *within 60 minutes*, within which time the patient's unit had to be notified if the physician were not available. The notification call had to be recorded in the computer and also entered into a telephone logbook. During the day and evening shifts, the calling was done by laboratory clerks; on the night shift, technologists did both the testing and the calling. The practice of the laboratory staff was to call the patient's unit, relying on unit staff to contact the physician.

The rerun results were automatically entered into the computer, were examined at once, and the new printout was attached to the original. If the critical value was verified, the technologist further documented the record and flagged the critical value on the printout. The technologist was then responsible for carrying the printout with the verified critical result to a slot set aside for first-time criticals. Normal operations did not require the technologist to record when the results were placed in the slot, so Clara needed to ask for help to record this. Table C3.1 shows the time from the rerun to the placement of the results in the slot as *Step 3*. It was the clerk's responsibility to retrieve the results from the slot and call in the results to the patient's physician or unit. The technologists were not obligated to inform the clerk when they placed critical results in the slot. The clerk was expected to contact the physician or unit and record the call by a coded entry in the computer so that the record would include the time when the call was made. Table C3.1 refers to the time from the results being placed in the slot to the time of the call recorded in the computer as *Step 4*. The clerk was also responsible for recording the call in a telephone logbook. There were no guidelines on whether the computer entry should precede the time in the logbook entry or the reverse, but Clara defined the logbook entry as the point at which *Step 5* ended. The time period of interest to the laboratory manager was the combined time for Steps 3 and 4.

Research Design

Clara and the client decided that a sample of 100 first-time criticals would be adequate. They agreed that data for entire days, even if not in unbroken sequence by date, was preferable to data for unbroken sequences that might have incomplete data for given days. This decision resulted in data for a discontinuous period of 11 days because data for days during which data were improperly collected were discarded. The technologists were enlisted to record on the computer printouts the times they first decided test values were first-time criticals and the time they placed the printouts with the verified results in the critical values slot.

The lead technologist was asked to record any times a test instrument or the computer were not working, but this never occurred. All times recorded by staff were to be taken from the same designated department clock. All other data were computer generated or retrievable from institutional data sources. Clara collected and photocopied all the printouts with Hgb and Hct criticals for each of the two shifts for full days until she had her base of 100. Later, data on attitudes and beliefs were collected through two staff questionnaires.

To facilitate staff cooperation, Clara and the client agreed that no staff would be identified beyond job title and shift, only summary data would be presented to management, and no person would be harmed as a result of the study—no data could tie any staff member to problem data.

Data Collection and Operational Definitions

The unit of study was the first-time critical, prior to verification, as found on the computer printout for a given day during the first two shifts. Specimen laboratory code numbers were treated as confidential; Clara assigned project codes to the specimens which, along with test dates, were used for identification in tables.

Critical values and *first-time critical values* were used as synonymous terms unless the actual distinction was important. "Laboratory technologist" and "laboratory worker" were used as interchangeable titles.

In seven instances, the time entered by the technologist for placement of results in the slot preceded the computer-generated time listed for the rerun. As this was impossible, Clara wrote in a time for placement in the slot that was the same time or later than the rerun, but earlier than the record of the call in the computer, and ignored the technologist's entry. None of these instances were associated with problem waits, and none affected the validity of the results with respect to the 60-minute time period criterion.

Final List of Possible Causes

Clara identified 25 possible causes from sources in the literature, interviews with staff members, her collaborator, and her own experience.

Work-related possible causes

1. Any step by job title that contributed to excess waits
2. Any step by job title that contributed to missing criticals
3. Specific shift
4. Specific test instrument
5. Heavy workload
6. Instrument malfunction
7. Computer down time

Subjective staff causes

8. Staff do not feel personally involved in reporting test results on time
9. Staff believe that management will do what it wants regardless of staff ideas

10. Staff believe that the problem is other people's fault
11. Staff believe that nothing much is affected if calls wait beyond 60 minutes
12. Staff believe that no one holds them responsible for the time criticals are called in

The way the work is organized

13. Technologists allow work to accumulate before they note test results
14. Technologists allow work to accumulate before they run retests
15. Technologists allow work to accumulate before they place rerun results in the slot
16. Technologists do not have to inform the clerk when placing results in the slot
17. Test instruments can be left idle while technologists are at lunch
18. No calls are made while the clerk is at lunch

Other institutional factors

19. No defined policy on how to sequence the work
20. No standards in manuals on work sequence
21. Standards not designed to report critical results rapidly
22. Timeliness of reporting criticals not used for staff evaluations
23. Staff do not get feedback on delays in reporting criticals to units
24. Laboratory workers do not ask clerks about the report status of criticals or tell clerks when they place critical results in slot
25. Documentation method to report criticals is too general to be efficient or is poorly designed.

Data Analysis

Clara determined whether a critical value was missed by comparing the staff's printout data and rerun reports on first-time criticals with a master list of computer printouts at the end of the day. Clara could see if any first-time criticals were missed or not rerun and therefore not reported to the physician or unit. The second key variable was the elapsed time for the sum of Steps 3 and 4. Clara recorded whether the elapsed time was within or over 60 minutes from the time of the rerun. The problem indicators were the number of missed criticals as a percentage of the criticals in the study, criticals over 60 minutes as a percentage of identified criticals, and average elapsed times for Steps 3 and 4. The indicators were also calculated by shift, date, and instrument used.

Criteria to Prove the Problem

Before data collection was completed, Clara and her client decided on three criteria to prove the problem: (a) if *any* critical values were missed and not rerun, (b) if more than 5% of the critical values for which there were records took more than 60 minutes from rerun to the record of the call in the computer (Steps 3 and 4), and (c) if the average time from the rerun to the record of the call in the computer was more than 60 minutes.

Results

Out of 100 criticals, there was elapsed time data for 97; 3 were missed. There were some missing data on another 7 criticals, so data on a total of 10 criticals were lost. Of the 90 criticals with complete data on the wait for Steps 3 and 4, 11 showed elapsed times of more than 60 minutes.

The problem was proved for two out of three criteria. Three percent of the critical values were missed and not rerun (proved) and there was a 12.2% rate of critical values that took more than 60 minutes for Steps 3 and 4 (proved); but the average time for Steps 3 and 4 was only 28 minutes (not proved). Here was another example of an unacceptable but relatively small number of cases affecting the rate being offset in the average by other extremely short waits.

With two out of three criteria exceeded, the client agreed that the problem was proved. The laboratory manager was surprised at the 12.2% wait rate, but dismayed at the missed criticals; she was now more interested than before in the next stages of the project.

Identifying Causes

Research Design

There were only 11 criticals with excessive waiting times, so Clara increased the problem group by including criticals with waits of 50 minutes or more, reasoning that good reporting should not cut at exactly 60 minutes and that the adjustment would provide a larger sample base for analysis. As a result, the problem waits were increased by 5. Clara had data for 16 criticals with 50 minutes or more for Steps 3 and 4.

Objective Cause Data

Clara already had data on the steps by job title, shift, instrument, instrument malfunction, and computer down time. To examine the extent to which *specific steps* were causes, and to deal with accumulation of work, she designed a table to show the data by step according to job title. In dealing with Steps 3 and 4, Clara decided to apply the criterion that each step would be assigned half the allotted 60 minutes and would be perceived as taking too long if it exceeded 30 minutes. Based on the criterion of 30 minutes for each step, Clara calculated excess wait rates. The rates were 2% for the technologists' Step 3 and 27% for the clerks' Step 4. The average wait was 3 minutes for Step 3 and 26 minutes for Step 4. For the 16 problem criticals, the excess wait rate for Step 3 was 6%; for Step 4 it was 100%. Average waits were 5 minutes and 82 minutes, respectively.

Clara applied the 30-minute criterion to all three of the technologist steps (Steps 1, 2, and 3, as shown in Table C3.1) and the two clerk steps (Steps 4 and 5). For Step 1, the excess wait rate was 24%. For Step 2, the rate was 12%. As reported above, the rate for Step 3 was 2%. Thus it appeared that a major portion of the physicians' wait came prior to the steps included in the mandated 60-minute maximum wait limit.

There were only two steps for the clerks. As indicated, Step 4 had an excess wait rate of 27%; for Step 5, reflecting the entry of the call into the logbook, the rate was 31%, showing that the logbook data were different and worse.

At this point, Clara realized that the clerks were not recording the same time for the call in the computer and in the logbook. The data showed that the time was the same in only 9 of 90 cases (10%). Clara concluded that the clerks were recording the *time they made the entry*, and not the *time they made the call*. Assuming that the earlier of the two recorded times was the true time of the call, the correct time appeared in the database in 75 cases (83%), when the computer time was the same or earlier than the logbook time. In 14 cases, the logbook time was earlier. Of these 14, only one case would have changed from a problem case to an acceptable case if the logbook time were correct. Its total wait would have gone from 226 minutes to 40 minutes. Clara concluded that, if clerks were recording the time they made the record and not the time they made the call, it put all the record keeping into question. It was not a cause of the problem, but it undermined the institution's ability to assess the problem and probably exaggerated it.

Returning to the cause data, Clara needed to verify whether technologists allowed work to accumulate in batches before they looked at the results, before running the retests, and before placing the verified results in the slot. She needed to verify whether technologists had to inform the clerk of results being placed in the slot, whether test instruments could be left while technologists were at lunch, and whether results accumulated in the slot while the clerk was at lunch. Some of these were to be verified by observation, some by interview, and some also with questionnaires.

Because Clara was not able to collect data on the total number of tests done by staff each of the 11 days, she was limited in how she could study workload as a cause. Clara decided to have an item on workload on the questionnaires and also create, as a further check on workload, data on the number of criticals found in a given day. It would have been helpful to have data on the number of staff on duty each day, but such data were not considered at the outset and could not easily be collected later.

To deal with instruments being left and no calls being made while laboratory workers or clerks were at lunch, Clara examined the existing data for the 16 problem samples by placing them in order by the time the results were placed in the slot. For each of the titles, Clara noted whether Step 3 or Step 4, respectively, was more than 30 minutes and whether the step fell within the lunch period for the job title.

The data showed that lunch was involved in 7 of the clerks' 16 problem tests and only one of the technologists' problem tests. To further support the evidence, Clara examined whether tests were done out of order after they piled up; that is, if they were taken from the top of the pile rather than from the bottom. For laboratory workers, only one sample was taken out of order with respect to the rerun time. It did not correspond to a lunch period and was off by only 1 minute. For the clerks, seven late criticals fell around the lunch hour, and seven entries of calls were entered in the computer out of order. Five were during lunch periods, suggesting that, after accumulating the results, the calls were made as they lay on the pile, last done first, rather than in order as they arrived.

Clara interviewed management to determine whether there was a defined policy on how to sequence the work, whether there were standards in manuals on work sequence, whether the standards related to getting critical results out rapidly, whether performance on timeliness was used for evaluations, and whether staff got feedback on delays in reporting criticals. This last cause was also represented in the questionnaires. In addition, Clara investigated the documentation method to report criticals to assess whether it was too general to be efficient or was poorly designed.

Subjective Cause Data: Questionnaires

Clara designed two staff questionnaires to investigate subjective causes, each with 10 questions. Figure C3.1 presents the "Laboratory Worker Questionnaire"; the "Laboratory Clerk Questionnaire" had the same or similar questions, which were given the same numbers in both survey instruments. Each asked the respondents to check or tell which statements they agreed with, disagreed with, or whether they did not know.

The instruments were successfully field tested with laboratory workers and clerks who were not involved with the laboratory tests being studied. Both Question 1s were used as icebreakers, asking whether there was a problem in the laboratory about getting initial critical values called to units within 60 minutes of the results being verified. This set the context for the other questions. (Fifty percent of laboratory workers and 83% of clerks thought there was a problem.)

To add to the limited data on workload, Question 8 for the technologists stated, "On the days there is a heavy workload I do not get some of the initial criticals to the clerk slot on time." The ending for the clerks substituted the words, "I may not call the units about some initial criticals on time." The belief that the problem was other people's fault was handled in the technologists' Question 9: "If the initial criticals are not getting called in on time it is not due to the way the laboratory workers carry out the work; it is something else." The

Dear Colleague,

I am trying to find a way to help the lab improve the number of initial critical values that get called to the units within the required time. You can help me by checking (or telling me) which statements you agree with or disagree with. Please note that no names are being used. The data will all be confidential.

	Agree	*Disagree*	*Don't Know*
1. We have a problem in the lab about getting initial critical values called to units within 60 minutes of the result being verified.	( )	( )	( )
2. Even if there were a problem, it is not a very important one, because nothing much is affected if the unit waits more than 60 minutes.	( )	( )	( )
3. I get little feedback about how many of the initial criticals I handle get called in on time.	( )	( )	( )
4. I do not get personally involved in the testing: if there are delays in reporting, it is part of the work.	( )	( )	( )
5. If I came up with a way to get the results out better, management would do what it wants anyway.	( )	( )	( )
6. No one holds me responsible for how soon the initial critical values are called in.	( )	( )	( )
7. If lab workers did not accumulate the retesting of criticals, the calls could be made sooner.	( )	( )	( )
8. On the days there is a heavy workload, I do not get some of the initial criticals to the clerk slot on time.	( )	( )	( )
9. If the initial criticals are not getting called in on time, it is not due to the way the lab workers carry out the work; it is something else.	( )	( )	( )
10. If the lab workers would ask the clerks about the time a call was made for their criticals, calls would be made sooner.	( )	( )	( )

Figure C3.1 Laboratory Worker Questionnaire

clerks' Question 9 ended, "it is not due to the way the clerks carry out the work; it is something else."

Question 10 for laboratory workers asked, "If the laboratory workers would ask the clerks about the time a call was made for their criticals, calls would be made sooner." Clerks were asked, "If the laboratory workers would tell the clerks each time a critical was put in the slot, the calls would be made sooner."

Criteria to Prove the Causes

There were seven work-related possible causes. A *step associated with a job title* would be proved to be a cause of *excess waits* if the number of criticals over 30 minutes for the step was more than 9% and if the average for that step among the 16 problem cases was greater than 30 minutes. A *step associated with a job title* would be a cause of *missing critical data* if the percentage of samples with missing data for the step was over 9%.

A *specific shift* would be a cause if its percentage of over-50-minute criticals for Step 3 or 4 was more than 10% higher in one shift, if the shift accounted for at least 10% of the total in the sample, and if its percentage share of problem cases was at least 10 percentage points greater than its percentage share of the sample. A similar set of criteria was applied to *specific instruments*.

Heavy workload would be a cause if there was a positive correlation between total criticals for a day and the number taking over 50 minutes for the two crucial steps. R was to be at least .4, significant at the .05 level or better, and at least 50% of the staff in the problem job title (which turned out to be the clerks) had to have supported this view, and at a higher rate than the nonproblem job title (laboratory technologists). *Instrument malfunction* and *computer down time* would be causes if they were present in at least 10% of problem cases.

There were five subjective causes. These would be proved if at least 50% of the staff in the problem job title responded in support of the view and responded at a higher rate than those in the nonproblem job title.

There were six possible causes related to the way the work was organized: (a) *Technologists allow work to accumulate before they note test results* would be proved if the accumulation were verified by observation and if more than 9% of total and problem criticals for Step 1 ran over 30 minutes. This would then be a cause for the overall physician wait. (b) *Technologists allow work to accumulate before they run retests* would be proved if the accumulation were verified by observation, if more than 9% of total and problem criticals for Step 2 ran over 30 minutes, and if at least 50% of the staff responded to the questionnaire in support of this. This would also be a cause for the overall physician wait.

(c) *Technologists allow work to accumulate before they place rerun results in the slot* would be proved if the accumulation were verified by observation and if more than 9% of total and problem criticals for Step 3 ran over 30 minutes. (d) *Technologists do not have to inform the clerk when placing results in the slot* would be proved if Clara verified that no such policy existed, if clerks were not being notified, if more than 9% of total and problem criticals for Step 4 ran over 30 minutes, and if at least 50% of the staff responded to the questionnaire in support of this. (e) *Test instruments can be left idle while laboratory workers are at lunch,* and (f) *no calls are made while the clerk is at lunch* would be proved if the situation were verified by observation, if more than 9% of Steps 3 or 4 ran over 30 minutes for the total and the problem group, and if at least 30% of waits over 30 minutes occurred around lunch hours. This would be reinforced if a substantial portion of those waits falling around lunch hours were taken in reverse order of the original time of the run.

There were seven other institutional causes. For (a) *no defined policy on how to sequence the work,* Clara would have to find no documented guidelines. For (b) *no standards in manuals on work sequence,* she was to find no mention of work sequences in manuals. For (c) *the standards are not designed to get critical results reported out rapidly,* there would have to be no time standards for the individual steps by job title (which would lull staff's awareness of their own share of the 60 minutes). For (d) *timeliness of reporting criticals is not used for staff evaluations,* an interview with management would have to support this.

For (e) *staff do not get feedback on delays in reporting criticals to units* and (f) *laboratory workers do not ask clerks about the report status of criticals or tell clerks when they place critical results in the slot,* the proof would be if at least 50% of the the staff in the problem job title responded to support this and at a higher rate than the nonproblem job title. For (g) *the documentation method to report criticals is too general to be efficient or is poorly designed,* the method used by staff would have to be judged to be too general to pinpoint individual staff participation in getting results out, would have to be vague about when and how to record the calls made, and would have to be shown to be only roughly related to official policy on who in the unit was to be called.

Results

Of the 25 causes studied, 8 were proved, 3 were partly proved, and 2 were proved in relation to the physicians' overall wait, for a total of 13 causes:

1. Step 4, done by the clerks, was proved to be the major source of waits beyond 60 minutes.
2. The *day shift* was partly proved to be more associated with the problem than the evening shift.

Subjective staff causes were:

3. *Staff do not feel personally involved in reporting test results on time.*
4. *Staff believe that management will do what it wants regardless of staff ideas.*
5. *Staff believe that the problem is other people's fault* (partly proved).

Proved causes listed under the way the work is organized were:

6. *Technologists allow work to accumulate before they run retests.*
7. *Technologists do not have to inform the clerk when placing results in the slot.*
8. *No calls are made while the clerk is at lunch.*

Proved additional institutional factors were:

9. *Standards are not designed to get critical results reported out rapidly.*
10. *Staff do not get feedback on delays in reporting criticals to units.*
11. *Laboratory workers do not ask clerks about the report status of criticals or tell clerks when they place critical results in the slot.*
12. *The documentation method to report criticals is too general to be efficient or is poorly designed* (partly proved).

If the total wait by the ordering physician were also considered,

13. *The two steps done by technologists, Steps 1 and 2, as shown in Table C3.1, would also be included.*

The proved and partly proved causes clustered around the clerk's Step 4, largely supported by lack of an individual time limit for the step, lunchtime accumulation of critical reports in the slot, not being alerted to the presence of reports in the slot, and an overly general and poorly designed method to report criticals. The subjective causes show distancing from the effects and skepticism about management's intent, as well as lack of communication by technologists.

When the client saw Clara's results, she was surprised at the number of proved and partly proved causes but felt intuitively that they were valid; she therefore approved the results.

Solutions

Feasibility Limits

When Clara interviewed the laboratory manager, she was given three limitations on proposed solutions. There could be no major costs incurred, no additional staff hired, and flextime could not be used, although starting times for work could be changed.

Choice of Solutions

Clara interviewed staff and received some creative suggestions. She also reviewed the literature, met with her collaborator, and considered her own ideas. After she selected a set of solutions, she brought them to staff to get their reactions. She then presented the best solutions to the client.

Clara dealt with the key clerk step, Step 4, by making a general policy suggestion. She stated that management needed to set separate policies for Step 3 and Step 4 to ensure that technologists and clerks were each aware of their own time limits. She suggested a written policy of 30 minutes for each step and inservice training for the clerks to ensure that their limit was understood. Clara suggested a new, more specific policy: to have part of the technologists' Step 3 include informing the clerk when an initial critical was placed in the slot and to write on the printout the time the results were placed in the slot, just as was done during the project. Technologists' inservice training would include emphasis on the need not to accumulate critical results, and each critical would be rerun and placed in the slot with the time entered as soon as noted.

Clara suggested that, when only one clerk was on duty during a lunch period, a laboratory technologist or the lead technologist be assigned to make the calls to the units. This was also to be covered in inservice training.

Standards would specify that entry of the call into the computer should come before entry into the logbook, that calls should be made in order of the time of the rerun, and that both entries should reflect the time of the call and not the time of the entry. Clara suggested that, if management considered it important that staff not accumulate samples before reading results and before reruns, written policy on the precise sequencing desired should be formulated and presented during inservice training.

The day shift's lead laboratory technologist was to be asked to do twice-daily checks to be sure that criticals were noticed, placed in the slot, and called in on time, so any problems, including missed criticals, could be noted, acted on, and additional training or other action provided.

For subjective causes, Clara suggested separate inservice training for laboratory technologists and clerks to explain the solutions and show management's commitment. Inservice training would explain the effects on patients when results are not received on time; case studies of criticals would be presented to show how the critical results are used in patient care and how important time is. Monthly staff meetings would also include case studies, would review how staff were meeting reporting standards, and would reinforce standards. Undermining conditions such as lack of a consistent policy on calling were also addressed. If current official calling procedures to have the physician called first were to remain, Clara suggested that this be part of inservice; if not, policy should be rewritten to reflect the call to the unit, as was then being practiced. To deal with Steps 1 and 2, Clara suggested that (a) when the laboratory technologist loads the instrument with 1 to 12 racks, one rack at a time should be dealt with as it is finished, and (b) the rack should be removed from the instrument and the results reviewed. Any results found to be initial criticals should be rerun at once on the backup instrument or by interrupting the current run, using the start button to continue the run. This would permit initial criticals to be moved through quickly, without adding much time to other specimens.

The laboratory manager agreed that there was a need to set a 30 minute limit for each step and thought it was a good idea to have staff inservice training. She agreed to new specifications for the technologist's step, that inservice training should cover the new rules, and that when only one clerk was on duty a laboratory technologist or the lead technologist should be assigned to make the calls, and this would be covered in inservice training. She also said that management considered it important that staff not accumulate samples before reading results and before reruns. She agreed on the sequence suggested by Clara and that it should be taught during inservice training.

The laboratory manager also agreed that standards should specify that calls should be made in order of their times of rerun, that entry of the call into the computer should come before entry into the logbook, and that the entries should both be for the time of the call. She deferred deciding about having the day shift's lead laboratory technologist do twice-daily checks until she concluded a review of the job's responsibilities. She did not agree that there should be separate inservice training for technologists and clerks because she believed that joint inservice training would help the staff see the overall connections between the steps.

She liked the idea of using case studies based on criticals in inservice training and monthly staff meetings and agreed that management should decide on consistent calling procedures regarding who in the unit would be called first, and this would be included as part of inservice training.

Implementing Solutions and Making Them Operational

The client was pleased with the simplicity and cost efficiency of the solutions, and it appeared that most would be implemented, especially as staff were already positively inclined towards them. Unfortunately, implementation was deferred when the entire department became involved in the uncertainties of budget cutbacks, early retirements, and retrenchment due to the fiscal crisis faced by the organization and health services generally.

However, because the staff involved understood the project and the causes of the problems, and because they had been involved in designing the solutions, they were able to implement many solutions themselves by changing some of their work behaviors and being conscious of how they carried out their own steps.

Note

1. Linda Q. Stevens was the internal consultant for this project.

Case 4

Time Spent in Rehabilitation
by Amputation Patients in a Municipal Hospital[1]

In this instance, a municipal hospital was concerned about the length of stay of rehabilitation patients. While not subject to prospective payment restrictions, similar cost pressures nevertheless existed. The case was unusual because of the large number of possible causes that were examined.

Proving the Problem

The Problem

A major municipal hospital's department of rehabilitation was concerned when its indicator data showed an unusually long length of stay for patients. This suggested the need for more intensive assessment, and patients recovering from amputations of the leg were selected for detailed study. Patients judged ready for rehabilitation were provided with assistive devices, including prostheses; they were discharged when they could ambulate unaided with assistive devices. The question was whether amputee patients at this hospital took longer than appropriate to complete their in-house rehabilitation. Dan, a staff physical therapist, offered to carry out the study, an attractive offer because there was a limited budget for data collection.

The Client

The clients were the clinical director of rehabilitation medicine and the director of physical therapy. Both were enthusiastic about the project because the problem was one they had been concerned about for a long time.

Importance

The fiscal implications for the hospital were obvious. In addition, when patients take too long to complete rehabilitation, it can affect their well-being and may impede medical recovery. A prolonged hospital stay negatively affects the achievement of high functional status, such as the ability to ambulate independently with a prosthesis, self-care activities, and return to normal living. This can lead to disappointment with the rehabilitation process and rejection of the assistive device.

Final List of Possible Causes

Dan believed that sources of delay could stem from the conditions existing when the patient was referred, the bedside care given, the rehabilitation program, patient education and self-care, the prosthesis, and the situation into which the patient would be released. After interviews with staff, a review of the literature, and talking with his collaborator, Dan selected 50 possible causes, including some related to the tendency of patients at municipal hospitals to experience more severe and chronic symptoms, reflecting socioeconomic risk factors.

Risk factors related to patients' medical condition

1. Whether patient has anticipated problems (AP)
2. Medical or psychological components of AP status (cardiopulmonary disease, diabetes, neurologic problems, fracture; depression, psychosis, attempted suicide)
3. Poor wound healing at the surgical site
4. Bad nutritional status
5. Weight status (overweight, normal, underweight)

6. If patient had problems with stump shape
7. Amputation above or below knee
8. Cognitive status (three degrees)
9. Days from surgery to rehabilitation

Causes related to demographics or socioeconomic experience

10. Sex
11. Age (under 40, 40-60, 61-70, over 70)
12. Type of insurance (none, Medicaid, private, Medicare, or Medicare and other)
13. Marital status
14. Whether patient has a permanent home
15. Number of people in the patient's household (self only, 2, more than 2)
16. Use of English (OK, not good [NG])
17. Language used
18. Coming from hospital or elsewhere
19. Whether patient has a job waiting

Causes related to inadequate support, care,
and education by the institution

20. Specific staff
21. Specific job title (activities carried out by PTs, OTs, RNs)
22. Staff experience in the department
23. Staff highest degree of education
24. Staff knowledge of how to care for amputee patients
25. Staff attitude towards problem of length of stay
26. Staff belief about the nature of the problem
27. Staff belief about consequences of the problem
28. Whether staff feel accountable for length of stay
29. Whether patient received pre-op education
30. Percentage rate of broken PT appointments
31. Whether patient knows how to care for stump
32. Whether patient is compliant with stump self-care
33. Whether in teaching stump shaping, the PT used printed materials, demonstrated, or asked patient to demonstrate back

34. Whether in teaching self-care, the PT used printed materials, demonstrated, or asked patient to demonstrate back
35. Whether in teaching use of prosthesis, the PT used printed materials, demonstrated, or asked patient to demonstrate back
36. Whether in teaching transfers to and from bed, chairs, and so on, the OT used printed materials, demonstrated, or asked patient to demonstrate back
37. Whether in teaching upper body use, the OT used printed materials, demonstrated, or asked patient to demonstrate back

Causes related to the prosthesis

38. Whether patient feels comfortable with prosthesis
39. Whether prosthesis was painful when received
40. Whether patient wanted prosthesis
41. Whether prosthesis is painful now
42. Whether patient has medical complications due to the prosthesis
43. Whether the prosthesis vendor delivered on time
44. Whether the prosthesis vendor delivered the correct prosthesis
45. Whether the prosthesis vendor delivered an ill-fitting prosthesis

Other institutional causes

46. Whether there is a defined policy related to care of amputation stumps
47. Whether there are standards in manuals on amputation care
48. Whether performance on amputation care and length of stay is used for evaluations
49. Lack of feedback to staff on length of stay
50. Documentation method or forms are too general about risk factors, poorly designed, or nonexistent

Research Design

Dan hoped to follow patients from arrival to discharge, but to have an adequate number of subjects within his time constraints, he included patients who were already discharged and were now in follow-up care. He interviewed current patients as they were discharged and recently discharged patients during outpatient follow-up visits. His sample included 53 patients with chart information, of whom 27 provided data during face-to-face interviews.

In the interview, Dan asked:

1. When you first had your surgery, and before you came to us for rehabilitation, did anyone teach you how to care for the surgery wound?
2. Please tell me what you did to care for the surgery wound.
3. Did you want your prosthesis when the time came for it?
4. Was the prosthesis painful when you got it?
5. Do you feel OK about having a prosthesis now?
6. Is the prosthesis painful now?

Operational Definitions

Dan defined anticipated problems (AP) that would make patients "sicker" and more likely to remain under treatment operationally as a set of medical conditions that could lead to more time in rehabilitation. This set included at least three out of five medical conditions, including cardiopulmonary disease, diabetes, neurologic problems, fracture, or another major disease condition; the set also included a diagnosis of depression, psychosis, or attempted suicide. The definition was accepted by management and staff; it covered conditions that could be found in chart information and therefore could be used to identify patients as they entered the study. The study included 30 patients with AP and 23 without AP.

Data Collection Instruments

Dan assigned code numbers to each patient and each staff member who provided care to the 53 patients. The department's staff included physical therapists, occupational therapists, and nurses. To prove the problem, Dan collected data by patient code for the date of admission to rehabilitation and the date of discharge; he then calculated elapsed days. Additional data covered possible causes and included data for every category of possible cause that could be obtained through chart information or the patient questionnaire. He used check sheets for categoric variables so the data collector could check the appropriate column. Staff information included experience in the department and educational attainment.

Criteria to Prove the Problem

The problem indicators were average length of stay and percentage of patients above specified lengths of stay. Dan reviewed the literature and interviewed professional staff in several hospitals to identify the maximum acceptable stay of amputation patients in rehabilitation. The limits seemed to be no longer than 24 days for patients with no exacerbating conditions and no longer than 30 days for AP patients. The issue of whether these limits were appropriate for a municipal hospital that served poor and indigent patients remained to be resolved.

Dan suggested that the average stay be no more than 2 days over the limit, based on group limits of 30, 35, and 24 days, respectively, for the total, AP patients, and non-AP patients. He suggested that allowable limits be no more than 10% of patients above 30 days overall, above 35 days for AP patients, and above 24 days for non-AP patients.

The 24-day limit for non-AP patients was easily accepted by the clients, but they agreed on 35 days for AP patients only after heated debate. The 35 days acknowledged that the municipal hospital served patients "sicker" than even the general concept of AP allowed, because the poor and indigent arrived with a greater number of neglected and chronic health conditions that compromised their rehabilitation prognoses.

Results

The results were dramatic and exceeded the clients' expectations. As Table C4.1 indicates, 86.7% of AP patients were above the limit and 65.2% of non-AP patients were above their limit, with a total rate of 77.4% above the limit. Average days were 77 for AP patients, 38 for non-AP patients, with an overall average of 60 days. This meant that AP patients were 42 days and non-AP patients were 14 days above acceptable average days in rehabilitation, even with separate limits taking AP status into account. Although both groups far exceeded the limits, the situation was much worse for the "sicker" AP patients. The

Table C4.1 Criteria for Proof of Problem and Results: Amputation Patients ($N = 53$)

Measure	Point Beyond Which Problem Exists (Percentage, Rate, etc.)	OKed	Actual Results			Source
Percentage of patients over the limit[a]						
With AP	> 10.0	x	86.7%		Proved	Table 1.9
Without AP	> 10.0	x	65.2%		Proved	
Total	> 10.0	x	77.4%		Proved	
				Average		
Number of days average			Average	Days Over		
stay is over the limit			Days	Limit		Table 1.9
With AP	> 2 days	x	76.8	41.8	Proved	
Without AP	> 2 days	x	37.6	13.6	Proved	
Total	> 2 days	x	59.8	29.8	Proved	

NOTE: AP = anticipated problems.
a. Limits: AP, 35 days; without AP, 24 days; total, 30 days.

clients were taken aback by the magnitude of the problem, even though they were both aware that there was one.

Identifying Causes

Objective Cause Data

Most of the objective cause data were collected during the proof of problem period. Other cause data, such as the percentage of physical therapy appointments missed (the number missed as a percentage of the number the patient had been expected to attend), were collected near the time of a patient's release. Observational chart data included whether the patient knew how to care for the stump (also reflected in the questionnaire), whether the patient was compliant with stump self-care, whether the patient had medical complications due to the prosthesis, whether the prosthesis vendor delivered on time and correctly, and whether the prosthesis fit correctly. All the data were arranged in tables by patient code, according to length of stay.

Subjective Cause Data: Interviews and Questionnaires

Dan interviewed staff to determine which of three teaching practices were used with each patient in relation to five areas of patient education. The teaching techniques were (a) use of printed material as follow-up, (b) use of demonstration, and (c) asking the patient to demonstrate back after seeing the demonstration. The teaching categories were (a) teaching patients how to shape the stump, (b) self care, (c) use of the prosthesis (these three taught by physical therapists), (d) how to transfer to and from bed, chairs, and so on, and (e) how to use the upper body (these two taught by occupational therapists).

Dan designed a staff questionnaire to test knowledge and attitudes. Physical therapists and occupational therapists were asked to respond to nine statements, choosing true, false, or don't know or agree, disagree, or don't know. To assure cooperation, the responses were identified only by job title. Staff knowledge of how to care for amputee patients was tested with three statements. The correct answer is shown in parentheses.

1. When an amputation stump shrinks or expands there is little that can be done to adjust the stump to fit the prosthesis. (false)
2. Detecting skin breakdown is the job of nursing, and rehabilitation staff do not have to account for it. (false)
3. There is a danger that in asking the amputee for so much rehabilitation activity, skin breakdown occurs. (true)

Staff attitude towards the length of stay problem was examined with one statement, "Whether amputees stay a long or short time in rehabilitation is not really the concern of the therapist." Staff belief about the nature of the problem was covered by two statements:

The length of time an amputation patient stays in rehabilitation can reflect causes other than the patient's medical condition. (true)
The length of time an amputation patient stays in rehabilitation can reflect medical causes and the quality of care. (true)

Staff belief about the consequences of the problem had one statement, "When an amputation patient stays a long time in rehabilitation this can be harmful to the patient" (true). Whether staff felt accountable was covered by the statement, "As far as I know, I am not expected to be concerned about how long it takes for a patient to be able to leave rehabilitation." Lack of feedback on length of stay was covered by the statement, "I get no feedback on the length of time amputee patients in my care remain in rehabilitation."

Dan also investigated institutional causes, such as whether there was a policy on care of amputation stumps; whether there were standards in manuals on amputation care; whether performance on amputation care and length of stay was used for evaluations; and whether the documentation method or forms were too general about risk factors, poorly designed, or nonexistent.

Criteria to Prove the Causes

With 50 variables to contend with, Dan adopted model criteria for the types of variable involved. For *dichotomous variables*, the percentage of patients over the limit had to be much higher in one category than in the other as a first condition. Also, the *t* test for the difference between the two means had to be significant at least at the .05 level, or the coefficient of correlation had to be .4 or more and significant, and/or the variable had to be included in a stepwise multiple regression equation to explain length of stay.

For *multicategory variables*, the average days in rehabilitation had to be highest among a subgroup, and the subgroup's percentage share of days in rehabilitation had to be more than five percentage points above its share of patients (a disproportionate share). This was also applied to specific staff.

For *continuous variables* such as days between surgery and the start of rehabilitation or the rate of broken PT appointments, the coefficient of correlation had to be .4 or more and significant at least at .05, and/or the variable had to be included in a stepwise multiple regression equation.

For *language*, inadequate (NG) use of English had to be proved, and one or more languages had to predominate among patients with the longest stays but not among those with short stays. For *specific job title*, care-related causes associated with specific titles had to be proved. For *experience in the department* or *educational level*, the staff most associated with the problem had to have a different pattern from staff least associated with the problem.

For *subjective staff causes*, more than 30% of the staff had to answer inappropriately or "don't know" to specific relevant questions, and staff more associated with the problem (higher ranks) had to do worse than those less associated with the problem (lower ranks). For *subjective patient causes,* more than 30% of patients had to answer in a manner to confirm the cause, with higher percentages for ranks 27 to 44 than for ranks 1 to 18.

Other institutional causes required that the conditions they referred to be verified in interviews with management or examination of documents.

Results

Eleven risk factors related to the medical and socioeconomic conditions of the patients were proved. Six proved causes related to inadequate support, care, and education by the institution; 5 related to the prosthesis; and 2 were other institutional factors. In the list below, those with asterisks were further corroborated through statistical analysis.

Proved medical and socioeconomic risk factors

1. AP status*
2. Diabetes and/or depression components of AP status
3. Poor wound healing at the surgical site*
4. Bad nutritional status*
5. Being overweight
6. Having problems with the stump shape*
7. Age, especially over 61*
8. Having Medicare and either private or Medicaid insurance (which made the stay possible and reflects age)
9. Being single and, to a lesser extent, being widowed
10. Not having a permanent home
11. Living alone*

Proved causes related to inadequate support, care, and/or education by institution

12. Two specific staff: one PT and one OT
13. In teaching stump shaping, the PT did not use printed materials*
14. In teaching self-care, the PT did not use printed materials*
15. Patient's rate of broken PT appointments*

16. Patient did not know how to care for the stump
17. Patient noncompliance with stump self-care*

Proved causes related to the prosthesis

18. The prosthesis was painful when received
19. The patient had medical complications due to the prosthesis*
20. The prosthesis vendor did not deliver on time*
21. The prosthesis vendor delivered an incorrect prosthesis*
22. The prosthesis was ill fitting*

Other proved institutional causes

23. Performance on amputation care and length of stay was not used for evaluations
24. Documentation method or forms too general about length of stay risk factors

Table C4.2 presents the results of t test and simple correlational analysis for 14 variables that proved to be significant on one or both statistical tests or were significantly included in an explanatory stepwise regression equation. (Bear in mind that not all causes were tested this way.)

Stepwise multiple regression built an equation with a multiple r of .854, significant at .00005. The variables, in descending order of importance, were *medical complications from the prosthesis* (simple r = .626), *the rate of broken PT appointments* (simple r = .563), *AP status* (simple r = .497), the *number of people in the household* (inverse; simple r = −.285), and *trouble with the fit of the prosthesis* (simple r = .442). *Poor wound healing* was also highly correlated with the length of stay (simple r = .599), but it was also correlated with medical complications from the prosthesis, and washed out.

Solutions

The clients were pleased with the results, which bore out many of their expectations. They set only one feasibility limit: no major outlay of funds. Dan interviewed the staff he had consulted about possible

Table C4.2 Results of Statistical Analysis: Significant *t* Tests and Coefficients of Correlation for Days in Rehabilitation and Causes

Cause Category	Number of Patients	Mean Days	*t*-Test F Value	Probability Level	1- or 2-Tailed	Coefficient	1-Tail Significance	Comments
			t-Test Results			Correlations		
Medical complications from prosthesis								
Yes	13	102.77	2.13	< .00025	1	.626	.001	Higher with complications[a]
No	40	45.82						
Poor wound healing at surgical site								
Yes	19	91.16	2.85	< .00025	1	.599	.001	Higher with poor healing[b]
No	34	42.26						
Percentage rate of broken appointments	53					.563	.001	Direct
Anticipated Problems								
AP	30	76.83	1.25	< .00025	1	.497	.001	Higher with AP[c]
No AP	23	37.57						
Fit of the prosthesis								
NG	28	76.14	2.05	.0005	1	.442	.001	Higher with ill fit[c]
OK	25	41.48						
Problem with stump shape								
Yes	29	73.17	1.83	.003	1	.376	.01	Higher with problem
No	24	43.62						
Age	53					.320	.01	Direct
Doing stump care								
Yes	31	50.10	1.15	.016	1	.294	not	Higher without care
No	22	73.45						

(continued)

Table C4.2 Continued

Cause Category	Number of Patients	t-Test Results				Correlations		Comments
		Mean Days	t-Test F Value	Probability Level	1- or 2- Tailed	Coefficient	1-Tail Significance	
Vendor delivery								
On time	36	52.03						
Late	17	76.23	1.01	.018	1	.289	not	Higher if late
Nutritional status								
OK	40	53.42						
NG	13	79.38	1.70	.019	1	.285	not	Higher if NG
Number of people in household	53					−.285	not	Inverse[d]
PT used written materials to teach stump shaping								
Yes	14	41.43						
No	39	66.38	1.21	.041	2	.281	not	Higher without materials
PT used written materials to teach self-care								
Yes	8	35.25						
No	45	64.16	1.29	.056	2	.264	not	Higher without materials
Vendor: RX								
Correct	40	54.12						
Incorrect	13	77.23	1.48	.033	1	.254	not	Higher with incorrect

NOTES: The F value is the ratio of the variences of the two samples. AP = anticipated problems; NG = not good.
a. This variable entered into stepwise multiple regression on days in rehab at the .00001 significance level.
b. This variable did not enter the stepwise multiple regression on days in rehab because it correlates at .488 with medical complications from prosthesis.
c. This variable entered into stepwise multiple regression on days in rehab at the .002 significance level.
d. This variable entered into stepwise multiple regression on days in rehab at the .007 significance level.

causes, explaining those that had been proved, and asked for suggestions. He went back to the literature and also considered his own ideas. The final list of solutions was approved by the staff he had been interviewing.

Dan grouped his solutions to reflect the clustered causes. To deal with *medical and socioeconomic risk factors*, he suggested that management review and change the criteria by which the department decides which patients are ready to be admitted to rehabilitation, including standards for patient stability. His point was that the department was admitting patients before they were stable enough to benefit from rehabilitation (perhaps reflecting pressures from prospective payment arrangements); this added to the stay and to the exaggerated AP status. To deal with this, he suggested having routine consultations done by appropriate medical specialists to deal with diabetes, depression, and other serious conditions. He also recommended that the hospital universally use glucometers to measure blood sugar levels instead of the old method (paper strips) still in evidence.

Dan proposed that bedside physical therapy be resumed for recent amputees being considered for transfer to rehabilitation because bedside care is an alternative to broken appointments for seriously ill patients. He noted that, now that risk factors were identified, there should be a way to flag patients at risk upon their entry to rehabilitation, and he asked that management design a preventive program for patients at risk.

Dan asked that a reevaluation of the nursing care of stumps be done under the direction of the head nurse and that regular inservice training on the care of amputees be instituted that would highlight recent developments. Dan proposed that the department use stump shrinkers instead of bandages for all amputee patients. He suggested a consultation upon admission with registered dieticians to deal with nutrition and overweight; he asked for regular consults with the staff psychiatrist and regular counseling supplied by counselors with a gerontology background.

Dan suggested that professional staff develop written materials for physical therapists to use with patients on the shaping of the stump and self-care and that patients' knowledge of self-care be assessed and reviewed periodically and raised in counseling sessions. To assist, Dan recommended that patient information be interlinked to permit counselors and psychiatrists to access self-care documentation. He suggested that staff's evaluations include their patients' self-care and length of stay. Dan also suggested greater involvement of social services, such as an admission interview to evaluate a patient's community support and social needs and to aid in establishing a support network.

To deal with *prosthesis vendors*, Dan proposed that the patient be attended by a physical therapist when the prosthesis was delivered, that the prosthesis should be tried out immediately, and that pain should be treated as a serious indicator, so that an ill-fitting or painful device would be rejected unless the problem could be cared for on the spot.

Dan suggested that the hospital make timely, correct delivery and rapid correction of painful or ill-fitting devices the basis for continued patronage of vendors, and that this be specified in the vendor contract. This would mean keeping records on these criteria for each vendor and reviewing them every few months. New vendors would be given 4-month trial periods.

In 1997, a JCAHO manual example from physical rehabilitation indicated that consideration should be given to patient satisfaction with the orthotic or prosthetic devices relative to fit and function. In this case, Dan was requiring immediate evaluation of the prosthesis as a form of prevention.

Implementing Solutions and Making Them Operational

By the time of his report, Dan had already influenced management to put vendors on notice with regard to their poor provision of service. The rest remained to be done at the time Dan left for a supervisory position elsewhere.

Note

1. Alexander S. Kagan was the internal consultant for this project.

Incomplete Laboratory
Referrals in an HMO Center[1]

In this case, the problem was missing information in the orders for patients' laboratory tests, but adherence to a current referral form proved to be an obstacle to improvement.

Proving the Problem

The Problem

Edna was the supervisor of a laboratory center in a health maintenance organization (HMO). When a physician required laboratory tests, referral forms were filled out; the patient took them to the laboratory center, where staff drew blood or took other specimens and sent them to a clinical laboratory for testing. Edna was concerned that the referrals were sometimes too incomplete for staff to be able to proceed with specimen taking.

The Client

Edna initiated the quality improvement project on her own authority, seeking approval from senior management. The clients were the center administrator and the regional administrator of the HMO. Edna took on the project because it dealt with a long-standing problem that never seemed to be resolved. Edna suggested to both administrators that she might be able to come up with successful solutions and got permission to go ahead with the project.

Importance

Many laboratory tests ordered for patients are urgent; some are related to imminent surgery. Thus there is concern when laboratory referrals arrive without enough information for them to be processed. However, Edna had to establish a link between incomplete referrals and consequences; she had to show that some types of omissions resulted in unacceptable delays in the laboratory work, and this became part of her project.

Relevant Steps

When a patient saw a physician, paperwork for laboratory tests began with a referral form. The HMO used a standardized official form, but some offices had been using an older, no longer official form that provided more details about the test being ordered, including whether the patient needed to fast before the specimen was taken. Referral forms were partly filled out in the clinician's office. The patient was then asked to take the referral to Reception, where a receptionist or medical assistant completed the information and prepared a specimen label by hand or had one generated by computer. The computer-generated label was a source of information for the laboratory if the referral form lacked identification data also called for on the label.

Patients were expected to bring the referral form and label to the laboratory when they came to have specimens taken. The patient could arrive at the laboratory later than the day the referral was filled out, depending on the reasons for the tests and the dates for further procedures. Edna's concern was with unnecessary delays once the patient arrived at the laboratory.

The information that the laboratory needed in order to proceed included the patient's full name, ID number, the tests ordered, the requesting physician's name, and for tests with fasting options, whether they required prior fasting. Although most data could be filled in by anyone in the office, only the physician could decide on the test and whether prior fasting was required.

Observation Units, Normal Loads, Quantities, and Time Frame

The laboratory center handled about 75 referrals per day, with patients arriving from 23 offices 5½ days each week. The unit of observation was the referral form that reached the central laboratory.

Operational Definitions

Because Edna had to identify whether there were delay consequences, she needed an operational definition of delay. She defined delay as the number of days between the day the patient arrived at the laboratory and the day the specimen was actually collected. Even if there were missing items, if the specimen was collected the same day, the delay was treated as zero, because the consequence to the patient was the overriding concern. If there was a delay, the total days of waiting included days during which the laboratory was closed.

Cases arose of patients with missing information not returning to the laboratory during the period in which the project was conducted. Total days of delay for such patients was defined as the most days accounted for during the data collection period of the project, 27 days; this did not account for the likelihood that the patient would not return at all. Therefore, total days of delay were underestimated. A separate count was made of patients who had not returned by the end of the data collection period to provide a sense of the magnitude of this consequence.

Final List of Possible Causes

In deciding on the possible causes, Edna was unable to find much information in the literature, but staff were enthusiastic and had several good ideas. The final list contained 21 possible causes.

Related to the institution

1. Any specific missing items on the referral form that produced delays

2. Any medical specialty associated with missing information
3. Any medical specialty associated with delays due to missing information
4. The official referral form did not ask for fasting orders
5. No defined policy on who fills out specific items of information
6. Performance on completion of referral information not used for evaluation
7. Supervisors do not hold staff accountable for complete referral forms
8. Lack of feedback on incomplete referrals
9. Patients are not told to go to Reception for additional referral form information
10. Patients do not go to Reception to have the referral form completed
11. Lack of use of the computer to generate the patients' labels

Related to staff

12. Specific physicians by office associated with delays
13. Specific office job titles associated with missing items
14. Perception that there is no policy on who fills out the referral form
15. Years of experience with the HMO
16. Knowledge of the importance and consequences of incomplete referrals
17. Attitude toward the problem is "It's not my job"
18. Attitude toward the problem is "It is not important because someone else will do it"
19. Attitude toward the problem is "I am too busy"
20. Attitude toward the problem is "This is a fair trade-off for other things that have to be done"
21. Staff do not feel accountable

Research Design

Edna's database was a 100% sample of all referrals brought to the center during 3 representative days. The 175 referrals that were collected represented 15 of the 23 offices, each identified by an assigned project code. Referral data included an assigned patient project code, the date of arrival at the laboratory center, and the coded ID number of the office. The office, once known, identified the physician and the medical assistant and/or receptionist. If any of the patients were delayed due to omissions in the referrals, the date the patient returned was recorded; 27 days was assigned if patients had still not returned when data collection ended. Additional data were collected in interviews with patients and management and in telephone interviews with physicians and staff.

Data Collection Instruments

The basic data were arranged by office and project codes. Data on causes included the medical specialty of the office, years of experience in the HMO for staff, and job title. Tables showed the presence or absence of information for each of the six items that were required for the procedure to go forward (first name, family name, patient ID, tests ordered, referring physician, and fasting orders if relevant). There were check-off columns to show whether the label issued was computer generated, whether the referral form was the official one (without an item on fasting orders) or the unofficial one (which had a place for fasting orders), whether there was any delay, and if so, when the laboratory work was done and the number of days of delay.

Tests were identified as those for which fasting orders might be required or those for which fasting orders were not required, so that tests that did require such orders became a subset of the larger group. There were 95 referrals for which fasting orders were relevant, 54% of the 175 referrals in the sample.

The summary data gave totals and subtotals by office, by whether the tests needed fasting orders, by whether the label was computer generated, and by type of referral form. There was summary data on the percentage of referrals with any of the six items missing, on missing items as a percent of the total, and on the percent with delays that had missing fasting orders.

Criteria to Prove the Problem

The criteria to prove the problem and its extent covered both missing items and delays. Table C5.1 shows the indicators and criteria, including the percentage of tests with essential items missing from the referral forms, the amount of delay caused by the missing items, specific information about tests that might require fasting, average days of delay, and the percentage of patients who did not return by the 27th day. There were 13 indicators with various criteria agreed to by the clients.

Table C5.1 Criteria for Proof of Problem and Results: Missing Referral Data

Measure	Point Beyond Which Problem Exists (Percentage, Rate, etc.)	OKed	Actual Results		Source
Percentage with any of the six essential items of information missing	> 5.00%	x	32.0%	Proved	Table 1.1
Percentage missing by item					
First name	> 4.00%	x	4.6%	Proved	
Family name	> 3.00%	x	4.6%	Proved	
Patient's ID number	> 3.00%	x	8.6%	Proved	
Tests ordered	> 3.00%	x	1.1%	Not proved	
Ordering MD's name	> 3.00%	x	4.0%	Proved	
Missing fasting orders as percentage of tests that require fasting	> 3.00%	x	50.0%	Proved	
Those with delay as percentage of those with any missing items[a]	> 3.00%	x	44.6%	Proved	Table 1.3
Average days of delay[a]					Table 1.3
Average of 175	> 0.02 days	x	2.2 days	Proved	
Average of total with missing items	> 0.22 days	x	6.8 days	Proved	
Average of those with delays	> 2.00 days	x	15.3 days	Proved	
Patients who did not return by October 24[a]					Table 1.3
As percentage of those with delays	> 1.00%	x	44.0%	Proved	
As percentage of those with missing items	> 0.01%	x	19.6%	Proved	

NOTE: Table shows 100% of sample of 175 referrals over 3 days.

a. A delay is counted in days: 0 if test was done on the same day, calculated as date when done minus date patient arrived for the work. Average days of delay is total number of days of delay divided by 175, or divided by the number who had delays, or divided by the number with any missing items. Total days of delay was approximated for referrals where the patient did not return. In such cases, the figure assigned is 27, accounting for the maximum number of days of data collection but not counting the likelihood that after such a delay the patient will not return.

Results

As Table C5.1 indicates, all the criteria to prove the problem except one were exceeded. Only 1% were missing the name of the test. The highest missing rate was for fasting orders, at 50% of tests that required such orders; 44.6% of referrals with missing items had delays, and these were all referrals with missing fasting orders. The average delay for patients with delays was over 15 days, and 44% of these patients did not return during the project. This established both the problem and its importance. The clients were convinced.

Identifying Causes

Objective Cause Data

Edna had already collected a good deal of the data on causes during the proof of problem phase. She now developed analysis tables and prepared to collect additional objective cause data. She ranked physicians and staff by their involvement with delays and missing data based on information already collected. Nonphysician staff ranks were calculated from data summarized by office. For each, (a) the percentage share of total referrals (indicating importance in the sample) and (b) the rate of missing items were calculated, excluding items that only physicians could supply. Disproportionate share by office was also calculated as (c) the percentage share of referrals subtracted from the percentage share of missing items. A positive number indicated a disproportionate share of the problem. A final rank was obtained by adding the ranks for each of the three factors and ranking the final sums. The lowest sum was rank 1; equal sums were assigned equal ranks.

Ranks for physicians were also calculated by office, but based on six variables. These included (a) percentage of total referrals, (b) percentage of total days delay, (c) percentage of total days delay minus percentage of total referrals, (d) rate of missing fasting orders, (e) rate of delay, and (f) percentage of fasting orders. The ranks were summed and given a final rank. In this calculation, all offices with no fasting tests were combined into one group, all of whom received the rank of 1, because only fasting tests had delays.

Subjective Cause Data: Interviews and Questionnaires

To determine if there were policies on whether the physician, medical assistant, or receptionist should fill out the referral form and whether supervisors hold staff accountable for complete referrals, Edna arranged telephone interviews with office personnel and physicians.

She asked the respondent, "Do you know whether there are any items on the referrals that *must* be filled in? Which are they?" and "Who does it?" She created tables on which she could check the title responsible for filling out the referral, including "no one," which was the response selected by each office. Edna also asked how the supervisor handled incomplete laboratory referrals, with places for her to check who was told, whether a report was sent, whether nothing was done, or something else. All the offices chose "nothing is done."

Edna interviewed management to investigate whether there was a policy on who fills in specific items on the referral and how many items must be done. There was no policy. She also learned that incomplete referrals were not dealt with in staff evaluations.

The research design also called for patient interviews to determine whether patients with incomplete referrals were told to go to Reception for additional information by office staff and whether patients actually went to Reception to have the referral forms completed. Four offices were chosen as sites: two with the worst delay records (highest ranks) were chosen and two with the next to lowest ranks. (Ranks 2 and 3 were used because rank 1 included offices that had no need for information on fasting orders). Edna went to each office to interview five patients with incomplete referrals as they left the physician, to see if they were being sent to the receptionist to complete the form and to see if they actually went to Reception.

Question 1 was designed to make sure that the patient had a referral form for a laboratory test: "Do you have a form you need to take for a laboratory test?" Question 2 was used to select only patients with forms that were incomplete at this point. "May I see the form?" If the form was complete, Edna would go on to another patient. If it was incomplete, Edna asked, "Were you asked to go anywhere to have this form completed?" The answer could be yes, no, or don't know. If the patient said yes, Edna asked question 4: "Where?" and noted if the answer was Reception. If that answer was yes, Edna asked Question 5: "Where will you go now?" and noted if Reception was named.

Edna designed a structured telephone interview to test causes such as staff knowledge and attitudes. It is presented in Figure C5.1. The opening statement explains the purpose of the interview and assures the confidentiality of the information. Nine questions covered possible

Phone or face-to-face interview: "I am doing a study of the way we deal with lab test referrals. The information I am collecting is designed to get people's opinions about the referral form information items. The data will be confidential; no names will be used. May I ask you a few questions?"

Office Code ____ *MD ( ) Receptionist ( ) Medical Assistant ( )*

	Agree	Disagree	Don't Know
1. It is not important to get all the information on the lab referral form while the patient is in the office because it can be picked up at a later stage.	( )	( )	( )
2. It is not my job to make sure all the information on the lab referral is filled out.	( )	( )	( )
3. If information on name, patient ID, ordering physician, tests, and fasting status are missing from the referral form, unwanted delays in testing can occur.	( )	( )	( )
4. I am not asked to account for the amount of information filled out on the lab referral forms I deal with.	( )	( )	( )
5. It is not important to write on the lab referral whether fasting is required before coming to the lab because someone will tell the patient.	( )	( )	( )
6. I am too busy to make sure all the information on the lab referral is filled out.	( )	( )	( )
7. Considering how busy this office is, not filling in all the lab referral information is a fair trade-off on doing other things.	( )	( )	( )
8. I get no information on whether our lab referral forms have missing information.	( )	( )	( )
9. I think that all offices should generate labels using the computer to assure that the lab gets the information it needs.	( )	( )	( )
10. I think that all referral forms should have a place to indicate whether a test requires fasting.	( )	( )	( )

(MD only)

	Agree	Disagree	Don't Know
11. If there were a referral form that allowed me to check off all tests ordered and whether fasting is required, I would be sure to fill it out.	( )	( )	( )

(Receptionist or medical assistant only)

	Agree	Disagree	Don't Know
12. If there were a list of tests showing which ones require fasting, I would be sure the information was on the referral form.	( )	( )	( )

Figure C5.1 Office Interview

causes. The 10th asked if all referral forms should have a place to indicate fasting orders. Question 11, asked only of physicians, asked for a response to the possible solution of there being a place on the referral form to check off tests ordered and whether fasting is required. Question 12, a parallel question, asked receptionists and medical assistants whether they would be willing to check that fasting information was entered on the referral form.

Criteria to Prove the Causes

With 21 variables to account for, Edna was able to use some models, but several criteria had to be tailor-made. For *any specific missing items* on the referral form producing delays, the missing rate for the item had to be greater than the overall rate and the item had to account for a major portion of referrals with delays. For any *medical specialty associated with missing information* and any *medical specialty associated with delays due to missing information*, the specialty had to be associated with the three highest-ranked offices based on missing information and with missing fasting orders, respectively, and could not be associated with the 3 lowest-ranked offices.

For *official referral form did not call for information on fasting orders*, the missing and delay rates for fasting orders had to be more than 10% higher for the official form. For *no defined policy on who fills out specific items*, institutional sources had to give no evidence on who should fill items out, and the item had to be a problem. For *perception that there is no policy on who fills out the referral form*, the response to the relevant question had to be that there was no such policy, but there would also have to be such a policy actually in existence.

For *performance on completion of referral information not used for evaluation*, the situation had to be verified through management sources. For *supervisors do not hold staff accountable for complete referrals*, the responses to the survey had to show that the 5 highest-ranked offices selected the relevant survey answer; for *lack of feedback on incomplete referrals*, physician and staff responses to the survey had to support the view, and the situation had to be shown to be true.

For *patients are not told to go to reception for additional referral form information* and *patients do not go to reception to have the referral form com-*

pleted, at least 20% of the patients with missing information who were interviewed had to have responded to support the causes, and this had to be higher for patients from higher-ranked offices.

For *the use of handwritten rather than computer-generated labels*, hand-written labels had to be associated with a higher rate of missing items, have a higher share of missing items than share of referrals, and account for at least 15% of referrals. (All the offices had the computers needed to generate labels.)

Specific physicians or offices associated with delays had to be among the 5 highest for the items on which they were ranked. *Specific office or job titles* had to be among the 3 highest for the items on which they were ranked, and the same job title had to appear for each, specifically, receptionist or medical assistant. For *years of experience with the HMO*, the pattern had to be similar for higher-ranked staff or physicians and not be present for lower ranks.

For *knowledge of the importance and consequences of incomplete referrals, attitude toward the problem is "It's not my job," "It is not important because someone else will do it," "I am too busy," "This is a fair trade-off for other things that have to be done,"* or *staff do not feel accountable*, more than 30% of respondents to the questionnaire had to answer the relevant one or two questions to support the attitude or knowledge, and the percentage had to be higher for staff in high-ranking offices.

Results

Only the referrals missing fasting orders resulted in delays, so Edna was interested in whether the official referral form, which did not call for information on fasting orders, made a difference. What complicated the situation was the fact that the medical director himself had designed the official form. Edna compared the rate of missing fasting orders for the two types of forms. For the official form, the rate of missed fasting orders was 68.8%; for the unofficial form, it was 11.1%.

Edna considered the use of computer-generated labels because they were a source of information that could provide data missing on the referral form.

Handwritten labels had higher rates and strongly disproportionate shares of missing items; they accounted for 17 percent of the referrals but up to 88 percent of missing items.

The results of the patient questionnaire showed a clear pattern. Not being asked to go to Reception and not going to Reception appeared with patients from offices with high ranks, except for one patient. Lower ranked offices had much higher rates of patients being asked to go to Reception and going than higher ranked offices.

Of the 21 possible causes investigated, 13 were proved or partly proved:

Related to the institution

1. Fasting orders produced delays
2. Internal medicine was associated with delays due to missing information
3. Internal medicine was partly associated with missing information
4. The official referral form did not ask for fasting orders
5. No defined policy on who fills out specific items of information
6. Performance on completion of referral forms is not used for evaluation
7. Supervisors do not hold staff accountable for completed referral forms
8. Lack of feedback on incomplete referrals for physicians
9. Patients are not told to go to Reception for additional referral form information
10. Patients do not go to Reception to have the referral form completed
11. Lack of use of the computer to generate the patients' labels

Related to staff

12. Three specific physicians by office were associated with delays
13. The receptionist job title was associated with missing items

The results pointed to *institutional causes* as the main source of the problems. Even though two proved causes related to staff, institutional issues were implicated: three specific offices and their physicians had the worst records for MD-generated information; they were associated with internal medicine and fasting orders. The job title linked with missing items was the receptionist, a title associated with offices of internal medicine.

Solutions

Feasibility Limits

The clients were convinced about the results and looked forward to the solutions. The feasibility limits they set were: no additional costs except for one-time costs and no additional staff.

Choice of Solutions

The same staff members Edna had interviewed on possible causes had interesting ideas about solutions. Edna incorporated some, and after getting their approval for her final list, Edna prepared a report that opened with this general statement:

> In studying the completeness of laboratory referral forms sent by participating offices, 15 offices were found to have sent referrals during the research period. Five specific items were associated with unacceptable rates of missing information; but only one item, whether fasting is required prior to the test, was found to be responsible for delays in processing, including patients not showing up again to have specimens taken.

Some of the proposals required policy changes. For example, Edna was adamant that, unless management agreed to the one-time cost of redesigning the referral forms, the problem of delays could not be solved. She noted that, when asked whether all referral forms should have a place to indicate whether a test requires fasting, 100% of all physicians and office staff in the 15 offices agreed that they should. She also showed that an unofficial form that asked for fasting had much lower rates of missing items and delays.

Edna suggested that the new form should be preprinted with the names of the most common tests, plus additional spaces to write in other tests, and should have a place to indicate whether fasting was required. Edna recommended that there be a policy on who fills in the fasting section. Preferably, this should be the physician, who would fill it in when selecting the tests. Alternatively, receptionists and medical assistants could be given a list of tests showing which generally require fasting or could check the physicians' completeness.

Edna supported this proposal by indicating that, when physicians were asked whether they would fill out such a form, 87% answered that they would, including 83% of those with the most problems on this item. When receptionists and medical assistants were asked whether, if they had a list of fasting tests they would be sure the information was on the form, 94% said they would, including 100% from the offices and the title with the most problems on this item.

Edna suggested that the laboratory center should send memos to the ordering physician when patients were delayed by lack of fasting orders, noting that there was feedback to staff but little to physicians. A form could be prepared for this purpose.

Other suggestions included the need for management to make clear in writing who is to fill out the items on the referral forms. She suggested that physicians should be asked to account for their own names, the tests, and whether fasting was required. Office staff should be asked to check for completeness and fill in patient information such as names and patients' IDs. They should also make sure patients know where to go upon leaving the physician, such as to Reception. Edna suggested that management require that the computer be used to generate patient labels, that offices have signs in appropriate languages telling patients what to do, where to go, explaining fasting (especially important), and telling how to get to Reception for completion of information. For patients judged to be confused, Edna suggested that escorts be provided.

Edna recommended that inservice training be designed for physicians and staff without singling out anyone for blame but that offices of internal medicine should be made to understand that the problems arise more frequently there because the nature of the specialty calls for fasting tests. The training would include the effects on patients when they are delayed due to information gaps and what happens, such as in the operating room, as a result. It would cover use of the new forms, who does what, sending patients to Reception, use of computer-generated labels, patient instruction sheets, and feedback procedures. Edna also recommended that both physicians and office staff be held to account for the completeness of their referrals, once responsibilities were made clear, and that evaluations should include this aspect of the work.

Implementing Solutions and
Making Them Operational

The staff had been very enthusiastic about the project and support-ive of the solutions. However, once the final report was presented, very little was done to implement the solutions. Edna was able to influence the design of pre-entered laboratory labels, which now automatically include all the patient ID information needed for the referrals, but the old official referral form without fasting orders is still in use. Edna was given a promotion that took her away from the problems of patient delays, and her voice is now silent about the issue. This is sad, because it is not likely that HMO "report cards" will deal with this. The use of indicators to assess HMO performance is associated with broader issues than those involved here.

Note

1. The internal consultant for this project wishes to remain anonymous.

Case 6

HMO Patients' Problems With Crutches and Canes[1]

In this case, process errors produced at one stage of treatment were noticed at a later stage. The case is unusual because the internal consultant worked at an occupational level not usually associated with the role of the internal consultant.

Proving the Problem

The Problem and the Client

Fran worked as a physical therapy assistant in an HMO group that had nine ambulatory care facilities, of which four provided physical therapy services. Fran was concerned about the assistive devices already in use by patients when they appeared for their first physical therapy visit as ambulatory patients. She believed that crutches and canes were often too high or too low and that canes were being used on the same side as the affected limb, rather than on the opposite side. The physical therapy administrator and the director of nursing (the clients) readily agreed to the project when it was proposed.

Importance

Fran was concerned because patients with incorrectly adjusted devices reported pain and other discomfort in parts of their bodies other than those referred for physical therapy treatment, apparently the result of incorrect adjustment or use of the devices. She believed that this could add to the length of treatments and the number of treatments needed.

The clients agreed on the importance of the problem. Crutches that are too high press against the armpit and push the shoulder upward as the patient walks, sometimes resulting in shoulder pain, weakness, numbness, and tingling sensations in the arms due to injury to nerves in the axilla. Eventual arm paralysis can result if this continues. The proper gait with crutches is a "swing-to-gait," which cannot be done with crutches that are too high. Hopping on the good leg, which is the remaining alternative, can result in hip pain, adding to the disability. Crutches that are too low force the patient to bend while walking, with armpits resting on top of the crutches for the swing-to-gait. This also causes pressure on the nerves in the axilla, with similar consequences. Another consequence may be loss of balance and falls, also possibly adding to the disability.

Canes that are too high or too low result in shoulder fatigue, but the major problem with canes is that, when they are used on the same side as the disabled lower extremity, patients have less endurance for walking, increased pain in the disabled leg, and hip pain where there was no pain before.

Relevant Steps

Patients first went to receive their assistive devices from a nursing department in one of the four equipped HMO centers, where they were fitted and instructed in their use. The patients could be seen by nurses, medical assistants, or a physical therapist, depending on the center.

Patients using *axillary crutches* were usually referred for their first physical therapy treatment from 6 to 8 weeks after the initial adjustment of the crutches. Patients using *canes* were usually referred for their first physical therapy treatment from 2 to 3 weeks after the cane length was selected and the patient was shown how to use the cane.

Operational Definitions

Fran's operational definitions for incorrect height of crutches or use of a cane and for experience of pain were tested as follows: Fran's judgments were matched in a field test of five patients against her supervisor's judgments. They were in close agreement without knowing each other's "calls" on these variables.

Final List of Possible Causes

Fran examined only three possible causes:

1. The location (center)
2. The staff, by job title, doing the fitting
3. The education of the staff on how to adjust or fit the assistive devices and teach patients how to use them

Research Design and Data Collection

The design for the study was for Fran to observe and follow patients with ambulatory devices who arrived for their first physical therapy treatment at her center. At the first visit, Fran judged whether a patient was properly or improperly fitted or adjusted, and she continued to collect data at each visit until the patient was discharged. The database included 61 patients who arrived during the test period. Each patient with crutches or a cane was asked:

> When you got your crutches (cane), at what location did you get it?" (The four locations were named, accounting for one of the possible causes.)
> When your device was given to you, who taught you how to use it? (The three job titles were named, accounting for the second cause category.)

At each subsequent visit, each patient was asked:

> Do you have pain/numbness or tingling in your hip (shoulder, arms)? (Yes or no.)

Symptoms were followed at each visit by the question:

> How much pain or numbness or tingling sensation do you still have? (The responses were "a lot"; "a moderate amount," "a slight amount," or "none at all.")

Data on the length of each visit and the number of visits until discharge were also collected. To obtain comparative data on the length and number of treatments, Fran matched patients with incorrect fit or adjustment with patients appropriately fitted or adjusted, as soon as an appropriate partner arrived in the study. Fran matched subjects by sex, age, nature of the disability, body weight, required gait, and type of ambulatory device. Given the constraints of time and the number of variables required for matching, only eight pairs were obtained: Five pairs were men with crutches, and three pairs were women with canes.

Criteria to Prove the Problem

Fran had 17 indicators and proof-of-problem criteria. Table C6.1 presents the indicators, criteria, and results. Fran had to prove that more than 5% of patients arrived at their first physical therapy treatment with crutches too high; no more than 5% with crutches too low; no more than 10% was allowed for incorrect use of canes.

To prove the outcome effect of the incorrect fit or use, Fran had to show that at least 10% of patients in each category of incorrect crutch fit or use of a cane reported symptoms that were not part of their original referrals. She also had to show that no more than 2% of patients correctly fitted with crutches or canes reported such symptoms. Fran had to show that, among matched pairs, those with improper fit of crutches or use of canes and symptoms would average at least two more treatments or 8 or more minutes per treatment than those with correctly fitted crutches or correct use of canes.

Results

As Table C6.1 indicates, Fran proved 14 of her 17 criteria. Of the 61 patients who arrived with ambulatory devices, 59% were incorrectly fitted or using the devices incorrectly. It was worst for use of crutches, with 61.8% of the 34 in the category incorrect: 41.2% were too high, and 20.6% were too low. Among 27 cane users, 55.6% were using them on the wrong side.

Symptoms not part of the original referrals were reported by 33.3% of patients with improper fit or use; crutches that were too high had a

Table C6.1 Criteria for Proof of Problem and Results: Patients With Ambulatory Devices on Initial Visit for Physical Therapy

Measure	Point Beyond Which Problem Exists (Percentage, Rate, etc.)	OKed	Actual Results	Source
Percent of patients with incorrect fit or use, by category				Table 1.1
Crutches too high	> 5%	x	41.2%	Proved
Crutches too low	> 5%	x	20.6%	Proved
Total crutches (34)	> 10%	x	61.8%	Proved
Cane use (27)	> 10%	x	55.6%	Proved
Total (61)	> 10%	x	59.0%	Proved
Percent of patients with incorrect fit or use reporting symptoms not part of original referral by category				
Crutches too high	> 10%	x	42.9%	Proved
Crutches too low	> 10%	x	14.3%	Proved
Total crutches (21)	> 10%	x	33.3%	Proved
Cane use (15)	> 10%	x	33.3%	Proved
Total (36)	> 10%	x	33.3%	Proved
Percent of patients with correct fit or use reporting symptoms not part of original referral by category				
Total crutches (13)	< 2%	x	0.0%	Proved
Total canes (12)	< 2%	x	0.0%	Proved
Total (25)	< 2%	x	0.0%	Proved
Average additional treatments or minutes in treatment for patients with incorrect crutch or cane adjustment and new symptoms, compared with patients with correct crutch or cane adjustments and without new symptoms				
	Averages		Averages	Table 1.2
Improper crutch fit and symptoms (5) compared	> 2 more treatments	x	Treatments +3	Proved
with proper crutch fit and no symptoms	> 8 more minutes per treatment	x	Minutes +3	Not proved
Improper cane use and symptoms (3) compared	> 2 more treatments	x	Treatments +2	Not proved
with proper cane use and no symptoms	> 8 more minutes per treatment	x	Minutes +1	Not proved

rate of 42.9%; those fitted too low had 14.3%. No patients with correct adjustments had additional symptoms. The symptoms added an average of three treatments for crutch users with symptoms.

The three criteria that were not proved were additional treatments for cane users with symptoms and additional minutes of average treatment time for crutch and cane users with symptoms.

Identifying Causes

Research Design

The clients were impressed with the results and agreed that a problem did indeed exist. Now Fran was ready to examine her three possible causes: center location, job title, and education of the staff related to fitting the devices. The work on the first two of the causes was to analyze the data already collected by arraying them by problem, location, and job title. All that still remained after that was to identify whether, where, and how each staff member was trained to fit the devices.

Criteria to Prove the
Causes and Results

The criteria to prove the causes were simply that the problem data be more associated with one or more of the locations, job title categories, or a lack of training. This meant higher error rates and a substantial and disproportionate share of errors.

The first two causes were found to be related to the third. In the one location where only physical therapists did the adjusting, there were no errors, but the physical therapist accounted for only 8% of the total. In the two locations that used medical assistants, the error rate was 100%, as it was for the job title (medical assistants were 43% of the total). In the location where medical assistants and nurses both did the work, the error rate was 47%; the nurses' error rate was 33%.

Proper education explained the physical therapy rate; lack of any education on the subject explained the medical assistants' error rate. It turned out that nurses were also not trained to fit the devices and instruct patients in their use, but at the center with mixed staff, there was a nurse who had learned how to do the work from an orthopedist with whom she had worked. She accounted for the 20 correct fits out of the total of 38 at that center.

Solutions

Fran had severe feasibility limits on any solution she might suggest. She could not ask that physical therapists do the fitting and instruction or that patients go only to centers with adequately trained staff; the feasibility limits prohibited additional workloads for physical therapists and the addition of any staff and required that all four centers must continue to fit and instruct.

Fran asked that the HMO provide inservice training to all staff who fit patients and instruct them in the use of ambulatory devices. The cost of training would be made up in fewer treatments and decreased symptoms.

Implementing Solutions and Making Them Operational

The director of nursing said that she would fund the training as part of her in-service budget for nurses and medical assistants. The physical therapy administrator said that he was willing to provide the training. By the end of the project, there was agreement that the solution would be implemented.

Fran demonstrated that, with the use of proper research and communications skills, staff in lower levels of the organizational hierarchy can make positive contributions to improved patient care. She had been able to bring attention to an aspect of patient care too minute to be picked up by the broader standards of accreditation review but which connected importantly with staff training, patient satisfaction, outcomes, and cost.

Note

1. The internal consultant for this project wishes to remain anonymous.

Case 7

Dealing With Hemolyzed Blood Samples
in a Hospital Laboratory[1]

In this case, the internal consultant found a set of nested problems. The original problem was thought to be too many hemolyzed blood specimens sent to the laboratory, but it eventually appeared that there was also a problem with the way the laboratory itself dealt with and reported hemolyzed specimens.

Proving the Problem

The Problem

Gwen was an assistant section manager in a special chemistry laboratory of a proprietary hospital. As part of the organization's increasing interest in quality improvement, Gwen was asked to study the incidence of hemolyzed blood specimens reaching the laboratory for testing. When a blood sample is taken for testing, it can become *hemolyzed*: The red blood cells can be broken, and hemoglobin (iron-containing pigment) is released into the serum (fluid part of the blood). The serum appears red instead of its normal yellow color. The client wanted Gwen to investigate whether there was too high a rate of hemolyzed blood specimens reaching the laboratory for testing.

Importance

When specimens are hemolyzed, they may create falsely elevated test results. If a laboratory has no choice but to use such a hemolyzed specimen, it is expected that it will comment on this in its report and indicate the degree of hemolysis (slight, moderate, or gross), as tests vary in their degree of sensitivity to hemolysis. The physician cannot understand the test results without being warned about the hemolysis.

If a specimen is too hemolyzed, the test should be cancelled and the specimen redrawn. This adds to the cost of the test, delays the results, inconveniences the patient, and poses an added risk of accidental needle pricks to staff; there is the temptation to run the test regardless of the degree of hemolysis. If the test is not cancelled, it is important to mention the hemolysis in the laboratory report.

The Client

The client, the director of the laboratory, asked Gwen to conduct the study. However, because the problem involved the quality of blood specimens sent to the laboratory, the quality assurance manager was also involved as a client.

Relevant Steps

Data collection was to start in the units where the blood was drawn because, to find the causes, Gwen needed to know when each blood specimen was drawn and the technique used, such as how the equipment and blood were handled and when (or if) the blood was put on ice. Additional steps in the laboratory involved assessment of whether hemolysis was present, whether this was within test limits, whether the test should be cancelled, testing, and the test report.

Gwen wanted to learn the rate of hemolysis in the specimens received but also wished to take into consideration each test's tolerance for hemolysis. She collected data on the degree of hemolysis allowed for each test so that she could find not only how hemolyzed the samples were but whether tests needed to be cancelled due to hemolysis.

Research Design and Details

The study focused on the smaller of two hospitals served by the special chemistry laboratory. Due to the volume of work, a week's worth of data was sufficient. To explore whether the problem existed at both the hospitals and to get results early enough to change the research design if needed, Gwen decided to evaluate specimens coming to the laboratory from both hospitals for a 5-day trial period. Then, having adjusted the design, Gwen would collect 7 days of data from the smaller hospital, including enough information on where the blood was being drawn to provide data on causes that could be linked to how the blood was dealt with in the units and in the laboratory.

The units of analysis were every blood specimen sent to the laboratory during the study period, identified by patient ID, the number on the requisition slip, the unit it came from, and whether the patient suffered from hemolytic disease. (If a patient has hemolytic disease, there is inevitable hemolysis and the test is not cancelled.) To avoid overwhelming the laboratory, data collection was split into a week for inpatient testing and a week for outpatient testing. With the 5-day field test, during which only laboratory data were collected, data for 505 specimens were collected during 19 days. No patients had hemolytic disease, so all the data were usable.

During the 5-day field test, Gwen discovered that some tests that should have been cancelled because of hemolysis were run. She also found that, among the tests that were run with unacceptable levels of hemolysis, the report to the physician often did not provide this information. This raised two additional problems and showed the importance of the field test.

The data from the units and the corresponding laboratory data were collected on the same day by the staff doing the work. Gwen had designed a table to be filled out by the staff who drew blood specimens. It explained what was being asked for and had columns for the date and time the blood was drawn, the patient ID, the staff member's ID, job title, and unit (location). It asked specifics such as whether the blood was hard to draw, whether it was put on ice, when, and what equipment was used to draw the blood. Gwen did not realize that, without field testing in the units, she would miss the fact that data on specimen collection were a burden to collect and that staff felt too busy to collect all the data asked for.

Gwen calculated the elapsed times from drawing the blood to when the specimen was put on ice, arrived in the laboratory, was spun down, and was tested. She collected chart data, including evidence of whether a test was cancelled if the specimen was judged to be hemolyzed and, for a test improperly not cancelled, whether the report informed the physician of the hemolysis. The late discovery of the two additional problems was not a disaster because much of the information was still available after the fact. Gwen went back to the reports in the charts to see what was cancelled in relation to the degree of hemolysis and the tests' tolerance. This was not the case with getting the data from the people who drew the blood, because staff could not be expected to remember specific conditions under which blood was drawn for particular specimens.

Final List of Possible Causes

Gwen identified 15 possible causes for the hemolysis problem, based on the literature in the field and staff suggestions. She added two causes for the lack of proper cancellation and reporting by the laboratory staff.

Patient risk factor

1. Patient has hemolytic disease

Technique used and staff-related

2. How the blood is taken (syringe, vacutainer, existing line)
3. Difficulty drawing blood
4. Pulling back too fast on syringe
5. Transfer of blood from syringe to vacutainer too forceful
6. Mixing tubes too hard
7. Blood put on ice too soon
8. Too much elapsed time before being tested
9. Lack of knowledge of technique or timing
10. Lack of staff concern
11. Specific job title
12. Individual staff member
13. Blood kept in laboratory too long before being spun down

Institutional factors

14. Specific location (unit)
15. Lack of written supervisory standards on hemolysis
16. Lack of supervisory standards on cancellations due to hemolysis
17. Inadequate laboratory record and requisition forms with regard to the presence of hemolysis

Criteria to Prove the Problem

The indicators to prove the problem of excess hemolysis were stated in two ways. Both reflected all the specimens sent to the laboratory, but the first took test sensitivity into account. *Warranted cancellation* was defined as the sum of tests that *were cancelled* due to hemolysis plus tests that *should have been cancelled* due to hemolysis and were not. The indicator was *the percentage of samples that warranted cancellation due to hemolysis*.

Specimens with unacceptable hemolysis were described in three test sensitivity categories: no hemolysis allowed, slight hemolysis allowed, and moderate hemolysis allowed. No test allowed gross hemolysis. The problem would be proved in each category if there was a warranted cancellation rate of more than 0.5%. Table C7.1 presents the criteria and the results.

The other indicator for proving the problem of excess hemolysis took all the hemolysis into account, regardless of test. This was the *percentage of total samples with hemolysis*, expressed regardless of test, in three categories: slightly, moderately, or grossly hemolyzed. The thresholds were more than 1% of total samples slightly hemolyzed, more than 0.5% moderately hemolyzed, and more than 0% grossly hemolyzed.

The indicator for the second problem was *the percentage of tests that should have been cancelled due to hemolysis and were not*. The proof-of-problem criterion was whether more than 1% of the tests that warranted cancellation were done anyway. For the third problem, the indicator was the *percentage of tests wrongly not cancelled for excess hemolysis with no notation of hemolysis in the laboratory report*. The criterion for this was more than 0.2% of tests wrongly not cancelled with no notation of hemolysis in the report (virtually none allowed).

Table C7.1 Criteria for Proof of Problem and Results: Hemolyzed Blood Samples

Measure	Point Beyond Which Problem Exists (Percentage, Rate, etc.)	Oked	Actual Results			Source

Percentage of samples that warranted cancellation due to hemolysis[a]

Percentage of samples whose tests should have been cancelled due to hemolysis			Wrongfully			Table 1.10
			Were Cancelled	Not Cancelled	Total	
First 5 days	> 0.5%	X	2.5%	2.5%	5.0%	Proved
The 14 days	> 0.5%	X	5.5%	11.0%	16.4%	Proved

Tests warranting cancellation based on test sensitivity groupings

The 19 days			Percentage of Test Groups			Table 1.10
None allowed	> 0.5%	X	7.6%	15.8%	23.4%	Proved
Slight allowed	> 0.5%	X	0.6%	0.6%	1.2%	Proved
Moderate allowed	> 0.5%	X	3.2%	0.0%	3.2%	Proved

The 19 days			Percentage of 505 Samples			Table 1.11
None allowed	> 0.5%	X	12.9%			Proved
Slight allowed	> 0.5%	X	0.4%			Not proved
Moderate allowed	> 0.5%	X	0.4%			Not proved

Percentage of samples by degree of hemolysis

The 19 days			Percentage of 505 Samples			Table 1.11
Slight hemolysis	> 1.0%	X	9.7%			Proved
Moderate hemolysis	> 0.5%	X	3.0%			Proved
Gross hemolysis	> 0.0%	X	1.0%			Proved

Percentage of tests that should have been cancelled due to hemolysis and were not

The 19 days	> 1.0%	X	65.2%			Table 1.10 Proved

Percent of tests wrongly not cancelled for excess hemolysis with no notation of hemolysis in the laboratory report

The 19 days	> 0.2%	X	93.3%			Table 1.10 Proved

a. No patients had hemolytic disease, so entire sample could be reported.

Results

Although the 5-day results underestimated the problem, analysis of the data showed similar problem levels in both hospitals. Table C7.1 shows the results for the 19 days. All the criteria to prove the excess hemolysis problem were exceeded. Expressed in terms of the degree to which the tests allowed varying degrees of hemolysis, the greatest problem turned out to be tests that allowed *no* hemolysis: 23.4% of such tests had samples with some hemolysis. For tests that allowed *slight* hemolysis, 1.2% had higher levels of hemolysis; for tests that allowed *moderate* hemolysis, 3.2% had higher levels (actually one specimen with gross hemolysis).

The data on the second criterion, which most directly reflected problems with the condition of the specimens, showed that 9.7% of the samples had *slight* hemolysis, 3% had *moderate*, and 1% had *gross* hemolysis, so all categories were a problem, with slight hemolysis the biggest problem.

As serious as these problems appeared, the two other problems were more serious. Gwen showed that 65.2% of the samples with unacceptable levels of hemolysis *were not cancelled*, largely samples for tests allowing no hemolysis (12.9% of the 505 samples). Even worse, of the tests that should have been cancelled but were not, 93.3% had no indication in the report that the blood had been tested with an unacceptable level of hemolysis.

The clients were convinced by the data, and the laboratory director indicated that Gwen would be allowed to institute any reasonable solution to solve the problems evidenced in the laboratory.

Identifying Causes

Objective Cause Data

Gwen examined 17 possible causes, including three for which there were objective cause data: whether the patient had hemolytic disease, specific job title of the staff drawing the blood, and specific location (unit). There was blood collection data for 383 tests on variables such as *job title* and *unit*, representing the 14-day sample.

The data on technique were extremely sparse. The database included 183 specimens with data on *how the blood was taken* (syringe, vacutainer, existing line), *difficulty drawing blood*, *elapsed time before being tested*, and ID data on the *individual staff* members. Because none of the 183 involved the use of syringes, there were no data on *pulling back too fast on the syringe* or *too forceful transfer of blood from the syringe to the vacutainer.* Only 25 specimens had data on *when blood was put on ice*, and only two had data on the *time until the sample was spun down.*

The problem variable was the degree of hemolysis of the sample, as that best reflected blood-drawing technique. Gwen calculated rank orders for the 11 staff, three job titles (phlebotomist, nurse, and hemodialysis technician), and 7 units involved during the test period by adding ranks for the respective hemolysis rates and ranks for disproportionate shares of slight, moderate, and gross hemolysis. The lowest hemolysis rates and the lowest proportionate shares of hemolysis had the lowest ranks. Equal numbers received equal ranks.

Additional information was collected on the adequacy of the requisition and laboratory record forms with respect to hemolysis, whether there was a lack of supervisory standards in the laboratory on cancellations due to hemolysis, and lack of written supervisory standards on blood drawing technique.

Subjective Cause Data: Questionnaire

Subjective causes included *lack of knowledge of technique or timing, lack of staff concern,* and *perceived lack of supervisory standards on hemolysis.* These were dealt with through a staff questionnaire, which was successfully administered to all 11 staff who drew blood during the test period. The questionnaire introduced the study, assured the staff of confidentiality, and asked for responses of true or false, or agree very much, agree a little, disagree, or don't know. The statements were:

1. When drawing blood, it makes a difference whether the specimen is hemolyzed and to what degree.
2. When drawing blood with a syringe, how hard you pull back on the plunger can affect whether the blood is hemolyzed.
3. When drawing blood into a vacutainer, how fast the blood comes out affects whether the blood is hemolyzed.
4. Having to dig around to find a vein can affect whether the blood is hemolyzed.
5. When using a vacutainer, shaking it vigorously can affect whether the sample is hemolyzed.

6. In transferring blood into a vacutainer from a syringe, the proper way is to inject the blood through the vacutainer stopper with the syringe needle.

7. In transferring blood into a vacutainer from a syringe, the proper way is to remove the stopper from the vacutainer and the needle from the syringe and then transfer the blood into the vacutainer.

8. For blood specimens that have to be put on ice, except for testing for ammonia, the blood must not be put on ice until it has clotted.

9. I am not always sure that I know the proper way to draw and handle blood.

10. When I draw a blood sample, getting the specimen drawn is my main concern; technique is standard and not a problem.

11. Standards for drawing blood are vague and not specified.

12. I do not get feedback on whether specimens I have drawn are hemolyzed.

Criteria to Prove the Causes

The patient has hemolytic disease was never involved because no patients whose specimens were in the sample had the condition. *Specific job title, specific staff member,* and *location (unit)* required that the unit, title, or individual be ranked among the top three in the category. In addition, for *job title,* the unit could not be the same for the three highest-ranked titles; for *specific staff member,* the unit or title could not be the same for the three highest-ranked individuals.

The lack of samples taken with syringes eliminated several possible causes. Another *method* could be proved if all the units using it had the highest rate of hemolysis and a disproportionate share. *Mixing tubes too hard* and *lack of staff concern* required that at least 60% of the higher-ranked "problem" staff would respond improperly to the relevant questionnaire item and at a higher rate than the lower-ranked staff.

Difficulty drawing blood had a double requirement: (a) the rate of hemolysis had to be higher for staff who reported difficulty than for those who reported no difficulty, and the rate for no hemolysis had to show the reverse, and (b) at least 60% of the higher-ranked, "problem" staff had to respond incorrectly to the relevant questionnaire item, and this had to be higher than for the lower-ranked staff. Similarly, *blood put on ice too soon* required that (a) the rate of hemolysis by category be higher for specimens put on ice too soon, or that the rate for no hemolysis would show the reverse, and (b) at least 60% of the higher-ranked "problem" staff would respond improperly to the relevant questionnaire item and higher than the lower-ranked staff.

Too much elapsed time before being tested also required that (a) the rate of hemolysis by category be higher for specimens that waited too long, and that the rate for no hemolysis would show the reverse, and (b) at least 60% of the higher-ranked "problem" staff would respond improperly to the relevant item and at a higher rate than lower-ranked staff.

Lack of knowledge of technique or timing required that for at least two out of nine statements dealing with knowledge on the questionnaire, at least 60% of the higher-ranked "problem" staff would respond improperly and at a higher rate than the lower-ranked staff.

Blood kept in the laboratory too long before being spun down required that the rate of hemolysis by category would be higher for specimens kept too long, or that the rate for no hemolysis would show the reverse.

Lack of written supervisory standards on hemolysis required that (a) hemolysis not be mentioned as a criterion for evaluation of staff who draw blood and (b) at least 60% of the higher-ranked "problem" staff would respond to support this view on the relevant questionnaire item and at a higher rate than the lower-ranked staff. *Lack of supervisory standards in the laboratory on cancellations due to hemolysis* required that staff evaluation criteria not mention cancelling tests for improperly hemolyzed samples. *Inadequate requisition and laboratory record forms with regard to hemolysis* would be proved if there was no place on the requisition form to indicate the hemolysis tolerance of a test and if the laboratory report form had no place to indicate the degree of hemolysis.

Results

Nine causes were proved or partly proved. The *dialysis unit* and *how the blood was taken* were both proved. In the dialysis unit, two needles were involved in drawing the sample from an existing line. *Putting blood on ice too soon, too much elapsed time before being tested*, and *blood being kept in the laboratory too long before being spun down* were proved or partly proved with very sparse data.

Lack of knowledge of technique or timing was also proved, although the general level of knowledge for all staff who drew blood was not high. *Lack of written supervisory standards on hemolysis* was partly proved; hemolysis was not mentioned as a criterion for evaluation of staff who drew blood. *Inadequate requisition and laboratory record forms with regard to the presence of hemolysis* was proved, as was *lack of supervisory standards in the laboratory on cancellations due to hemolysis*.

Solutions

The clients were convinced by the data and ready to seriously address the solutions. Their only limitation on the solutions was that they not be too costly.

Gwen was encouraged by the staff she consulted about solutions to propose a policy of reinforcing adherence to correct procedures through education of both the staff who drew blood and laboratory staff through periodic data collection and analysis and three changes in documentation. Staff supported her final list of solutions.

1. Requisition forms were to be redesigned to allow the time for important steps in the process to be entered, as a way of reminding unit staff of timing.
2. Requisition forms would show hemolysis limits for tests, as a reminder to laboratory staff.
3. Laboratory report forms were to be redesigned to show the degree of hemolysis of the sample.
4. Manuals for laboratory staff would include hemolysis test tolerances and limits. The manual for staff who draw blood would include specific procedures for specimen collection.
5. Unit staff evaluations would include performance on drawing blood; laboratory staff evaluations would include proper cancellation and reporting.
6. There would be inservice training on technique for all staff involved in drawing blood, with special emphasis on finding an acceptable way to draw blood in the dialysis unit and teaching it.

These recommendations were in line with JCAHO standards, which ask the organization to assure that specimens for laboratory tests be satisfactory and that written procedures be in place for specimen collection.

Implementing Solutions and Making Them Operational

Gwen had approval to plan and implement solutions for the laboratory at once. She got approval to alter the report forms, revise the manuals, conduct inservice training for the laboratory staff, and pay closer supervisory attention to the reports. She was able to get approval for the clinical chemist to present an inservice educational program for all staff who drew blood that covered drawing, transferring, and handling blood specimens, including the consequences of having poor specimens. Written guidelines were amended as appropriate. Plans were made to evaluate the solutions 6 months after they were implemented. The organization was now in a position to adopt new indicators to monitor and document the quality improvement process on the units and in the laboratory.

Note

1. Karen Moskogianis was the internal consultant for this project.

Errors in Filling Prescriptions in a Hospital Pharmacy[1]

Sometimes problems or opportunities for improvement appear at the interface between departments. In this case, complaints from nursing stations about medications delivered by the pharmacy pinpointed an area needing attention.

Proving the Problem

The Problem and the Client

Hope was an office manager in the pharmacy of a voluntary hospital. The pharmacy management was concerned about reports from nursing stations that patients' medications arrived with errors; when Hope expressed an interest in quality assessment, she was asked to find the causes of the problem and come up with some solutions. As the office manager, Hope was somewhat removed from actual pharmacy operations, but she was interested in quality improvement. The pharmacy director was willing to help Hope understand the day-to-day operations of the pharmacy and was willing to participate as the client.

Relevant Steps and Terms

It was necessary for Hope to learn the language of the pharmacy to understand its operations. The pharmacy containers used to fill medication orders were labeled with information including the patient's name, ID number, unit, and bed, and were referred to as *patient bins*. The medications to fill the bins were taken from three *pick bin* stations, normally one bin to a medication. The pick bins were filled from *supply bin boxes*, the original shipping containers in assigned locations in the storage area.

Medication orders were filled in the pharmacy and sent to the nursing units. The bins were filled daily with any medications ordered by physicians, aside from *floor stock*, which was normally found at the nursing units. Such items were not supposed to be listed in orders to the pharmacy nor kept in the pharmacy pick bins. Staff filled and delivered floor stock separately.

Physicians' handwritten orders to start, change, or discontinue medications were sent to the pharmacy, were reviewed by one of seven pharmacists, and were entered into the pharmacy's computer, which was used to print out each day's *medication fill lists*. These daily medication fill lists specified patient ID number, unit, and bed. The medications were identified by medication name, status, type, dosage, route, frequency, units per dose, fill (par) units, order number, a place for the *bin filler* to record how many units were placed in the bin (which had to match the par number), and places for the filler and *checker* to sign off. The original medication orders were discarded after 7 days.

The pharmacy used 486 patient bins. Pharmacy technicians filled 396 of the patient bins; pharmacists filled an additional 90. Pharmacists checked the technicians' work, but the filling by pharmacists was not checked. Hope decided to evaluate the accuracy of two days' worth of filling and checking. She identified four lettered bin groups, totalling 486 bins; they would produce a total of 972 observations.

A, with 174 bins, was filled by Technician 1 and checked by Pharmacist 1
B, with 191 bins, was filled by Technician 2 and checked by Pharmacist 2
C, with 31 bins, was filled by Technician 3 and checked by Pharmacist 3
D was composed of four subsets:

16 bins filled by Pharmacist 1
14 bins filled by Pharmacist 2
37 bins filled by Pharmacist 3
23 bins filled by Pharmacist 4

Final List of Possible Causes

Hope interviewed the pharmacy staff to get ideas about possible causes and reviewed the relevant literature. She compiled a list of 43 possible causes based on these and several others she became aware of as she conducted the study. Some possible causes were factors related to staff, but most referred to work conditions and procedures and were therefore institutional.

Factors related to staff

1. Specific staff
2. Specific job title of filler
3. Years experience in pharmacy
4. Educational level
5. Language barrier
6. Not committed to quality
7. Feeling rushed
8. Not feeling accountable
9. Spotting a problem but not asking about it

Specific types of errors in patient bins

10. Medication missing in bin or wrong medication
11. Medication present without order
12. Units per dose wrong
13. Medication expired
14. Form of medication wrong
15. Floor stock found in bins

Factors related to work situation

16. Specific bin groups (nursing units)
17. Specific medications
18. Requisition missing when accuracy was checked
19. No check of accuracy of computer entry of requisition
20. Handwriting on requisition not legible
21. Incomplete requisition

22. Contraindicated medication
23. Requisition administered on unit for first dose and bin not filled
24. Bins not filled by first being emptied
25. Inadequate lighting
26. Inadequate space to fill or check patient bins
27. Wrong medication in pick bins
28. Similar names
29. Similar look
30. Similar package
31. Medication does not have its own pick bin
32. Medications missing or below par in supply bins
33. Wrong medication in supply bins
34. Check of patient bins not signed off
35. Pharmacists' bins not checked
36. Check of patient bins does not catch errors
37. Bins not checked by first being emptied
38. Incident reports only record serious errors
39. Data discarded too soon
40. Talking among staff during filling or checking
41. Work interruptions during filling or checking
42. Bin assignments change each week
43. Inadequate feedback on accuracy

Research Design and Data Collection

Hope chose test days so that the staff would be dealing with the same bins on each of their two observation days. She watched and checked the work of each of the three pharmacy technicians on two discontinuous days before the pharmacists checked their work. She also checked the work of the four pharmacists who filled bins. Hope evaluated the accuracy of the three pharmacists who checked the technicians' work on two other days, after their checks and corrections were completed. Unfortunately, time did not allow Hope to check the checkers on the same day she evaluated the bin fillers' work. Because the pharmacists were not checked, there were no checkers to evaluate.

Errors found in patients' bins both before and after checking were categorized as (a) missing medication or incorrect medication, (b) incorrect units per dose, (c) whether expired, (d) incorrect form of medication, and (e) the presence of a medication without an order. A medication was correct if it had none of these errors. Hope also noted whether the checker initialed the medication fill list as required; missing initials could mean no check was made.

If the medication was missing or wrong, no further errors were noted. A given bin could have multiple medications and errors. These were recorded separately, by error type, which could add to more than the total number of bin fills because there could be more than one type of error in a bin. In the aggregated data, total correct and incorrect added to the number of bins because there was no double counting with respect to correct and incorrect designations. For each bin, Hope collected data on the ID number of the physician, whether the order form was legible, whether there was an order on file; whether the order was ongoing, contraindicated, new, or to discontinue; the name of the medication if there was a problem; whether the medication was floor stock; and whether the corresponding bin fill was correct.

At the end of each day of the study, Hope checked the accuracy of the medication fill list by comparing it with any new orders sent to the pharmacy. This allowed her to evaluate the legibility of the orders. Hope also examined every fourth pick bin in one of the 3 pick bin stations. She checked bins for correct medications and for unlabeled, wrong, expired, or missing medications and also for mixed doses, mixed forms, or wrong units per dose. Causes such as similar name, similar look, similar packaging, or wrong bin were noted so the explanations could be compared with errors in patient bins.

Hope also checked closed boxes in designated locations in the supply bin area. There were to have been 5 boxes present for each medication's appointed location. Hope noted wrong medications and how many boxes were missing from the par requirement of 5 for the location. Hope also examined incident reports for 6 months and noted what was dealt with in the reports.

Criteria to Prove the Problem

There were 20 separate proof-of-problem indicators, broken down by type of error; these covered the total as well as technician bin groups A, B, and C before and after being checked and the unchecked pharmacist bins in group D. These are shown in Table C8.1.

Table C8.1 Percentage of Pharmacy Bin Fills With Errors

| | Groups A, B, C[a] | | Group D[a] | | |
	Before Check[b]	After Check[b]	No Check[b]	Sent to Units	Problem Status
Criteria to prove the problem	> 1.0	> 0.0	> 0.0	> 0.0	
Total	9.2	9.5	12.2	10.0	Proved
Wrong or missing medications	5.5	0.8	5.0		Proved
Medications without order	1.9	1.6	1.7		Proved
Wrong units per dose	1.3	6.2	5.0		Proved
Expired dates	0.3	0.0	0.0		Not proved
Wrong form	0.3	0.8	0.5		Partly proved
No record of checker's initials	—	1.1	—		Proved

a. Bin groups A, B, and C were filled by pharmacy technicians before the check and then were checked by pharmacists. Bin group D was filled by pharmacists and not checked.
b. Checked error rates can exceed unchecked rates because checkers were not evaluated on the same day as pharmacy technicians.

As only the technicians' work was checked, and the problem was the accuracy of what left the pharmacy and arrived at the units, the percentage of errors allowed for A+B+C before checking was 1%, but for A+B+C after checking and for D, no errors were allowed. The zero criterion was also set for missing initials to designate that checking was done.

Results

As indicated in Table C8.1, every criterion to prove the problem was exceeded except for expired dates and the wrong form in bins filled by the technicians. The overall error rate for medications reaching the units was 10%; the highest error rate for fills going to the units was in the wrong units per dose category, followed by medications present without orders. Pharmacists had trouble with units per dose, wrong or missing medications, and medications without orders.

The irony of the pharmacists' work not being checked was that they had higher error rates overall and for wrong units per dose and wrong form; they actually approximated the unchecked errors of the technicians in other categories. It was hard to estimate the effect of the pharmacists' accuracy checks, because data on filling and data on checking were collected on different days. However, there was no evidence of low rates for checked bins. The checkers also failed to initial their checks about 1% of the time.

The client was impressed with the results and glad to have data on accuracy.

Identifying Causes

Subjective Cause Data: Questionnaire

There were 43 possible causes to assess. Most were already accounted for by data collected during the proof-of-problem stage. To deal with subjective causes, Hope administered a questionnaire to the three technicians and four pharmacists whose work she had studied. Respondents were asked to agree or disagree or indicate true or false for:

1. My job is centered around getting patient bins filled as quickly as possible.
2. My job is centered around getting patient bins filled as accurately as possible.
3. I get very little feedback on whether my work filling bins is accurate.
4. I sometimes feel so rushed at work that I don't even know if I am being accurate.
5. I would be more accurate if I could do the same bins for a month at a time rather than change every week.
6. When I do not find the medication I need in the pick bin, I do the best I can with what is there.
7. When I find a problem with a medication fill list order, I take it to the pharmacist who entered the order into the computer.
8. My supervisor pays little attention to how accurately I fill the patients' bins.

Statement 9 asked for ideas about solutions:

9. I would like to improve the way the work is done in filling the bins. (If yes) I would suggest the following:

Criteria to Prove the Causes and Results

Nine possible causes related to staff. Two were proved. For *specific staff* and *job title*, Hope ranked the staff members or titles according to error rate, disproportionate share of errors, and proportion of the work. The criterion was whether any staff member or title ranked highest in all three factors. No single staff member, whether technician or pharmacist, stood out. Neither the technicians nor the pharmacists accounted for most of the errors. *Years of experience in the pharmacy* showed no pattern in relation to staff arrayed by rank. *Language barrier* did not apply; only one staff member had a language barrier. *Educational level* was proved. Hope found that higher-ranked staff had less education; this showed up within both technician and pharmacist titles.

Subjective staff factors were evaluated in relation to answers on the questionnaire. A cause would be proved if more than 50% answered to support the cause and if staff ranked highest in errors were more associated with the attitude than those ranked lower. *Staff not being committed to quality* was associated with Statements 1, 2, and 9; *feeling rushed* was associated with Statement 4; *not feeling accountable* was associated with Statement 8. Statements 6 and 7 were associated with *if spotting a problem, not asking about it.* Only *feeling rushed* was proved.

Six specific types of errors were evaluated. Four were proved. Specific types of errors in patients' bins were causes if a particular error accounted for more than 5% of errors, excluding errors of floor stock appearing in bins. *Missing or wrong medication, medication present without order, wrong units per dose,* and *floor stock found in bins* were proved. With regard to floor stock, Hope discovered that staff violated the prohibition and placed floor stock in bins when floor stock ran out, to save time. Floor stock actually accounted for 26% of errors.

Twenty-eight other possible causes related to the work situation. Fifteen were proved: (1) *Requisition missing when accuracy was checked* was proved; 36% of incorrect bin fills had no record of the order, and there was no other way to check the accuracy of the fill list. It turned out that orders often came orally and were not followed up in writing. (2) *No check of accuracy of computer entry of medication order* was proved, because there was no way to check the accuracy of the fill list. Related to this, (3) *data discarded too soon* was proved; the only record against which to check the bins was the fill list; records were missing or discarded after 7 days.

At least 50% of staff reported (4) *little feedback on accuracy*. (5) *Bins not filled by first being emptied* and (6) *bins not checked by first being emptied* were both proved. Hope observed this practice during her study, and there was a 1.9% rate of medications present without orders before checking and 1.6% after checking. Related to this, (7) *inadequate space to fill and check patient bins* was proved. Hope noted that the computer took up most of the counter area where fillers and checkers worked; two fillers asked for redesign of the work area to provide more space in response to Statement 9, and the checkers' error rate was 9.5%. (8) *Work interruptions during filling or checking* caused by phone calls about the orders was also observed, and this was mentioned by two fillers in response to Statement 9.

(9) *Wrong medication in pick bins* was proved; the pick bin check showed that there were wrong medications in 100% of the pick bins, and wrong medications was actually proved as a cause. (10) *Medications missing or below par in supply bins* and (11) *wrong medication in supply bins* were both proved: 71% of supply bins showed medications below par or missing, 51% were in the wrong location, and 57% of staff answered "true" to Statement 6. (12) *Incident reports only record serious errors* was proved: There were only 7 incident reports in 6 months, yet Hope noted many phone calls from units requesting corrections for medications, and no records were kept on the phone calls.

(13) *Pharmacists' bins are not checked* was proved: The unchecked pharmacist bins had an error rate of 12.2% and accounted for 18.5% of the bins. (14) *Check of patient bins does not catch errors* was proved; the error rate after the check was 9.5%. Related to that, (15) *check of patient bins not signed off* was proved: Bins that were supposed to be checked had error rates of 9.5%, and 1.1% of bins showed no sign of an error check.

The largest group of proved causes related to the *institution*: Work conditions undermined accuracy. There was inadequate work space for inputting data into the computer, for filling bins, and for checking bins. As a direct result, bins were not emptied before filling or when being checked for accuracy. This may have accounted for medications without orders in patients' bins. *Wrong medications in supply bins* were partly due to floor stock being placed in bins as a way of saving the time needed to fill them on the units; this problem was compounded because staff did not know the floor stock for each area or floor.

The causes related to staff show that they felt rushed and harassed by having to answer the phones while they were filling bins. Staff felt that they got little feedback on accuracy. Also, because the staff with less education had more of a problem with errors, they may have needed more training.

Solutions

Feasibility Limits

The client was again convinced by the results because they made sense to him and supported his impressions. The feasibility limits he set for Hope were no major costs; any costs had to be one-time costs; no additional staff; reassignments might be considered; and quality standards must be met.

Choice of Solutions

Hope came up with 11 solutions, some of which were suggested by staff when they filled out the questionnaire; she had very positive feedback when she asked for reactions to her final list.

1. Make copies of the medication orders when they are brought to the pharmacy and retain them. Follow up on oral orders.
2. Assign one pharmacist to check the bins filled by the pharmacists.
3. Enforce the policy of doing complete checks and signing off for them.
4. Maintain records for use in evaluation.
5. Have the engineering department design a counter top to allow the computer to be off the work area needed to empty bins before filling and checking.
6. Once the space is available, enforce the correct method of emptying bins before filling and checking.
7. Assign one staff member to check and correct pick bins once per week.

8. Post which medications are floor stock above or near the appropriate bin groups, and provide orientation to the staff.
9. Assign a pharmacist to be the designated one to answer phones in rotation so that staff filling bins are not interrupted.
10. Provide feedback on accuracy through use of records and periodic checks similar to those done in the study.
11. Provide inservice training and orientation on these policies.

By the time Hope was ready with her final report, the solution of assigning a pharmacist to answer the phones had already been approved and implemented. The other solutions were awaiting further deliberations.

JCAHO standards and guidelines were not specific enough to pick up the work-related dysfunctions in the pharmacy. Attention seems to be focused more on the safe preparation and accurate administration of drugs and less on accuracy before transmission to nursing stations. This project dealt with the interface between the pharmacy and nursing and was able to decrease the problems facing the staff who administer the drugs by increasing the accuracy of what was delivered. The data collection experience provided a prototype for the development of pharmacy indicators and moved the department towards more regular monitoring of quality.

Note

1. Gisela Perez was the internal consultant for this project.

Case 9

A Labor-Management Health and Safety Committee[1]

In this case, a committee organized to deal with occupational health and safety issues in a municipal agency was not functioning; as it turned out, the health and safety issues of the large staff were not being addressed.

Proving the Problem

The Problem

Ira was a deputy assistant director in a large municipal agency. He had recently been assigned to represent management on a labor-management health and safety committee formed a year earlier. The committee's mission was to deal with environmental health and safety issues at all the local offices of the agency. To his surprise, Ira found that few problems ever came before the committee.

The agency was mandated, under the state's Public Employee Safety and Health Act and the "Right to Know" law, to inform all employees of their right to work in a safe, nonhazardous environment. The committee's disuse was seen as a symptom that the intent of the act and the law was not being fulfilled. Ira believed that not only was the Committee not being used, local office environmental health and safety problems were probably not being dealt with as well.

The Client

The director of the agency asked Ira to investigate why the committee was not functioning as expected. The committee comprised eight union and eight management representatives, with a cochair for each subgroup. The cochairs of the committee were included as clients so both labor and management would have representatives to approve project criteria and solutions.

Research Design and Data Collection

To prove the two problems, Ira had to identify what environmental health and safety problems existed at the local offices and then learn how they were being handled. After that, Ira would explore causes for the nonuse of the Committee.

The Agency had about 100 local offices in 50 locations, covering six different functional divisions. Because the offices for each function were similar to one another, Ira decided to use a sample of six offices representing each of the six functions. With the cochairs' approval, Ira chose three criteria to select one office from each of the six divisions. The criteria were to ensure (a) that the greatest number of people would be involved in the sample of six offices, (b) that the greatest number of problems could be uncovered, and (c) that the problems would be a representative cross section.

Once the offices were selected, Ira arranged to meet staff at each of the six offices and identified a person who would know about office conditions and who could represent the union point of view, such as a union steward or delegate. He located a similarly knowledgeable representative of management, such as an office manager. He met with the individuals to discuss the project and requested their participation. When he had agreement, he noted the date and the individuals' names, and he assigned ID codes.

Ira drew up a preliminary list of possible health and safety problems by meeting with his collaborator and experts in the field, and by carrying out a review of the literature. He took the preliminary list to specialists at the National Institutes for Occupational Safety and Health (NIOSH) for their opinions. They helped consolidate the list and judged it comprehensive, understandably worded, and well designed.

The list was approved by the two committee cochairs; Ira then designed and field tested a questionnaire. It asked the two respondents at each office to examine the list, add to it, and evaluate the seriousness of the problems at that office. Question 1 was "Is this a problem here?" and listed 44 possible problems that might have affected the safety of staff in the offices, with a place to fill in any other problems. In answer to the question, the respondent could check whether the item was a major or minor problem at that office, was not a problem, was not applicable to the office, or that the respondent did not know. One item was added to the list as a result of field testing in an office that was not part of the sample.

Ira judged whether a problem existed at a local office based on survey responses. A problem was defined as an item that either the labor or the management representative of the office selected as a major problem, or that both selected as a minor problem, or that both indicated they did not know about, as this was a problem in itself.

The second question on the questionnaire asked the respondent where he or she went if a problem was reported for an item, with the choice of checking off going to the union, going to management, going to the labor-management committee, or filling in another option. Figure C9.1 is the final form of the survey. It was successfully field tested and then administered to the 12 representatives.

Criteria to Prove the Problem

The indicator to show whether there were unsolved problems at local offices was the number of items judged to be problems by representatives in the sample of six local offices. The criteria to prove the problem were, overall, more than 10 categories identified as problems and, for any office, more than 2 categories identified as problems.

The indicator for the second problem, that health and safety problems were not being taken to the labor-management committee, was the percentage of either group of representatives or of both groups who did not mention the committee as a place to go with problems. The criterion was more than 40% not mentioning the committee.

Dear colleague,
We are attempting a survey of health and safety issues found at agency offices. Please answer the following questions truthfully. Please add to the list below if there are problems at *your* office that are not already on it.

	1. Is This a Problem Here? (Check what applies)				2. If a Problem Reported, Where Do You Go? What Do You Do?		
Office ID: A ( ), B ( ), *C ( ), D ( ), E ( ), F ( )* *Respondent ID* _____	*Yes, Major*	*Yes, Minor*	*Not Applicable*	*Do Not Know*	*Go to Union*	*Go to Labor-Management Comittee*	*Write in Other*
Peeling paint							
Lead in paint							
Ventilation not adequate							
Fume hoods inadequate							
Not cleaned regularly							
Bathrooms unsanitary							
Leaky plumbing							
Drinking water not adequate							
Hazardous flooring							
Improper electrical grounding							
Misuse of extension cords							
Inadequate relief when using video display terminals (VDTs)							
Not enough fire exits							
Fire exits blocked							
Roof leaks							
Inadequate handicapped access							
Chemical hygiene plan not in place							
No "Materials Safety Data Sheet" on site							
Inadequate toxic materials training							
Poor infectious materials disposal							
Poor infectious materials handling							
Poor infectious materials training							
Poor sharp materials disposal							
Poor sharp materials handling							
Poor sharp materials training							
Exposed friable asbestos							
Suspected exposed asbestos							
Inadequate fire evacuation plan							
Sputum induction machine enclosure							
Not wearing dosimeter badges							
Centrifuges missing safety globes							
Not using special gloves							
Not using special goggles							
Employees not inoculated for measles, mumps, rubella							
Employees not inoculated for Hepatitis-B virus (HBV)							
Employees not screened for tuberculosis							
Lack of a security officer							
Smoking regulations not enforced							
Lack of security outside building							
Noise pollution							
Air pollution							
Muggings							
Drug traffic							
Lack of rest facilities for staff							
Fill in any other problems							

Figure C9.1 Survey of Office Health and Safety Problems

Results

Union representatives identified 25 major problems, 73 minor problems, and did not know about 46. Management representatives identified 27 major problems, 52 minor problems, and did not know about 33. There was agreement on 63% of the items. An overall problem rate of 36.7% was found, as defined earlier.

Thirty-one categories qualified as problems using the agreed-upon definition. There were 12 problems that both representatives designated as a major problem, 28 that one of the representatives designated as a major problem, 29 that both representatives designated as a minor problem, and 28 about which neither representative had knowledge. Six problems were identified by only one office; all the other problems appeared in from two to six offices. The three found in each office were lead in paint, irregular cleaning, and unsanitary bathrooms. No office had fewer than 11 problems; one office had 22, and the average was 16 problems per office. This project problem was proved.

When answering the second question, respondents mentioned three additional options used only by management people: going to security, going to the police, and handling the problem personally. The responses showed that union people went to the union with 20% of the problems, but management never went to the union. Management representatives went to management with 93% of the problems, and union people went to management with 80% of the problems. There was a higher agreement rate here (almost 74%). *None* of the representatives chose the option of going to the labor-management committee; that health and safety problems were not being taken to the labor-management committee was proved. The clients were fully convinced that both problems were proved.

Identifying Causes

Final List of Possible Causes

It was not necessary to collect cause data while work on proving the problem was underway. After the problems were verified, Ira developed a list of 10 possible causes for nonuse of the committee:

Related to management

1. There was no system to get an office's health and safety problems to the attention of the committee.
2. The committee had not told people it existed.

Related to local office labor and management leadership

3. Labor or management people did not know which issues were to go to the committee.
4. The committee did not know what to do about the problems.
5. The union did not support the committee.
6. Management did not support the committee.

Related to staff

7. Staff did not know that they had a right to ask for help on health and safety issues at work.
8. Staff believed that health and safety issues were not important.
9. Staff believed that there were few health and safety issues at the office.
10. Staff believed that, even if reported, it wouldn't make any difference.

Subjective Cause Data: Questionnaires

The causes of the committee's nonuse were investigated with two questionnaires. Because behavioral issues were involved, it was important to have staff members' opinions. Figure C9.2 was designed to elicit responses to 12 questions. It opened with the information that "we" are trying to learn staff's ideas about the committee; it indicated that, as an employee of the agency, the respondent had the right to work in a safe and nonhazardous environment; it then described the committee.

The respondent was assured that the survey was anonymous. After acknowledging that the labor-management health and safety committee had not been receiving requests from agency offices to settle health and safety issues at the offices, it asked, "What do you think the reasons are?" and presented 11 reasons. The reasons were to be categorized as an *Important Reason*, a *Partial Reason*, or *Not a Reason*. Question 12 asked for any additional reasons.

Dear colleague,
We are attempting to find out what ideas staff have about a labor-management health and safety committee that has been set up by the agency. As an employee of the agency, you have a right to work in a safe and nonhazardous environment. The committee has been set up to deal with health and safety issues at the offices. Please answer the following questions truthfully. This survey does not ask for your name.

The Labor-Management Health and Safety Committee has not been receiving requests from agency offices to settle health and safety issues at the offices. What do you think the reasons are?

Check off the reasons you think are most important and any others you think are partial explanations.

	Important Reason	Partial Reason	Not a Reason
1. Staff do not know about the committee.	( )	( )	( )
a. This is the first time I have heard about it.	Yes ( )	No ( )	
2. Staff do not know they have a right to ask for help in dealing with health and safety issues at work.	( )	( )	( )
3. Health and safety issues are not very important.	( )	( )	( )
4. There are very few health or safety issues at this office.	( )	( )	( )
5. Even if we reported the issues, it wouldn't make any difference.	( )	( )	( )
6. The labor or management people here do not know what issues can go to the committee.	( )	( )	( )
7. The committee probably doesn't know what to do.	( )	( )	( )
8. There is no system to get our office's problems to the attention of the committee.	( )	( )	( )
9. The union doesn't support the committee.	( )	( )	( )
10. The management doesn't support the committee.	( )	( )	( )
11. The committee has not told us it exists and we do not know anything about it.	( )	( )	( )
12. Anything else? (Fill in)	( )	( )	( )

_____

Office Code _____

Figure C9.2 Survey of Attitudes Concerning the Joint Labor-Management Health and Safety Committee

Ira selected a subset of three of the six offices as the survey population, choosing the three with the largest staffs to be the respondents. These had 18, 13, and 11 staff, respectively. The 42 staff members were 66% of the total staff in the six offices. The field test was carried out in a different office. The questionnaire was administered to all the employees at work on the day assigned; none were left for another day.

A second questionnaire was designed for the 12 committee members. It asked essentially all the same questions, but from the committee's point of view. Field testing for the second survey was done with a few executives but not by anyone on the committee. The version for members of the committee addressed the committee members as such and asked for anonymous responses. It also stated that the committee had not been receiving requests and asked, "What do you think the reasons are?" followed by similar reasons and options.

Approval for the questionnaires came only from the director, to avoid contaminating the cochairs' responses. The two questionnaires covered all the causes that were being studied and allowed those responding to add others. There were 40 responses from staff and 9 from committee members, of whom 5 represented management and 4 represented unions. No additional causes were entered in response to Question 12.

The reason with the highest rate of *Important* from staff was the response to Question 11, "The committee has not told us it exists, and we do not know anything about it" (97.5%). Committee members seemed unaware of this; only 11% chose it as important. The related reason, that "Staff do not know about the committee," had a 95% rate from staff and a 67% rate from committee members. On the other hand, only 10% of staff indicated that they were hearing about the committee for the first time. The second highest rate for *Important* chosen by staff was Question 8, "There is no system to get our office's problems to the attention of the committee" (95%). Only 22% of the committee members chose this answer.

Committee members' favorite choice for *Important* was Question 2, "Staff do not know they have a right to ask for help in dealing with health and safety issues at work" (90%; this was also chosen by 75% of staff).

The cause with the smallest staff selection as *Important* was Question 3, "Health and safety issues are not very important" (25%). None of the committee members selected this reason.

Staff and committee members had little agreement on Question 4, "There are very few health or safety issues at this office." Only 32.5% of staff chose this as *Important*, but 77.8% of the committee members chose it as applying to all the offices.

Faith in the system was low. Staff had an 80% Important rate for Question 5, "Even if we reported the issues, it wouldn't make any difference." The committee understandably had greater faith; only 22% chose question 5 as important. For Question 7, 52.5% of staff thought that the committee "probably doesn't know what to do" was an Important reason; this was agreed to by 44.4% of committee members, suggesting that the committee might not really have known how to function.

Staff had an 85% Important rate for Question 6, "The labor or management people here do not know what issues can go to the committee." Committee members had a rate of 55.6%.

Among staff, 70% chose as Important that (9) "The union doesn't support the committee," and 60% chose as Important that (10) "The management doesn't support the committee." Committee members had rates of 33% and 67% for the questions, seeing less opposition from unions than the staff did, even though 5 of the 9 respondents represented management.

Criteria to Prove the Causes

The criteria for most causes required that more than 50% of staff and the committee select Important and/or Partial for a question appearing on both questionnaires. For three causes, the criteria did not include the opinions of the committee members. One was that staff did not know about the committee and that the committee had not told staff it exists. The second was that respondents were hearing about the committee for the first time. The third was "Staff do not know that they have a right to ask for help on health and safety issues" (Question 7). The criterion for these was that more than 50% of staff choose these as Important or Partial reasons.

Results

The causes that were proved are as follows:

1. There is no system to get an office's health and safety problems to the attention of the committee.
2. Staff do not know about the committee, or the committee had not told staff it existed.

3. Labor or management people do not know which issues go to the committee.
4. The committee does not know what to do about the problems.
5. The union does not support the committee.
6. Management does not support the committee.
7. Staff do not know that they have a right to ask for help on health and safety issues at work.
8. Staff believe that even if problems were reported, it wouldn't make a difference.

Causes that were not proved were the belief that health and safety issues are not important and that there are few health and safety issues at the office. No other cause was suggested by the respondents.

Solutions

Ira did not seek feasibility limits for his solutions because he was dealing with an agencywide problem and preferred to develop an overall policy and plan. Ira talked with six representatives who had been most involved in the project and felt he got a good cross section of ideas, which he included in an integrated system. Feedback from 10 representatives was positive. The only concern was that implementation might not start soon enough.

To address the key management cause, Ira suggested that a health and safety officer be designated for the agency. Reporting to this individual would be a health and safety officer assigned to each building. These local officers would be the liaisons to the committee from each location.

Each local health and safety officer would be linked to a particular person on the committee. All involved would be trained in what to do and how to do it. The committee member for a particular division would be involved in employee training in that division, covering the specific health and safety problems identified for the division, as shown by Ira's project. The committee members would be trained to do this work beforehand and would be asked to recommend budget allocations to remedy problems.

Ira suggested a special meeting with the unions that would involve top-level officers from each division. Each union would have a health and safety officer present to ensure union input on who the local health and safety officers would be and who would be sent to the committee. There would also be a special meeting with management people at the office and division level to make sure they were convinced that the agency backed this effort. They would be asked for their input on who the local health and safety officers would be and who would be sent to the committee.

To reach staff, a letter describing the committee, its mission, members, and meeting dates would be distributed to all employees, signed by the director of the agency. There would be annual training sessions for all employees covering general "Right to Know" law and Public Employee Safety and Health Act provisions and mandates. Sessions would explain how to spot problems, how to deal with or prevent them, and how to use the local health and safety officer and the committee to get results. A contract with a local public college that trained professionals in this field was suggested to help keep costs down.

Implementing Solutions and Making Them Operational

Ira was designated as the agency's health and safety officer. He was given the power to initiate corrective measures for the problems he uncovered, especially because the agency was subject to citations and fines if corrective measures were not taken. He had the support of the director and the cochairs of the committee, who were impressed by the results of the project.

Ira knew that implementation of the solutions could take a year or more. He helped design a plan to develop a training curriculum and hire a trainer or approach the college, and he planned to stagger the training over a year so that all employees could attend. He also helped design a plan to remedy at once some of the defects uncovered in the report, using in-house resources and available funds. The design is now in place and functioning.

Note

1. Robert M. Debbie was the internal consultant for this project.

Nurse Attendance at Mandated Classes in an Outpatient Department[1]

In this case, the internal consultant was a catalyst. Changes were implemented even before the study was completed.

Proving the Problem

The Problem and Importance

Jan was a head nurse in a freestanding outpatient department of a municipal hospital. Staff involved in patient care were required to attend six continuing education classes per year provided by the hospital. Jan initiated her project because she thought that staff were probably not attending each of these classes once a year as mandated, and probably were not attending the first time classes were scheduled by the Department of Staff Development. The classes were:

1. Acquired Immune Deficiency Syndrome (AIDS) and HIV Infection
2. Infection Control
3. Risk Management and Quality Assurance
4. The Patient's Bill of Rights and Patient Relations
5. Fire Prevention and Safety
6. Occupational Hazards

The Client

The project involved three clients. The nursing supervisor of the Outpatient Department initiated the study, but the director of nursing, a more senior member of management, and the supervisor of staff development were consulted as well; the Department of Staff Development was in charge of continuing education.

Observation Units, Normal Loads, Quantities, and Time Frame

The Outpatient Department, located in its own building, was staffed by 36 registered nurses (RNs), 11 licensed practical nurses (LPNs), and 12 nurses' aides (NAs). Jan had planned to collect retrospective class attendance data for 12 months in 1991 and concurrent data for the first 3 months of 1992. Key variables were to include the attendance of each staff member by class, dates assigned to attend, whether attended, dates classes were scheduled, and when announcements went out, as well as information about the staff, including job title, demographics, shift, educational level, and experience in the department.

Scheduling and attendance data were the province of the Department of Staff Development, but Jan found that Staff Development had no record of how many classes were held, who was scheduled, or how far ahead staff were notified. There were no records on assignment, posting, or attendance, except for a log, which was kept haphazardly. The supervisor was reluctant to release *any* data, fearing it could be a source of embarrassment; Jan had to seek attendance records from the Department of Human Resources and Training. Their data covered only the number of classes given and who attended but not who was scheduled. Thus, for 1991, Jan had data only on the classes her staff attended.

To Jan's surprise, however, once she overcame the staff development supervisor's fear that the project would harm her, Staff Development began to collect the needed data in the way originally hoped for. As a result, Jan *could* get detailed current information for the period after March 10, 1992. Jan had affected the way data were collected, but this only helped to provide data through March 31, 1992, because then Jan's data collection would end.

The improvement in data collection came about when outpatient staff were asked to attend classes at the main building of the hospital, where the practice was to offer a day containing five classes held one after the other. Anyone coming late would miss all five classes, and everyone assigned was expected to stay for all five. Jan therefore had two time periods to consider: all of 1991 and from January 1 through March 10 in 1992 for limited information, and March 11 to 31, 1992, for more detailed information.

Final List of Possible Causes

Jan identified 18 possible causes based on her own ideas, a literature review, and staff interviews; responses to a staff survey added one more cause.

Related to staff

1. Specific staff
2. Specific job title
3. Staff absent due to lateness and not being allowed to attend
4. Staff on vacation for time scheduled
5. Staff think classes are boring
6. Staff do not feel secure or comfortable about taking classes
7. Staff do not feel they learn in class
8. Staff think they already know the material
9. Staff do not like attending class with people in other titles
10. Staff do not think classes are important
11. Staff do not feel accountable for attendance

Related to institution

12. Specific classes
13. Supervisors do not allow staff to attend when there is no one to cover clinic; short staff or no relief staff available
14. Classes not offered
15. Classes not scheduled during clinic hours
16. Staff notified too late
17. Staff not scheduled

18. Scheduling done without checking staff availabilities
19. Scheduling done at random without checking need

Data Collection

Jan assigned ID numbers to staff and job titles and used check-sheet tables to record attendance and nonattendance at the six classes. The classes given during the March 11 through 31, 1992 period were in the five-per-day format in which someone coming late would miss all five classes. Although 10 classes were scheduled, one of the six mandated classes, Patient Rights, was not given at all during the period, and only eight of Jan's staff were assigned. Data for this period covered each class presented, the date, time, posting information, number scheduled to attend, number who actually attended, percentage who attended of those assigned to attend, and whether staff availabilities were checked. Staff data included which staff were scheduled, job title, class, date, time, whether a staff member attended or was absent, and reasons for not attending.

Criteria to Prove the Problem

The first problem indicator, shown in Table C10.1, refers to the percentage of staff who attended all six classes in 1991. The other indicators for 1991 refer to the percentage of required classes attended. This latter indicator reflects the number of *attendances* required. For example, for 55 staff, 330 class attendances were required. The indicators for 1991 refer to 14 categories of staff, title, and class. The threshold criterion for each was set at less than 100% attendance, which was the mandated criterion.

A second set of 7 indicators for March 11 through 31, 1992 refers to those attending class as a percentage of those actually assigned. This was the only time period for which such data existed. A uniform criterion of 80% was assigned to all classes because not everyone might have been able to attend a given class, and there were 9 months remaining to the year.

A third set of 14 indicators covered the entire first quarter of 1992, with indicators comparable to those for 1991. However, the threshold for each was 40% attendance, because the period was only the first

Table C10.1 Criteria for Proof of Problem and Results: Attendance at Mandated Classes

Measure	Point Beyond Which Problem Exists (Percentage)	OKed	Actual Results		Source
Percentage of staff attending mandated classes, 1991:					Table 1.2
Attended all 6 classes	< 100	x	5.5	Proved	
Percentage attended	< 100	x	45.5	Proved	
RNs					
Attended all 6 classes	< 100	x	9.4	Proved	
Percentage attended	< 100	x	50.0	Proved	
LPNs					
Attended all 6 classes	< 100	x	0.0	Proved	
Percentage attended	< 100	x	25.8	Proved	
NAs					
Attended all 6 classes	< 100	x	0.0	Proved	
Percentage attended	< 100	x	51.4	Proved	
Percentage of staff who attended:					
HIV	< 100	x	52.7	Proved	
Infection Control	< 100	x	50.9	Proved	
Risk Management	< 100	x	7.3	Proved	
Patients' Bill of Rights	< 100	x	50.9	Proved	
Fire Prevention and Safety	< 100	x	50.9	Proved	
Occupational Hazards	< 100	x	60.0	Proved	
Percentage of staff who attended mandated classes, March 11-31, 1992:					Table 1.4
Total	< 80	x	70.0	Proved	
HIV	< 80	x	70.0	Proved	
Infection Control	< 80	x	70.0	Proved	
Risk Management	< 80	x	70.0	Proved	
Patients' Bill of Rights	< 80	x	0.0	No classes	
Fire Prevention and Safety	< 80	x	70.0	Proved	
Occupational Hazards	< 80	x	70.0	Proved	
Percentage of staff attending mandated classes Jan. 1 through March 10, 1992:					Table 1.7
Attended all 6 classes	< 40	x	5.1	Proved	
Percentage attended	< 40	x	24.0	Proved	
RNs					
Attended all 6 classes	< 40	x	8.3	Proved	
Percentage attended	< 40	x	28.7	Proved	
LPNs					
Attended all 6 classes	< 40	x	0.0	Proved	
Percentage attended	< 40	x	19.7	Proved	
NAs					
Attended all 6 classes	< 40	x	0.0	Proved	
Percentage attended	< 40	x	13.9	Proved	
Percentage of staff who attended:					
HIV	< 40	x	27.1	Proved	
Infection Control	< 40	x	32.2	Proved	
Risk Management	< 40	x	11.9	Proved	
Patients' Bill of Rights	< 40	x	15.3	Proved	
Fire Prevention and Safety	< 40	x	27.1	Proved	
Occupational Hazards	< 40	x	30.5	Proved	

quarter. A cushion was allowed, after which the next three quarters would cover the other 60%.

Results

As Table C10.1 indicates, each of the criteria to prove the problem was surpassed. Only 5.5% of staff attended all six classes in 1991, and only 5.1% attended during the first quarter of 1992. The percentage of required classes attended by staff was 45.5% in 1991 and 24.0% for the first quarter of 1992. In 1991, the percentage of assigned classes attended ranged from 51.4% for NAs to 25.8% for LPNs. No individual class did better than 60% (Occupational Hazards); Risk Management had the lowest, with a 7.3% attendance rate. The new changes after March 11 produced a rate of 70% attendance for eight staff assigned to five classes, which was under the rate of 80% set as the cutoff.

When Jan presented her results to the three clients, only the director of nursing was surprised; she expressed concern, advising the others to work on improving attendance. The stage was set for Jan to continue.

Identifying Causes

With most of the objective cause data collected, Jan arranged the staff attendance data in rank order of classes attended for the total test period: Lower ranks were associated with nonattendance, zero attendance was rank 1, and higher ranks were associated with higher attendance.

Subjective causes were dealt with in two nearly identical questionnaires for the nursing staff and their supervisors. Jan obtained an 80% response rate, with losses due only to staff not being present when the survey was administered. The questionnaires did not ask for the respondent's name. Jan put the respondent's code number on the back of the questionnaire, allowing her to relate the responses to the respondents' attendance.

Question 1 of the staff questionnaire listed the classes and asked the staff which ones they attended in 1991 and in 1992. The question was an icebreaker; it set the stage, was not threatening, and reminded the subjects of what the classes were. This question was also used to assess how reliable the answers might be, as Jan already had data on the classes attended.

The other questions were introduced by: "The following are reasons for not going to the classes. If you have missed any, check how important the explanations below are for you. They can be a main reason, part of the reason (not the main one), or not a reason at all." There was also a *Don't Know* choice. The supervisors' questionnaire had similar material "explaining why staff do not attend mandated classes." The reasons presented were

1. Classes are boring.
2. I do not feel comfortable in the classes.
3. I don't learn in class.
4. I already know the material.
5. I don't like to be in class with people in other jobs and titles.
6. I would go, but my supervisor says I am needed in the clinic.
7. The classes are not a priority for me.
8. When I am scheduled, I get pulled away because there is no coverage for me in the clinic.
9. No one checks on whether I go, so why bother?
10. Other (with space to write).

There were 49 respondents: 47 staff and the 2 supervisors. It was fortunate that only 1 respondent each was lost from the smaller groups of LPNs and NAs; the RNs lost 10 out of 36, a higher percentage loss but better borne by the larger group. The result of the staff accuracy check for Question 1 showed that staff were 40% accurate for 1991 and 94% accurate for 1992, which covered a shorter period, closer in time. Staff with higher attendance had better accuracy rates than those with lower attendance; it may be easier to remember an event than a nonevent.

Criteria to Prove the Causes

Jan set about to determine the criteria that would prove the 19 possible causes. *Specific staff* was to be proved if less than 10% of staff affected the average number of classes attended by at least one class, shown by recalculation without them. *Specific job title* would be proved if any title were more than one class below the average for both years. *Staff absent due to lateness and not being allowed to attend* could only be proved with data from March 11 to 31, so only one latecomer not allowed to attend class was the criterion. A similar criterion applied to *staff on vacation for the time scheduled*.

Staff think the classes are boring, do not feel secure or comfortable about taking classes, do not feel they learn in class, think they already know the material, do not like attending class with people in other titles, do not think classes are important, and *do not feel accountable for attendance* were all reflected in the questionnaires. The criteria were that at least 40% of staff with the lowest attendance must select the cause as a main reason or a partial reason in response to the appropriate question(s), that this rate be higher than that for the staff with the highest attendance, and that at least one supervisor must agree.

Specific classes would be proved if any had an attendance rate more than 10 percentage points below the aggregate average. The items *supervisors do not allow staff to attend when there is no one to cover clinic* and *short staff or no relief staff available* refer to the same cause. This cause would be proved by a combination of criteria: Data from March 11 through 31 would show this as a reason for at least one absent staff member, and at least 40% of staff with the lowest attendance would select the cause as a main or a partial reason in response to the appropriate questions; the rate had to be higher than that for staff with the highest attendance; and at least one supervisor had to agree.

A group of causes relied on the data from March 11 through 31. *Classes not offered* would be proved if any class were given less often than the others; *classes not scheduled during clinic hours* would be proved through inspection of class hours. *Staff notified too late* had to show posting less than one week in advance. *Staff not scheduled* was a response to the survey. The criterion for a write-in cause was that it had to be named by at least 7 staff.

Scheduling done without checking staff availabilities and *scheduling done at random without checking* were to be proved through interviews with nursing supervisors and the supervisor of staff development.

Results

Nine causes were proved, as follows:

Related to staff

1. The job title of LPN
2. Staff absent due to lateness and not being allowed to attend

Related to institution

3. The specific class: Risk Management
4. Supervisors do not allow staff to attend when there is no one to cover clinic; short staff or no relief staff available
5. Classes not offered (Patient Rights)
6. Staff notified too late
7. Staff not scheduled
8. Scheduling done without checking staff availabilities
9. Scheduling done at random without checking need

The main cause seemed to be that supervisors did not allow staff to attend class when there was no one to cover the clinic because of shortage of staff and no available relief. The other causes showed a pattern that reinforced this: Scheduling had been overlooking the circumstances in the department, such as notifying staff too late, scheduling without asking supervisors about staff availabilities, scheduling at random without checking with supervisors, and, as it turned out, scheduling classes on days that relief staff were not available. Jan added a tenth cause: the lack of an adequate record-keeping system.

Solutions

Jan's feasibility limits were to incur no major costs and suggest no additional staff. Her solutions were approved informally by the staff members she asked for feedback. She started with the need for a system of planning and record keeping on class attendance. Jan preferred a computerized system that would allow supervisors access to attendance data by staff ID, class, date, the class offered, and when assignments were made. However, she was willing to accept a procedural manual and paper records.

Jan asked to have Staff Development announce classes, but she wanted the supervisor to be the one to assign staff to the classes, drawing on the same database Staff Development used. Jan thought that classes should be given before, during, and after clinic hours, on days relief staff were available, and should reflect the staffing needs of the supervisors, who would be consulted. Supervisors would have access to staff records and would distribute the assignments personally, with adequate notice. Jan expected her solutions to cut down on meeting times because supervisors would not need to meet as often with Staff Development.

Although she did not like the five-class method for scheduling, Jan suggested that, if they had to continue, latecomers should be admitted to all the classes following the one for which they were late. Jan preferred that staff be assigned to the classes they needed, not in five-class groups. She suggested that classes should be given and assigned based on the number of staff needing them. Jan did not single out the title of LPN because LPNs were a small part of the staff and the problem was widespread; the solutions applied to every title.

Jan's long-range solution was to have classes taped for viewing, so small numbers of staff could attend when there was coverage to relieve them. Class discussions could be included, and brief exams could be given afterward.

Implementing Solutions and
Making Them Operational

At the point at which Jan was to make her final report on solutions, the supervisor of staff development was already conferring with nursing supervisors in the Outpatient Department on the availability of staff and was already keeping accurate records on staff attendance and reasons for nonattendance. She developed a data collection form similar to the one used by Jan. Posting was being done at least a week ahead and included the names of staff, the date, the place, and the time.

Staff were making a more conscious effort to attend classes the first time they were scheduled. This was partly due to their positive response to being involved in the project and partly because they had been able to discuss the importance of the classes and their effects on patient care and their own safety. They were also being held accountable for absences. These early changes suggested that the additional solutions offered by Jan would be well received; the clients were looking forward to the final report.

In 1991, the JCAHO had standards requiring that nursing be provided with ongoing education designed to improve staff competence and that participation be documented. By 1997, guidelines asked for a process to ensure that the programs be appropriate to staff members' patients. Current issues would probably also include the appropriateness of one-size-fits-all educational programs, the relationship of content to patient care quality, and the need to measure the success of the educational programs in behavioral terms.

Note

1. The internal consultant for this project wishes to remain anonymous.

Compliance With Discussions and Documentation
of Advance Directives in a Home Care Agency[1]

◆

This case dealt with compliance regarding Advance Directives (ADs) on the part of nurses engaged in home health care. The issue of ADs and how to present them is still the subject of widespread dissatisfaction.

Proving the Problem

Background, Importance, Relevant
Steps, and Operational Definitions

Kim, a registered nurse at a certified home health care agency, worked as part of a team of 14 nurse coordinators. Each nurse coordinated and administered care to about 30 patients and supervised the home health aides. Kim was concerned about the extent to which patients had discussions with nurses about ADs and whether patients' records documented their choices.

An *Advance Directive* is a legal statement by the patient indicating treatment wishes in the event the patient becomes incapacitated. An AD may be a health care proxy, a living will, and/or a consent to or request for a "do-not-resuscitate" (DNR) order conveying the patient's preferences.

A *health care proxy* or similar document, or a form of durable power of attorney, delegates another adult as *health care agent*, with the authority to make health care decisions on behalf of the individual signing if

274

that individual becomes incapable of making his or her own health care decisions.

A *living will* is a document that contains specific instructions concerning an individual's wishes about the type of health care choices and treatments he or she does or does not want to receive. It does not designate an agent to make such decisions.

A *DNR order* is a document in which the individual consents to or requests not to be resuscitated under specific conditions. Under such an order, health care providers are told not to attempt cardiopulmonary resuscitation in the event the person suffers cardiac or respiratory arrest. This request can be part of a health care proxy or a living will, or it can stand alone.

The federal government and the State of New York require that certain procedures regarding patient health care decision making be carried out to ensure each adult patient's right to participate in decision making about his or her health care and to prevent discrimination based on whether the patient has or has not executed an AD. The JCAHO considers ADs to be a patients' rights issue. The laws require hospitals, nursing homes, hospices, home health agencies, and other home care facilities to provide information to their patients regarding each patient's right to direct treatment and execute an AD. The organization is also required to ask each adult patient whether or not he or she has an AD. As a result, home health agencies generally adopt specific procedures. In this case, Kim's agency required that

1. As part of admission procedures (when the case is opened), each adult patient must be given a specified kit containing information about ADs, including models and forms. The patient has the option of asking that the material be given to the health care agent, a family member, or a primary caregiver.

2. Each patient or selected surrogate must be asked if the person has an AD; the response must be documented in the medical record.

3. If the patient has an AD, this must appear on the patient's Kardex file and must include name, telephone number, and other information about any designated health care agent. [A stamp had been created that listed the three ADs, with a place to circle the decision, yes or no; to show when copies were received or the AD revoked; proxy information; and the date of the initial entry.]

4. The nurse must request a copy of any AD and incorporate it into the medical orders section of the patient's medical record.

5. If the patient has a DNR order, the nurse must notify a coordinator, who must then apply a red stick-on dot to the front of the patient's chart.
6. If the patient does not have an AD, the nurse discussing this with the patient is to refer the patient to the information provided.

Other details were related to changes in ADs, how to execute DNR orders, the point at which ADs take effect, and how to deal with the situation at such time as the orders become applicable as specified.

The Problem

Kim thought that, to carry out the spirit of number 6 in the above standards, nurses should *discuss* the ADs with patients, not just leave the material, and explain that patients could opt to not have a proxy or a living will placed in the chart. Kim believed that not all nurses were discussing ADs with their patients or a responsible person on the initial visit; that when an AD was chosen, a copy was not always put in the chart; and that the red dot for DNR orders was not always on the record.

The Client

The agency's regional administrator approved Kim's use of time to conduct the study; she and the director of quality assurance, the clients, allowed Kim to solicit the help of staff to collect data. Because the questions were of continuing concern, the clients looked forward to seeing the results.

Observation Units, Normal Loads, Quantities, and Time Frame

For the proof-of-problem data, which would cover whether ADs were being discussed and to see if existing ADs were properly present and documented in the patients' charts, Kim obtained retrospective and concurrent data from the nurse coordinators in her team. Each supplied 15 patient charts, which produced 205 usable records. Each nurse coordinator selected 15 charts with the most recent admission dates, starting from when the project began and going backwards in time until 15 charts were selected. The period of time allowed for documentation of ADs was a minimum of 21 days after intake; this was allowed for a patient with an admission date that coincided with the start of the project and ended with the end of data collection. All nurses had until the end of data collection, so they had increasingly longer times depending on patients' intake dates.

Kim reviewed charted progress notes and the stamped form to ascertain whether discussions took place, reviewed initial and ongoing orders to check DNR status, checked Kardex files, and inspected the front of charts to see if red dots were there for patients who selected DNR orders. Kim collected staff data for 51 nurses, including the nurse coordinators, who worked with the 205 patients at some time during the study.

Criteria to Prove the Problem

The clients agreed to five indicators and criteria to prove the problems.

1. At least 95% of patients had to have *had discussions about Advance Directives.* This applied to all three types of ADs, as they were all discussed together.
2. At least 95% of patients who chose a *proxy* had to have *documention* in their charts. Proxy documentation included either the actual proxy or an indication of who the proxy was and how to reach him or her.
3. At least 80% of patients who chose a *living will* had to have *documentation* in their charts. (The patient had the option of not providing a copy of the proxy and living will; the living will was often held by lawyers.)
4. No less than 100% of patients who chose *DNR orders* had to have *documentation* in their charts.
5. No less than 100% of patients who chose *DNR orders* had to have charts with *red dots* affixed to the cover.

Results

Table C11.1 indicates that the criterion to prove inadequate discussion was met. Only 38% of the cases had evidence of discussion. All four criteria to prove the documentation problem were also met. Only 31% of the 16 who chose proxies had copies in their charts, only 17% of the 12 who chose living wills had copies in their charts, and only 17% (one) of the 6 who chose DNR orders had a copy in the chart. Most shocking was the fact that none of the 6 who chose DNR orders had a

Table C11.1 Criteria for Proof of Problem and Results: Advance
Directives

Measure	Point Beyond Which Problem Exists (Percentage, Rate, etc)	OKed	Actual Results		Source
Percentage of 205 patients with whom a discussion of Advance Directives was held					
Proxy	< 95.0%	x	38.0%	Proved	Table 1.3
Living will	< 95.0%	x	38.0%	Proved	Table 1.4
DNR	< 95.0%	x	38.0%	Proved	Table 1.5
Percentage of patients who chose an Advance Directive and had the document in the chart[a]					
Proxy[b] (of 16)	< 95.0%	x	31.3%	Proved	Table 1.3
Living Will[c] (of 12)	< 80.0%	x	16.7%	Proved	Table 1.4
DNR (of 6)	< 100.0%	x	16.7%	Proved	Table 1.5
Percentage of patients who chose DNR whose charts had a red star (of 6)	< 100.0%	x	0.0	Proved	Table 1.5

a. Due to the nature of the project, *in the chart* means in the chart by the end of data collection, which
gave 21 days or more, depending on the intake date.
b. The proxy documentation includes either the actual proxy or an indication of who the proxy is
andhow to reach him or her.
c. For the living will, it is up to the patient to supply the document for the chart.

red dot affixed to the front of their charts. The clients were convinced
and were anxious to start correcting the situation.

Identifying Causes

Final List of Possible Causes and Research Design

Kim had separate lists of possible causes for inadequate discussion
of ADs and inadequate documentation, although there were major
overlaps. Kim found a great many causes in the literature that stressed
subjective factors on the part of patients. Staff, on the other hand,
stressed inadequate preparation of staff as well as patient resistance.
Kim therefore included objective, subjective, and institutional factors.
Figure C11.1 shows the possible causes side by side, so the overlaps or

Lack of Discussion	*Lack of Documentation in Charts*

Objective Factors

1. Language barrier	1. Language barrier
2. *Specific staff*	2. *Specific staff*
3. Specific job title (coordinator or staff nurse)	3. Specific job title (coordinator or staff nurse)
4. Staff member's years with agency	4. Staff member's years with agency
5. Staff member's level of education	5. Staff member's level of education
6. Whether patient had a terminal condition	6. Patient does not want the documents in the chart
7. Patient refused to have discussion	7. *Patient doesn't have the documents*
8. *Patient is incompetent, requiring nurse to get in touch with surrogate; that was too difficult* (Staff response; not objective data)	8. Family/friends or others dissuaded or delayed the patient
	9. Patient has no one to be proxy
	10. *Nurse did not follow up*

Subjective Factors

9. *Nurse thinks the physician should be the one to do the discussion*	11. *Nurse thinks the physician should be the one to get the documents*
10. Nurse does not understand material	12. Nurse does not understand material
11. Nurse believes patient does not understand material	13. *Nurse believes patient does not understand material*
12. Nurse does not know of the policy on discussion	14. *Nurse does not know of the policy on documentation*
13. *Nurse believes orientation is lacking or inadequate*	15. Nurse believes orientation is lacking or inadequate
14. *Nurse believes it is too much work*	16. *Nurse believes it is too much work*
15. *Nurse thinks discussion is not important*	17. Nurse thinks documentation is not important
16. Nurse does not believe in Advance Directives	18. Nurse does not believe in Advance Directives
17. Nurse believes coordinator should be the one to do the discussion	19. Nurse believes coordinator should be the one to document
18. *Nurse does not feel accountable for having the discussion*	20. *Nurse does not feel accountable for documentation*
19. *Nurse believes policy on discussion is unclear*	21. Patient feels confused by the documents
20. Nurse thinks choices will result in worse or less care	22. *Patient does not know what he or she wants in document*
21. *Nurse thinks the intake day is not the time to have discussion*	23. *Patient feels it is too early for death-related decisions*
22. Nurse believes it negatively affects patients' morale	24. Patient believes superstition that it will hasten death
23. Nurse believes it delays recovery	
24. *Nurse feels uncomfortable with topic*	*(continued)*

Figure C11.1 Possible and Proved Causes for Problems With Advance Directives

Lack of Discussion	Lack of Documentation in Charts
Institutional Factors	
25. No defined policy on discussion	25. No defined policy on documentation
26. *Unclear standards about discussion in manuals*	26. *Unclear standards about documentation in manuals*
27. *Performance on discussions not part of staff evaluation*	27. *Performance on documentation not part of staff evaluation*
28. *Materials not in appropriate languages*[a]	28. *Materials not in appropriate languages*[a]
29. *Supervisors do not hold staff accountable or provide feedback*	29. *Supervisors do not hold staff accountable or provide feedback*
30. *Lack of communication on policy from central office*	30. *Lack of communication on policy from central office*
31. *Lack of systematic organization to ensure discussion* (agreed to by management, not supervisors)	31. Lack of systematic organization to ensure documentation
	32. Documentation method or forms nonexistent
	33. *Documentation method or forms judged too complex by professionals*

NOTE: Causes in italics were proved or partly proved as actual causes.
a. The materials were only in English; this was an issue for only three patients in the sample.

Figure C11.1 Possible and Proved Causes for Problems With Advance Directives (Continued)

counterpart wording is evident. There were 31 possible causes for lack of discussion and 33 for lack of charting.

Objective, patient-related data on the causes for lack of discussion were available for the 205 patients, but to deal with subjective patient-related causes for lack of discussions and lack of documentation of ADs chosen by patient, too few patients had discussions to evaluate and fewer chose ADs, making the study of documentation impossible.

Kim needed interviews with patients who had had the opportunity for discussion, and she decided on a sample of 30 patients to get an idea of possible deterrents. She enlisted the nurses to comply with AD discussions and to conduct structured interviews with 30 new patients who were not part of the original 205. As the purpose was to get data on patients' attitudes towards the ADs, it was important to have respondents who were exposed to the discussions as intended on intake so that they could respond knowledgeably to the questions about the discussions and charting the documents. The sample size was limited to 30 because it was necessary to work with new admissions, and time was running out.

Kim designed a staff survey and a patient interview protocol. To avoid contamination of the staff data, she administered the nurses' questionnaire before asking them to comply with discussions and interview new patients. The staff questionnaire was completed by the 14 team members and an additional 6 nurses who had at least two patients in the study, for a total of 20 nurses. The questionnaire explained the purpose of the study and explained that confidentiality would be guaranteed. Answers were *True, False,* and *Don't Know.*

1. In this organization, nurses are expected to talk to new home care patients about Advance Directives (AD) on the first intake day.
2. In this organization, after a patient chooses to have a proxy, nurses are responsible for seeing that the information about who the proxy *is* is in the patient's chart.
3. In this organization, after a patient chooses to have a living will, nurses are responsible for seeing that the living will is in the patient's chart.
4. In this organization, if a patient chooses DNR orders, the orders must be in the patient's chart.
5. In this organization, if a patient chooses DNR orders, the chart must have a red stick-on star or dot.
6. I received adequate orientation about how to handle ADs.
7. I do not handle ADs.
8. I do not believe in ADs.
9. I do not handle ADs on the first intake day.
10. I find the AD material too hard to understand.
11. When a patient is incompetent, it is too hard to find a surrogate with whom to discuss ADs.
12. I do not consider it good for patients' morale to discuss ADs.
13. I think that the AD material is too difficult for the patients to be able to deal with.
14. I think that the AD discussion delays the patients' recovery.
15. I am afraid that AD orders lead to less care being given to the patient.
16. Doctors are really the ones who should discuss the ADs.
17. The primary coordinators are the ones who should discuss ADs, regardless of whether a primary coordinator is the intake nurse.
18. ADs should not be discussed on the intake day.
19. This organization's policy on ADs is unclear to me.

20. Nurses work too hard to also have to deal with ADs.

21. ADs are not of major importance when compared with all the other things that nurses have to do.

22. It is personally too hard for me to deal with ADs.

23. I do not believe that the organization really expects me to deal with the ADs because they do not follow up on it or give me feedback on it.

24. In my experience, there is no really organized way in which ADs are supposed to be handled or followed up; not enough communication on this.

25. I received adequate orientation about how to handle AD documents in patients' charts.

26. The documents used for ADs are not all available for me to give to the patients.

27. I have not seen the red stick-on stars or dots with which to mark charts of patients who choose DNR orders.

28. I think that the AD material is too difficult for me to use to help the patients get ADs executed.

29. I think that the AD material is too difficult for the patients to use to get the documents they want.

30. Doctors are really the ones who should make sure that, if a patient wants ADs, the documents are charted.

31. The primary coordinators are the ones who should make sure that, if a patient wants ADs, the documents are charted.

32. If a patient chooses an AD, it is unclear to me whether I have to be sure the document gets into the patient's chart.

33. Nurses work too hard to also have to deal with getting AD documents into patient's charts.

34. Getting AD documents into patients' charts is not of major importance, given everything else nurses do.

35. I do not believe that the organization really expects me to deal with getting ADs into patients' charts because there is no follow-up or feedback about it.

36. In my experience, there is no really organized way in which ADs are supposed to be charted or followed up; not enough communication about this.

To determine whether *refusal* of the Advanced Directive discussion was a cause, any patients who refused the discussion while being approached were included, increasing the respondents until 30 interviewed patients were represented. Only one patient refused during the attempts to interview, bringing the total to 31. Among the 30, 4 had a terminal disease, 3 were not competent and required discussion with a surrogate, and none had a language barrier. The technique was face-to-face interviews, with nurses filling out a prepared questionnaire. The nurses first filled in basic data checks such as

1. Ask the patient: "Did you discuss Advance Directives on the intake day?"
2. Ascertain: Did the patient agree to have the discussion?
3. Ask the patient: "Before our last visit, had anyone talked to you about proxy, living will, and do-not-resuscitate orders?"
   If "yes," a. Who? b. Where? c. How long ago?

The nurses were asked to help patients understand that no names would be reported and that the purpose of the questions was to give them a chance to express their opinions with *yes, no,* or *don't know* answers as follows:

4. Did you find our talk about proxies, the living will, and orders about "do not resuscitate" confusing?
5. Did you find it OK to discuss these things on your first day?
6. Would you have preferred to wait a few days?
7. Do you feel ready to make these decisions?
8. Do you have the documents you need to get a proxy? To make a living will?
9. Do you have someone to ask to be your proxy?
10. Would you want your proxy in your chart?
11. Would you want your living will in your chart?
12. Did you find our talk about proxies, the living will, and orders about "do not resuscitate" upsetting?
13. Did you think that it would affect your care in a bad way?
14. Were you afraid that
    a. You wouldn't be able to change your mind?
    b. Your life would not be protected as much?
    c. It could bring on the worst?
    d. Anything else?
15. Did you think that your doctor, rather than I, should have been the one to talk about these things with you?
16. Did you know whether you wanted a person as your health proxy?
17. Did you know whether you wanted a living will?
18. Did you know how you felt about being resuscitated?

19. Did you change your mind since we last met because of talking things over with other people?
20. Do you want to tell me anything about the discussion and your decisions?

Criteria to Prove the Causes

There were a large number of possible causes, but only a few models were needed to select criteria to prove them. For *causes of lack of discussions*, objective cause data for the first set of 205 patients were first divided into two groups: those who had discussions and those who did not. Most criteria required that a given variable, such as language difficulty, must (a) appear more in one group (such as those who did not have the discussion) than the other, (b) be disproportionately distributed in that group, and (c) represent a major portion of that group. For variables represented by one or more items on the staff questionnaire, at least 40% of nurses with the least compliance had to answer questions in support of a cause, and the percentage had to be greater than for nurses with the best compliance. The same criteria applied to causes of *lack of documentation*, which were calculated separately from compliance with discussions. For the patients' interview instrument, which dealt with both problems, at least 30% of the respondents had to answer yes or no in support of the cause, depending on the question.

Results

The results appear in Figure C11.1. Proved and partly proved causes are in italics. Sixteen causes were proved for lack of discussion and 16 for lack of documentation. There were overlaps in 9 variables, of which 5 were institutional causes. Many patient attitudes and beliefs that had been mentioned in the literature were not proved; the results suggested that negative patient beliefs were not as important as has been thought, at least for this population. The proved causes pointed to practical difficulties, primarily ones that could have been cleared up if the initial discussions had been done and the material handled well.

Kim noted that, unlike the expectations about them among staff, patients tended to understand the ADs and were willing to talk about them; patients did not superstitiously read death-creating powers into the ADs.

Solutions

Management set three *feasibility limits* for Kim. No major costs could be incurred, but one-time costs were acceptable; no additional staff could be hired; and Kim could not suggest overutilization of existing staff or managers.

After discussing solutions with staff, and based on the number of causes and the complexity of the problem, Kim and her collaborator felt that she should write a position paper, followed by an integrated program. To that end, Kim came up with three major principles:

I. Staff should have access to policy about ADs and should know that management is serious about carrying it out.

II. Staff should have the opportunity to learn about and explore feelings about ADs discussions and follow-up charting.

III. The ADs were designed to allow patients the right to control their own health care even if incapacitated; although AD compliance is required by law, the informing motive must be the spirit of the ADs. This means that unless patients can have access to knowledge, time to decide, and the means to make informed choices, ADs are a mockery.

To support these principles, Kim suggested the following:

1. The AD policy should be presented in writing to each staff member, with a supply in each manager's office; it should be incorporated into clinical and procedure manuals.

2. Orientation should include policy on AD discussion and charting and should cover ideas and misconceptions about the issues involved. If possible, role-playing the patient trying to discuss and carry out the steps after choosing the three directives should be part of orientation.

3. Every 6 months, staff should be involved in group refresher training and discussion, including updating on new developments in the field.

4. Scheduling should take account of the time needed to have the discussions with patients and also with family members who need to be involved.

5. Supervisors should routinely pay attention to whether AD discussions are being held and whether documents are in the charts; record keeping on RN performance should make it possible to discuss AD compliance as part of staff evaluation, which should now cover AD compliance. This would include random checking of the charts of coordinators and intake nurses; follow-up memos would be problem solving in tone rather than accusative.

6. Management should assess the languages in which the documents are needed and arrange to obtain the appropriate language versions. The AD literature should also have the telephone number appended for audio tapes that can be selected by phone according to language; volunteers should be available to connect people with rotary phones or to help staff who need language help in the initial discussion.

7. Management should replace the red stick-on dot requirement with a red ink designation or stamp, which is much safer. When the patient selects DNR, the RN should write the order for submission to the MD, and must inform the business staff in an approved, standardized manner. These clerical personnel must be responsible for marking the chart in the designated way in red. They must be provided with inservice on this to be sure that they understand the how and why of it. Staff supervisors should check on compliance and provide feedback. In the instructions to staff, it should be noted that the new red designation (stamp) is to be placed wherever the red stick-on was originally designated and as described above.

8. As long as current policy is in place, intake nurses will be responsible for AD discussions on intake day, but the coordinators must be responsible for follow-up on the patient's being comfortable with decisions and seeing to charting the documents, particularly DNR and appropriate information on living will and proxy.

9. Staff meetings should deal with the content of this report and the steps to be taken by management among those offered above. This will show willingness to help but also hold staff accountable. Prior to this a specialist should help design a program to allow staff to explore their own feelings. The historic relationship of AD to patients' rights and issues of ethics should be discussed so that staff can feel part of an ongoing development and movement in health care.

10. Current staff should be given the opportunity to take the new orientation on ADs.

11. The new steps should be discussed with staff, and input to improve the steps should be encouraged.

12. Management should agree to allow meetings to discuss the options of having AD discussions on the day or session after intake or after rapport is established. The question of whether any of these ideas are

viable should be explored; if none of the ideas are viable, staff should be able to see why not.

13. Patients should not be rushed into decisions for or against ADs until they feel comfortable and informed.

14. The nurses must feel responsible for allowing time for discussions and following up later, or for arranging to talk with family members, rather than just leaving the material. This requires sensitivity training as part of the orientation described above.

15. Specialized volunteers should be trained and be on call to follow up on discussions with patients who cannot decide on the first day. RNs should be asked to record the status of AD discussions in the chart so follow-up can be monitored. This should include obtaining AD documents for patients who want them. The phone-in tapes should be able to answer many of the questions patients might raise. The volunteers might help to reach the surrogates who are hard to get hold of.

16. Patients who wish to discuss ADs with their physicians should be able to do so by having RNs write an order for this.

This plan has yet to be fully carried out, but the staff involved in Kim's team have been more careful to carry out discussions about ADs and to follow up with documentation. They are more attuned to the spirit as well as the letter of the policy and its intentions. There will be renewed effort in this area in coming years.

Note

1. The internal consultant for this project wishes to remain anonymous.

Case 12

Use of a Reminder Letter to Encourage Follow-Up Visits[1]

This case dealt with the problem of patient noncompliance, well known in the literature. A reminder letter solution had already been selected, but the internal consultant attempted to verify the extent of the problem and other risk factors before evaluating the success of the intervention.

Proving the Problem

The Problem

Lee was a clinical nurse in a medical practice office associated with a major voluntary hospital in New York City. The office was a comprehensive ambulatory care facility specializing in breast cancer. Lee worked in one of four collaborative practices that together treated over 800 women per year. Her office was headed by a surgical oncologist; staff included a medical secretary, an office manager, and Lee.

Lee had been concerned about the extent to which patients did not comply with follow-up visits during the postoperative phase of their care for breast cancer, and she was interested in investigating whether reminder letters would help. Lee planned to prove the problem, experimentally evaluate the use of a reminder letter as an intervention, and explore the significance of other risk factors obtainable through office records. This meant that risk factors would be studied along with evaluation of the follow-up letter.

The Client

The client was the surgical oncologist in whose office Lee worked, who was very receptive to the idea of the project. Lee also obtained the approval of the director of ambulatory care practices and the director of nursing research at the hospital center so that she would have access to chart data and eventually be able to ask for approval to make the solution operational.

Importance

After a woman is treated surgically for breast cancer, postsurgical follow-up visits are considered essential. In addition to the danger of recurrence, there are emotional, medical, and psychological after-effects to deal with and options to consider at various points. Follow-up appointments are recommended every 3 months for the first 2 years following surgery, every 6 months for the next 3 years, and once a year from then on.

The literature indicates relatively low rates of follow-up visits. Noncompliance rates for cancer patients appear to range from 19% to 50%, depending on the study. There are few predictors. Follow-up compliance has generally been found to be influenced by the atmosphere in the clinical setting, whether the patient's condition continues to be serious, and whether patients are reminded of their next appointment. There have been good results with nurse-initiated reminder letters, especially when the probability of missed appointments is above 20%. Many dental and gynecological practices routinely contract with agencies that provide a reminder service. Some sources consider it a patient's right to be reinforced about the need for continuing examinations. All this suggested the value of evaluating the reminder intervention.

Research Design to Prove the Problem

The retrospective database to prove the problem was chart records on the postoperative visits of 100 cancer patients with surgical dates from January through October of the prior year. The due dates for follow-up visits ranged from April of the prior year to July of the current year, covering the 3-month, 6-month, and 9-month visits. Lee defined noncompliance operationally as not calling for an appointment more than 4 weeks after the actual date for the visit.

A single data collection instrument for the retrospective study included all the data needed to prove the problem for the three visit periods. Arrayed by project ID numbers for 100 patients, the table showed the dates of surgery and had three banks of data for the three visit periods. Each bank had a column to show the due date, the date of the actual visit, and whether the patient did or did not arrive within 4 weeks. Due dates were adjusted to the date of the previous visit.

Criteria to Prove the Problem

The problem indicator was the percentage of patients out of all those who were due to call for appointments who still had not called more than 4 weeks after the due date. The criteria to prove the problem for the 3-, 6-, and 9-month visits were set respectively at more than 4%, more than 3%, and more than 5% noncompliance; these criteria were approved by the clients.

Results

The results proved the problem. Noncompliance reached 22% and 29% respectively for the 3- and 9-month visits and an alarming 46% for the 6-month visit. This reinforced Lee's original decision to evaluate the follow-up letter with patients due for the 6-month visit. The severity of the problem for the 6-month visit was new information for the clients, who were not aware of the great differences among the visit periods.

Identifying Risk Factors

Final List of Possible Risk Factors

Lee wanted to know whether there were factors easily determined from office records that could predict compliance. She investigated the relationship between compliance and eight risk factor groupings:

1. Receipt of the reminder letter as an intervention
2. Marital status (single, married, divorced, widowed)
3. Age (20-29, 30-39, 40-49, 50-59, 60-69, over 69)
4. Number of children under 18 (0, 1, 2, more than 2)
5. Place of residence (Manhattan, the other boroughs of New York City, or outside New York City)
6. Diagnostic category or reasons for the surgery (prophylaxis, intraductal insitu, lobular insitu, infiltrating ductal, infiltrating lobular, Paget's disease, inflammatory breast cancer)
7. Cancer stage (0, I, II, III, IV)
8. Type of surgery (lumpectomy, lumpectomy with axillary node dissection, total mastectomy, modified radical mastectomy without immediate reconstruction, modified radical mastectomy with immediate reconstruction, radical mastectomy)

Research Design

For several reasons, the 6-month visit was chosen to study the predictive effect of a reminder letter and other risk factors. This is a time when the surgical areas are generally healed, enabling the physician to perform a thorough physical examination. At this time, recurrence is most likely. This is also a time to assess shoulder and arm range of motion and reinforce hand and arm protections to prevent lymphedema, a persistent arm and hand swelling. This is when additional tests may be ordered, such as mammography. It is also when patients are likely to begin resuming their work, family, and social lives, which is a partial explanation of why the 6-month follow-up visit had twice the noncompliance rate of the 3-month visit.

The follow-up letter, shown in Figure C12.1, was designed by Lee in collaboration with her client, the oncologist. It was intended to be friendly and personal but to still read as an official letter, with the weight of the physician behind it; it was designed to explain benefits rather than threaten risks, to be more informal than scientific in language, to be in English for the trial, and to be sent on the office's letterhead stationary. This kind of detailed and personal letter is not the type of letter usually sent out by commercial agencies that send reminders.

The field test was successful and inspired comments such as, "Don't you have a system to do this already?" "I am so glad you are doing this; I forget a lot" and "I can't believe you don't do this. My dentist does this."

(On letterhead)

Inside Address   Date

Dear _____ :

It is nearly 6 months since you were treated by Dr. _____ for breast cancer, and
it is now time for your 6-month check-up. The check-up includes a physical
examination of your incision(s), an assessment of your range of motion in the
shoulder and the arm, and a review of the preventive measures to avoid swelling of the arm and hand. Usually, the doctor will suggest some additional tests,
such as mammography.

We invite you to raise any questions you may be having about your care or the
follow-up period at this visit.

Please call Dr. _____ 's office soon to make the appointment; we look forward
to seeing you. The number is (___) ___-___.

Very truly yours,

Dr. _____
and Staff

Figure C12.1 Follow-Up Letter

Data Collection

The database for the experiment with the follow-up letter and to
study risk factors was women whose 6-month visits were due during
the first 6 weeks of the 10 weeks Lee had to conduct the study. The first
6 weeks were used to accumulate patients and collect data. The final 4
weeks were needed to allow the last of the subjects 4 weeks to comply
or be judged noncompliant. Unfortunately, this gave Lee a control
group of only 20 who received no letter and 20 in the experimental
group, who received a reminder letter.

Lee assigned ID numbers to the 40 patients who were due for their
6-month visits by the end of November of the current year in the order
of their surgery. Odd numbers were assigned to the experimental
group; even numbers were assigned to the control group. This equal-
ized the effect of different external factors related to events by date,
such as the announcement in October of the new address of the office.
One patient's date fell just outside the first 6 weeks. The patient still

had not called when data collection ended, but because this was a bit short of the 4 weeks allowed for calling, she was eliminated from the control group, to which she had been assigned, leaving 20 in the experimental group and 19 in the control group.

The experimental group of 20 were sent the reminder letter approximately 2 weeks before they were due for their visits. The control group of 20 received no letter. The office secretary was the chief data gatherer.

The secretary had a master list of the patients being studied. As patients called for appointments, she checked to see if the patient was in one of the two groups. If she was, the secretary filled in the information called for by asking two questions: "Did you receive a letter reminding you that you are due for a check-up visit?" If the answer was yes, the secretary asked, "Would you have called without the letter?"

The data collection form had columns to note if any letter was returned and not delivered (none were), the dates of the appointments and calls, comments, and a choice of *would have, would not have,* and *maybe* for answers to the second question. (If any patients in the experimental group had called and said that they did not receive the letter, they would have been counted as in the control group.) There were 26 calls; 17 had received letters, and of those, 14 said they would not have called without the letter.

The summary data showed that the noncompliance rate was 15% for the experimental group and 53% for the control group. Of the compliant, experimental patients (70% of the experimental group), 82% said that they were affected by the letter.

Lee assigned patients to 5 ranks:

Rank 1: Each experimental patient who called and said that the letter made a difference.
Rank 2: Each experimental patient who called but did not say the letter made a difference.
Rank 3: Each control patient who called.
Rank 4: Each control patient who did not call.
Rank 5: Each experimental patient who did not call.

The ranks were assigned so that data could be studied by compliance characteristics as well as, and in combination with, experimental or control status. Ranks 1, 2, and 3 covered compliant patients.

Lee arrayed the risk factor data for the 39 patients by rank. For each multicategory risk factor group, Lee calculated the distribution across the 39 in the study (such as 20 received the letter and 19 did not; 51.3% and 48.7%, respectively). She did the same for the compliant group (ranks 1, 2, and 3) and the noncompliant group (ranks 4 and 5). Among compliants, 17 received the letter and 9 did not (65.4% and 34.6%). Among noncompliants, 3 received the letter and 10 did not (23.1% and 76.9). Proportionality for a category was calculated as its percentage share of the rank group minus its percentage share of the total. For example, receiving the letter was disproportionately represented in the compliant group (65.4% minus 51.3%, or 14.1 percentage points); not receiving the letter was disproportionately represented in the noncompliant group (76.9% minus 48.7%, or 28.2 percentage points).

Criteria to Prove the Risk Factors

If a category's percentage share of the compliant or noncompliant ranks minus its percentage share of the total was *positive* or *negative* by more than 10 percentage points for one of the compliance groups and not the other, the category was considered a possible risk factor. It was then subjected to more rigorous statistical tests such as correlation analysis, *t* test, and stepwise multiple regression analysis. The factors warranting further study were

1. Receiving the letter
2. Being married
3. Being widowed
4. Age
5. Living near the office (Manhattan)
6. A diagnosis of infiltrating ductal cancer

The second-level criteria were a coefficient of correlation above .3 and significant at the .05 level or better and/or *t*-test results significant at .05 or better, and/or inclusion in a stepwise multiple regression equation to explain compliance.

Results

Only two coefficients of correlation were more than ±.3 and significant; they were *receipt of the letter* (.399), a positive factor for compliance, and *being widowed* (−.378), a risk factor. The *t* tests for these two variables were the only ones significant at the .05 level or better, and these were the only variables included in a multiple regression equation, which reached an *r* of .499, significant at .006. These were the only factors considered proved. Being married was weakly related to compliance, a positive factor, with an *r* of .290 and *t*-test significance at .073.

Compliance appeared to be most affected by the follow-up letter. Lee had hoped to explain noncompliance by other factors easy to identify from office data, but the only risk factor to emerge was being widowed. Neither factor was able to explain more than 14% to 16% of the variation, and together in a stepwise regression equation no more than 25% of the variation.

Because one patient equals 5% in a sample of 20 patients, Lee realized that it would be well worth following this study with a long-term investigation involving larger numbers of patients, with a variety of follow-up visit periods, and with personal interviews and tracking.

A Solution

Feasibility Limits

Lee was told that, to be made operational, a reminder letter would have to be adopted by the entire Division of Ambulatory Care Practices because the manual search for patients and their due dates was burdensome to implement even with only the 6-month visit. An administrative decision would involve all the follow-up visits. The feasibility limits reflected the fact that the solution would have to be computerized, at least to note the dates and to print out the names of patients with visits coming up in the next 2 weeks. The limits were that any changes in computer-based files must have Hospital Center approval and that specific office changes be within the operating budget.

Choice of Solutions

Lee suggested that a reminder letter be used throughout the four ambulatory care cancer practices affiliated with the hospital and that a computer program be developed or an existing agency be used that would identify each patient's next appointment and generate a letter 2 weeks before the visit date.

Due dates for visits would be calculated from the date of surgery and updated to account for slippage in arrival dates; returned letters would initiate a search for change of address or would signal a problem. Lee wanted to develop specific letters for the 3-month and 9-month visits because they have unique functions, just as the 6-month visit does, with a generic letter for all later visits. She preferred that staff activate the computer and have the in-house capability of stamping and sending the letters, but she recognized that the letter might be put in the hands of a commercial agency. Lee believed that staff would be more sensitive and alert to errors in the system than a commercial agency.

Lee wanted to consider the possibility of paying special attention to the needs of widowed women by providing information or counseling about support systems. Because the hospital already sponsored support groups, Lee thought that the physician or nurse could have discussions about these with the patients.

Implementing Solutions and Making Them Operational

Evaluation

The follow-up letter was evaluated separately as a solution and as a positive factor. To be judged a success, the 6-month noncompliance rate of the experimental group had to be lower than that for the 100-patient chart study sample and lower than that for the control group, both by at least 20 percentage points. Anything less would not justify implementation.

Results

The criteria were met. The letter accounted for a noncompliance rate of 15%. It was 31 percentage points less than the 100-patient sample and 38 points less than the control group. The letter was judged a success even though it did not wipe out the problem entirely.

Unfortunately, at the time Lee completed her study, return visit compliance was not a high priority for the hospital. However, after 2 years, administrators came back to Lee to examine her results again and to reconsider a reminder letter and other suggestions. Other organizations were increasingly using outcome indicators for ambulatory care, including the use of reminder letters.

Note

1. Anne M. Walsh was the internal consultant for this project.

Use of an Internal Audit in an Intermediate Care Facility[1]

In this case, an existing internal quality assurance audit was evaluated. The analysis of the data resulted in the design of a new one, and the new audit was evaluated.

Proving the Problem

Max was the residence director in an intermediate care facility (ICF) that provided services to mentally retarded and developmentally disabled adults. ICF facilities provide a range of services, including medical, social, recreational, clinical, and nutritional care and help in daily living needs. Residence staff provide 24-hour coverage in three shifts.

The Problem

Max's agency managed 14 ICF residences. To help ensure that each residence house met standards and complied with state regulations, the organization had developed an internal auditing process that it administered about 3 months before each scheduled external state audit. Max believed that the internal audit was not properly identifying citable problems and was therefore not functioning to minimize citations for the agency's residence houses. He proposed to prove that and to design a new one that would be more sensitive.

Quality audits are conducted by state authorities at least once each year to ensure the quality and safety of the services provided. The audits evaluate residences for specific aspects of quality. The standards, referred to as "483 Tag Numbers," are numbered guidelines that describe the content of regulations and citable situations to be evaluated during a site visit. They begin with the prefix 483 and cover client protections, facility staffing, active treatment services, client behavior and facility practices, health care services, physical environment, and dietetic and nutritional services. Site visitors look for violations or omissions, which are cited under the specified tag numbers and are reported in a "Statement of Deficiencies," which must be responded to by the residence with a plan and targeted dates for correction.

The Client

The client was the agency's quality assurance specialist; he directly supervised most of the residence directors. He decided that the project was sufficiently important to appoint Max to the quality assurance team that assisted in internal audits.

Importance

Citations mean that the residents of a facility are not receiving proper care or protection. Having to wait for an external audit to find violations means that residents have to wait longer to have their care or protection improved, and accumulation of citations threatens decertification of the facility. Moreover, waiting for external audits is passive. A good internal audit can be a proactive influence with regard to overall functioning and can stimulate facilities to provide optimal care. It can mean continuous quality improvement rather than just quality compliance.

Relevant Steps, Observation Units, Normal Loads, Quantities, and Time Frame

Max decided to study the audits of the 2 prior years. Because there were massive numbers of regulations to deal with, Max decided to study *Client Protections* and *Health Care Services* because they represent a large part of the citations of an established facility and reflect day-to-day operations and the health concerns of the residents. To demonstrate that citations were a problem, to identify the residences in which they occurred, and to pinpoint the nature of the violations, Max designed tables to describe the residences, identify the citations over 2 years, and evaluate the experiences of the residences. The descriptive information about the residences permitted Max to decide which residences and tag numbers to study.

Max listed the tag numbers and categories covered by Client Protections and Health Care Services. Client Protections was covered by tag numbers 122 to 157; Health Care Services by tag numbers 319 to 405. Of the 123 tag numbers involved, Max identified 107 that applied to facilities in his agency. These became the master list he used to tabulate the tag numbers that were cited. Thirteen tag numbers were cited in the 2-year period: one under Client Protections and 12 under Health Care Services, with a total of 35. The tags with the greatest share of citations were number 130: Ensure privacy in treatment and personal needs; 324: Provide immunizations; 325: Routine screening laboratory examinations; and 336: Ensure that nursing reviews take place quarterly.

Each of the 14 residences housed from 4 to 18 residents, with a total of 142 residents. Five of the residences had no citations. Three residences with the highest citations per resident were identified. Max now had enough information to decide which tag numbers and which residences to study. To study the predictive nature of the old internal audit, Max studied all 35 citations in the nine residences with citations. To design a new audit instrument, Max considered all 107 tag numbers, with attention to the 35 citations. Max hoped to consult all the residences to obtain inputs and suggestions from staff, but he gave priority to the three problem locations.

The next step was to examine whether the existing internal audit could pick up violations before they were cited. Max created a table listing the 35 citations by tag number, residence, and abbreviated category content, with columns to organize the data into six diagnostic categories:

1. The tag number and audit question, if there was one that applied
2. Evidence that a relevant audit question applied to the citation

3. Whether no question applied to the citation
4. If a question applied, could the answer spot the problem cited?
5. If a question applied, *did* the answer spot the problem cited?
6. If a question applied, was it too unclear or unspecific to spot the problem?

As an example, tag number 130 in Residence 1 applied to privacy in treatment and personal needs. The audit question was "Do clients have privacy during treatment and care of personal needs?" The actual citation was that four residents' bedrooms had clear, see-through panels on the doors. Max judged that the audit question was not specific enough to pick up the violation.

Tag number 322 in Residence 8 applied to preventive and general care and annual physical examinations. The audit question was "Do clients receive preventive and general medical care as well as an annual physical?" The actual citation was that medical appointments were not made. Max judged that the audit question could predict the violation. In fact, it did not.

Criteria to Prove the Problem

The first problem to be proved was whether there were too many citations. The indicators and criteria were (a) more than 28 citations for the agency's residences in the 2-year period, (b) citations per resident more than 0.2 for the 2 years, and (c) more than zero residences with citations per resident above 0.2.

The second problem was whether the internal audit could pick up the citations actually made over the 2-year period. The problem would be proved if more than 10% of the 35 citations were not covered by audit questions. For citations covered by audit questions, there would be a problem if less than 90% were worded so they could predict the citations, if less than 85% of the citations were predicted, and if more than 10% had questions not specific enough or too unclear to predict the citations.

A third problem would be proved if more than 10% of the citations showed no evidence that their content was subjected to internal audit even though there were audit questions available for use.

Results

Excessive citations was proved. There were 35 citations (more than 28); citations per resident averaged 0.23 (a bit more than 0.20), and 4 residences exceeded the 0.2 maximum allowable rate (more than 0). Max had thought that clients' functional levels might influence citation rates, but the data showed that higher-level functioning residents were in the two highest and three lowest-rated residences.

The inability of the internal audit to pick up citations was proved. Seventeen percent (more than 10%) of the 35 citations were not covered by audit questions. Only 48% of citations covered by audit questions were worded so they could predict the citations (less than 90%). None of the citations were predicted, and 52% had questions not specific enough or too unclear to predict the citations (more than 10%).

There were no questions for 6 citations and questions that could have predicted the citations for 14. Of the 29 citations that had applicable questions, 15 had questions that were not specific enough or unclear. Max also found that some audit questions had incorrect tag numbers or were incorrectly worded with respect to their counterpart tag numbers.

There was evidence that no internal audit was applied in 48% of the citations (more than 10%), even though there were audit questions available. The audit was not always used in the three problem residences.

Causes

To design a new internal audit as a solution, Max examined the characteristics of the 35 citations. He tried to create descriptive phrases for the citations that he could quantify and attribute to general causes. This would tell him what an internal audit had to address. Max listed each of the 35 citations by tag number, residence code, a summary of the language of the tag number, and a summary of the language of the citation. Max attempted to apply a consistent set of descriptive phrases explaining what had gone wrong that could be listed under (a) wrong or missing aspects of documentation, (b) staff problems, or (c) the institution.

If the cause was *documentation*, it implied that the item was wrong or missing in client charts but that a policy was in place. *Staff problems* implied *staff error in carrying out duties* or *duties not carried out (missing)*. If the cause was *the institution*, it implied that the institution had *wrong policy* or that *the needed policy was not in existence (missing)*.

The analysis showed that missing staff actions accounted for 60% of the citations, followed by staff error (14%), missing policy (11%), and missing documentation (9%).

Max determined that the existing audit instrument had questions for only 22 tag numbers among the 107 that were applicable under Client Protections and Health Care Services and that most were just a rewording of the regulation in question format. They were also confusing, because compliance responses were sometimes yes and sometimes no, depending on the wording.

A Solution

Max decided to examine all the relevant 107 regulations under the tag numbers and categories covered by Client Protections and Health Care Services and to select those for the new audit that would benefit the clients and the institution. As Max was undertaking a new audit for Client Protections and Health Care Services, he decided to take special notice of tag numbers that reflected issues of client independence because it was becoming an important issue among residential programs, and he hoped to anticipate new directions in internal auditing in the field of mental retardation. About 28 tag numbers dealt with independence issues such as self-medication, access to keys, participation in social or religious activities, and exercise of rights as United States citizens.

Max also decided to eliminate tag numbers dealt with elsewhere in the audit system, to group tag numbers that overlapped in content, to break up tag numbers into components when several separate activities were involved, and to have the answer *yes* always indicate compliance with regulations.

The questions Max and others in the residences developed for the new instrument took the 35 citations and issues of independence into account. The product was both generic and agency specific. The style created could easily be applied to additional tag numbers, and existing questions could be revised easily, making the instrument flexible.

Figure C13.1 presents excerpts from the new audit. It opens with a rationale and instructions for its use, including advice on how to deal with questions that do not apply to the agency's clients. Tag content is described with questions that help to determine whether there is compliance with the regulations. The first part of the instrument asks general questions that refer to residential issues such as staff training, the structure of the facility, infection control, and some issues of independence. The second part is client specific. Spaces are available to list 18 residents by initial or code number. The auditor is asked to review clients' records and check *yes* for compliance, *no* for noncompliance, or leave the question blank if clients are not capable of performing the activity.

Implementing Solutions and Making Them Operational

The new audit was jointly created and reviewed by the client, directors, assistant directors, case workers, and a residential counselor. There was a high level of commitment to the instrument, even though its predecessor had not been well accepted. The field test was successfully carried out by an assistant director in one residence; this was someone who had performed several audits with the old instrument.

Evaluation Design

The evaluation design called for the concurrent administration of both the old and the new audit instruments at three residences, with the client and Max working together as an audit team. The data sources were client records and interviews with assistant directors, direct care workers, and residents. On the same day, first the old and then the new audits were administered. The old audit was done first because the larger number of items in the new instrument would be more of a contaminating factor than the other way around.

Dear Colleague,

The following questions have been designed to help prevent citations after auditing by regulatory agencies. The questions are grouped by the type of responses requested, but each also notes the Tag Number involved.

It is recommended that, in the instances where client charts are involved, you review 100% of the charts; we have supplied space for up to 18 clients per facility. When questions refer to clients who can understand or clients who are capable and your clients are not able to understand or are not capable, leave the questions unanswered.

	Yes	No
Tag 122		
Have all staff attended inservice training during the last year on clients' rights?	( )	( )
Tag 127		
Have all staff attended inservice training during the last year on prevention of client abuse?	( )	( )
Tag 128		
Is there evidence that team meetings deal with minimizing use of drugs and no use of restraints?	( )	( )
Tags 129 and 133		
Is there evidence that team meetings deal with providing clients with privacy and private time with individuals of their choice?	( )	( )
Tag 130		
a. Is there a screen for clients during examinations or when without clothing?	( )	( )
b. Are staff aware that the client should close the bathroom door?	( )	( )
c. Are clients who can understand aware that the client should close the bathroom door?	( )	( )
d. Are all doors to bathrooms and bedrooms made so that they cannot be seen through?	( )	( )
e. Is it staff policy to redirect clients when they are engaging inappropriately in intimate behavior?	( )	( )
Tags 134 and 135		
Can clients who are capable receive mail unopened? Can they have private access to a phone?	( )	( )
Tag 144		
Is the turnaround time for writing or returning calls to clients' families and friends less than 2 days?	( )	( )
Tag 327		
Is TB control in the form of adherence to universal infection control techniques and PPD testing for staff and clients done annually?	( )	( )

Tag 123

a. Is there a record in client's chart that the client or correspondent has been informed of rights and house rules?

Client

Yes

No

Figure C13.1 Internal Audit for Intermediate Care Facilities Dealing With Client Protections and Health Care Services (Excerpts)

(continued)

Tag 124
a. Is there evidence that the   Client
   client or correspondent   Yes
   was informed of client's   No
   medical condition,
   treatment, and risks?

Tag 125
a. Is there evidence that the
   client has been encouraged   Yes
   to register to vote, to vote,   No
   and be informed, if capable?

Tag 126
a. Is there evidence that the
   client has been encouraged   Yes
   to and/or does manage own   No
   finances, if capable?

Figure C13.1 Internal Audit for Intermediate Care Facilities Dealing With Client Protections and Health Care Services (Excerpts)

Data Collection

Forty-seven tag numbers were evaluated in three residences with the old and new audits. The data collection forms listed the tag numbers and asked whether the old audit had a question to cover the tag number. If the internal auditors found problems in a residence with any tag number using the old or new audit instruments, the specific tag number was checked off and totalled in appropriate columns. The total citations were entered in a bank of columns for each residence and for the grand total. Additional columns showed how many problems were found with the new audit that matched those found with the old audit and the number of additional problems found with either audit.

Success Criteria

The criteria for the new internal audit's success were that all citable problems found with the old audit had to be found with the new audit and that the new audit had to find additional citable problems. Max had hoped to include that any subsequent external audit would cite problems found by the new audit that were still not corrected when the external audit was conducted, but time did not allow this because the next audit was not yet due.

Results

Summary data indicated that 10 items were found with the old audit and 32 with the new audit. The new audit produced total overlap with items found with the the old audit; 22 additional items were uncovered with the new audit. All the criteria for the new internal audit's success were met.

There was no time to test whether subsequent external state audits cited any problems found by the new audit that were still not corrected, but there was great effort to correct the problems uncovered by the new audit, and that in itself made it valuable.

This seemed to be the beginning of a success story on implementation. However, there was a reorganization of the agency soon after this, and the new management did not implement the new audit, having relegated quality to a relatively low priority. Max left the facility, became the executive director at another agency, and was chosen to help develop a quality assurance instrument for state-monitored facilities.

Note

1. Errol Seltzer was the internal consultant for this project.

Use of Data on Unusual Occurrences
in an Emergency Medical Service[1]

This case is an example of continuous quality improvement. The internal consultant investigated an opportunity to improve service by using data already being collected, and all involved were committed to the idea.

Proving the Problem

The Problem and Client

Nick, the internal consultant, was in charge of staff in the operations office of a large emergency medical service (EMS). He knew that the department accumulated reports, called Unusual Occurrence Reports (UORs), about nonroutine problems in the service, but he had never seen any use made of them to identify trends or patterns of problems or to plan preventive measures. He asked whether he could use the reports to identify and correct preventable problems and was encouraged to proceed by the client, the chief of EMS operations.

UORs are filled out by EMS staff when they encounter situations that interfere with patient care, interefere with the performance of staff duties, or could possibly negatively affect the routine operation of the ambulance service. At the time he began, Nick did not know what characteristics described the bulk of unusual occurrences in the EMS or whether any were serious problems.

Importance

The EMS was constantly under review by the public and other agencies. Because the service is in the business of saving lives, any improvement in operations is of immediate importance for the public and the service itself.

Categories, Observation Units,
Normal Loads, Quantities, and Time Frame

Instead of steps, Nick had to deal with categories of UORs and decide which to select for study. Nick found a bewildering number of institutional categories assigned to UORs. There was a total of 720 UORs for the year Nick studied. The existing categories did not provide sufficient numbers in any category for Nick to select several large enough to study and generalize about. Nick grouped the UORs into 25 categories according to the nature of the occurrence, including whether quality of care was involved and with an *other* category for miscellaneous items. The entire group was arranged under 11 broad categories, as shown in Table C14.1.

Operational Definitions

The first major contribution of the project was Nick's creation of an operational definition of *severity of consequence* for the UORs; it was later adopted by the service. Because he was most concerned about patients, Nick classified UORs as having *major* or *minor* consequences based on the likely severity of consequences for humans, as determined by the service staff.

No distinction about severity of consequences was current in the classifications of the UORs at that time. Nick's definition of *major* was "consequences likely to result in very serious physical harm, permanent damage, or worse." *Minor* applied to "consequences likely to result in less than very serious physical harm." The definitions were simple and proved to be reliable in use.

Table C14.1 Proof of Problem: EMS

| | Limits | | Results | | |
	Number Per Year	Percentage of Major Consequences[a]	Number per Year	Percentage of Major Consequences[a]	Proved
Category					
1. Interference with the provision of care	> 30	> 2%	101	16%	x
2. Inappropriate provision of care	> 5	> 2%	38	18%	x
3. Delay in providing care	> 5	> 2%	44	18%	x
4. Equipment interference with care	> 10	> 2%	86	14%	x
5. Problems with staff members (not care related)	> 18	> 2%	36	0%	
6. Attacks on staff and equipment	> 36	> 2%	128	0%	
7. Care provision problems due to other caregivers	> 10	> 2%	14	7%	x
8. Dangerous conditions for staff	> 5	> 2%	49	10%	x
9. Problems with documentation	> 36	> 2%	118	0%	
10. Prisoner in need of care due to taser (electric shock)	> 6	> 2%	15	67%	x
11. Other	> 36	> 2%	91	8%	x
Total	> 197	> 2%	720	9%	x

SOURCE: Project Table 1.1.
a. Consequences for humans, based on service members' estimation.
  Major = consequences are likely to result in very serious physical harm or permanent damage, or worse.
  Minor = consequences are likely to result in less than very serious physical harm.

Data Collection Instruments

Because the project was to work with existing UORs, the data for the project were already collected. The tables Nick produced were used to group the data and to identify the consequence levels as either major or minor.

Criteria to Prove the Problem

To determine whether problems existed, Nick and the client agreed that the indicators would be expressed in terms of the 11 broad categories and the grand total. The criteria to prove the problem would be whether limits for each on the number of incidents for the year were

exceeded and whether the percentage of incidents with major consequences was exceeded. As Table C14.1 shows, the absolute limits for
categories varied to reflect the content of the categories. Limits ranged
from over 36, for *attacks on staff and equipment*, to over 5, for *inappropriate
provision of care*. The individual limits added to 197 UORs per year, and
this became the limit for the grand total. The criterion for percentage
with major consequences was set at over 2% for all.

Results

Eight of the 11 categories and the grand total proved to be problems. Each category exceeded its incidence limit, and only three had
acceptable rates of major consequences. Table C14.1 shows that the
category with the largest number of UORs was *attacks on staff and
equipment*, with 128. But this did not relate to patient care. The largest
category with consequences for patients was *interference with provision
of care*, with 101 UORs. It was 14% of the total and had a 16% rate of
major consequences. The category with the highest rate of major consequences was *prisoner in need of care due to taser (electric shock)*, at 67%;
but, with 15 cases, it was only 2% of the total. *Equipment interference
with care*, with 86 cases, was 12% of the total and had a 14% rate of major
consequences. Thus the two categories selected for study were *interference with provision of care* and *equipment interference with care*. Within
these, the subsets selected for study were *interference with patient care*
and *equipment failure*.

Identifying Causes

Final List of Possible Causes

Nick used the descriptions of the occurrences in the reports to
come up with a set of possible causes. He then interviewed 10 staff
members and reviewed the literature, which suggested 12 new possible causes. He worded causes in terms that would cover any related
occurrence; that is, the terms were free of reference to any specific
occurrence. For *interference with patient care*, Nick named 21 possible
causes that could be investigated through research using existing

Table C14.2 Possible Causes That Could Be Verified Using Existing Data

Interference With Patient Care	Equipment Failure
1. Patient problem medical or trauma	1. Patient condition medical or trauma
2. Caller information on patient's condition inaccurate	2. Caller information on patient's condition inaccurate
3. Caller information on patient's location inaccurate	3. Specific equipment or aspects of condition inaccurate
4. Crime at the scene	4. Age of equipment
5. Physical or weather hazards	5. Overuse of equipment
6. Language barrier or ability to communicate	6. Missing equipment
7. Patient drunk	7. Technology (whether state of the art)
8. Patient on drugs	8. Maintenance history
9. Escort drunk	9. How maintenance is carried out
10. Escort on drugs	10. Staff abuse of equipment
11. Family interference	11. Staff performance skill
12. Patient's physician interference	12. Specific title (stand-in for training or equipment differences)
13. Bystander interference	13. Years in service
14. Bystander physician interference	14. Specific ambulance staff (crew)
15. Specific ambulance staff (crew)	15. Shift
16. Shift	
17. Other agency interference	
18. Animal interference	
19. Hospital staff interference	
20. Staff attitude towards people	
21. Staff differences regarding diagnosis or treatment	

records in the agency (see Table C14.2). For *equipment failure*, Nick had 15 possible causes, shown in the same table.

Data Collection

This study relied on organizational data and the skill of the consultant in interpreting accumulated past material not specifically designed for the purpose for which it was now being used. As such, although the data were objective, there were subjective aspects to the extent that Nick made judgments about the events.

The unit of observation was the individual occurrence, coded by year, location, and number. Nick added a project ID number because he wanted to have consecutive ID numbers for his tables. There were 38 reports dealing with *interference with patient care* and 69 dealing with *equipment failure*. Aside from the UORs themselves, additional data sources were supervisors' cover letters, employee statements, ambulance call reports, unit activity logs, and staff evaluations. Some equipment had related correspondence.

For *interference with patient care*, Nick organized the data, including the incident ID, a brief description of the incident, and a cause category. For *equipment failure*, Nick included the incident ID, a brief description of the incident, the type of equipment, the type of failure, the equipment ID, and age in years. In all the descriptions, Nick consistently used the same language to describe the same situation, such as "the manufacturer returned equipment sent for repair saying there is no problem," "unit dumped charge internally," and "rear seal blew out of unit." Nick organized equipment failure by type of equipment to make aggregate analysis possible by equipment type. Objective cause data related to staff included code sheets containing staff IDs, titles, crew number, shift, and years of service by project ID number for all the staff involved.

Criteria to Prove the Causes

Nick developed criteria to prove the possible causes and obtained the approval of the client. There were 21 possible causes for *interference with patient care*. The most common criterion was that the cause had to appear in more than 8% of the incidents. For either *medical condition* or *trauma condition* to be a risk factor, one or the other condition had to have more than 52% of the UORs of the most important cause category and at least 50% of the total of 38 (69 for equipment failure). For *specific ambulance staff* to be a cause, a crew member had to be associated with two or more UORs and have a record of two or more reports of negative attitude towards people or be so evaluated by Nick two or more times. (A similar criterion applied to equipment failure.)

For one of the three *shifts* to be a cause, its percentage share of total UORs and UORs with the most important cause had to be highest and at least 2 percentage points higher than its share of calls. (This also applied to equipment failure.)

For *staff attitude towards people* to be a cause, more than 8% of the staff associated with the 38 UORs had to show the problem in either the UORs themselves or be so judged by Nick's reading of the report.

For *equipment failure*, in addition to the overlaps with *interference with patient care*, the possible causes included *specific title*, which was a stand-in for training or equipment differences. To be a cause, specific titles had to be associated with specific types of equipment and cause data and be associated with training, one title had to predominate and do so disproportionately, and/or a specific crew makeup by title had to predominate among UORs but not in the service as a whole. For *years in the service* to be a cause, a particular number of service years had to be more associated with more UORs than others, and the numbers had to grade up or down with years of service.

For *staff abuse of equipment* or *staff performance skill* to be a cause, staff with two or more UORs had to show some evidence of performance problems. For *specific equipment* and *aspects of equipment* to be causes, specific types of equipment had to account for more than 12% of the total, and for such equipment, specific aspects of the equipment had to account for at least 10% of the UORs for the equipment and 8% of the 69 total UORs. For *age of equipment*, being more than 6 years old had to account for more than 10% of any equipment's UORs, more than 8% of the total of 69, and a department expert had to judge age to be a factor.

For *overuse of equipment, missing equipment, technology* (whether state of the art), or *maintenance history*, the cause had to account for more than 10% of any type of equipment found to be a cause and 8% of the total of 69. For the *way maintenance is carried out*, biweekly maintenance had to be shown not to have been carried out for equipment shown to be a cause.

Results

The results showed six proved and two partially proved causes for *interference with patient care*. *Family interference* was the most important cause, with 47% of the UORs, followed by *other agency interference*

(21%). *Patient's physician interference* and *bystander interference* each had 13%. *Interference by hospital staff* and *inaccurate caller information* were partially proved at 8%.

Medical condition, rather than *trauma*, was a patient risk factor, accounting for 100% of family interference and 82% of the total of 38 incidents. *The third shift* (which ran from 4:00 p.m. to 12:00 midnight) was a cause. Its share of total UORs was 50%. Its share of family interference was 56%, and its share of service calls was only 39%.

For *equipment failure*, six causes were proved and one was partly proved. The most serious equipment failures were in *SAED defibrillators*, with 39% of the total, followed by *bag valve masks* (20%) and *Lifepack 5s* (19%). Within SAED defibrillators, the most important causes were *no preventive maintenance* (100%), *the manufacturer returned equipment sent for repair saying there is no problem* (56%), *no analysis function* (56%), *no shock* (22%), *past failure history* (18%), and *battery failure* (18%).

Within bag valve masks, *broken parts* accounted for 57% and *leaks* 43%. For the Lifepack 5s, *no preventive maintenance* accounted for from 85% to 100%, with *part failure* 69% and *battery failure* 23%.

Medical condition was a risk factor, with 100% of the most problematic equipment UORs and 97% of the total incidents. *Caller information on patient's condition was inaccurate* was partially proved; it was 11% of the most common equipment cause, but only 6% of the total.

The third shift was a cause. Its share of total UORs was 52%; its share of the second, third, and fourth most important equipment was highest, and its share of service calls was only 39%.

Emergency medical technologist (EMT) crews were associated with the most common UORs, those involved with SAED Heart Start defibrillator equipment and bag valve masks. They were the only title assigned to SAEDs. EMTs received no continuing education and less training. Their share of bag valve mask UORs was 71%, compared with a 76% share of service crews. The UORs probably reflect both different equipment and different training.

Maintenance history was a cause of 20% of SAED failures and 13% of equipment with past failures. *The way maintenance is carried out* was proved because a bimonthly maintenance plan was absent for SAEDs and 95% of Lifepack 5s.

Solutions

Feasibility Limits

Nick's feasibility limits were: The solutions could not decrease the level of care being rendered, could not increase off-service time for line units, or require major costs, and any costs had to be one-time costs.

Solutions and Implementation

Nick eliminated three of the causes that could not be prevented: (a) whether a patient's condition is medical rather than trauma, (b) the caller providing inaccurate information about the patient's condition, and (c) the shift (one could not change the circumstances that make the shift from 4:00 p.m. to 12:00 a.m. the most likely time of interference with patient care or equipment failure).

The rest of the causes were productively discussed with staff and related departments because there was widespread commitment to finding solutions. To deal with *interference with patient care by family, their physicians, and bystanders,* social and psychological sensitivity and crisis management training were suggested for crews to teach them to better handle these situations. Management accepted this solution and expected to follow with implementation.

For *interference by other agencies and hospital staff,* an interagency focus group was suggested that would draw on the agency people who were actually involved in the occurrences. The focus group would discuss their respective concerns and how to avoid a recurrence. This was favorably received and was to be further explored with the agencies involved.

With regard to *equipment failure caused by past failures and poor maintenance,* Nick suggested the installation of a preventive maintenance program, because there was none at that time. Nick learned that the EMS was currently designing such a program; Nick's data added support for its implementation. Nick did not deal with the semiautomatic external defibrillator cause in which *the producer did not find problems in returned equipment.* He suggested that preventive maintenance be used to deal with failure of analysis and shock functions.

Nick was able to find a major solution for *battery failure.* At the time of the project, the SAED battery charger had an indicator light that showed if the battery was being charged, but there was no indicator to show when the battery was *fully* charged. This could compromise the readiness of the battery in the field. Nick suggested the purchase of a battery charger with a dual light indicator, one to indicate charging in progress and one to indicate when the battery was fully charged. This suggestion was enthusiastically accepted and implemented by the Department of Technical Services and was applied to all EMS stations. The solution was even within the feasibility limits, because it was not Nick's department that paid the bill.

The bag valve masks suffered from *broken parts* and *leaks.* Nick suggested that the manufacturer be contacted and asked to deal with the problems. At that time the BVM packaging was a sealed cardboard box, which afforded no prior inspection and within which the BVM was compressed to save room. If the BVM was expanded with too much force, this could cause a tear and leak in the equipment. The manufacturer agreed to supply the equipment in a clear plastic bag, fully expanded and ready for immediate use.

The Lifepack 5s suffered from *part and battery failure.* Nick expected preventive maintenance and new battery chargers to solve these problems. *Staff titles* were expected to be taken care of by solutions implemented for the equipment.

This project was judged to be an outstanding success.

Note

1. Jerry Gombo was the internal consultant for this project.

Appendix 1

Outline for the Written Project Plan of Work

Introduction

The introduction puts the project in context. Provide a title and a brief overview of the institution, the situation, and some background. If appropriate, indicate who will function as an internal consultant and how interest in the project came about. You may give a brief history to explain the context in which your problem exists and tell what led you to suggest or be asked to do the project.

Problems

Problem Statement

State the broad problem so anyone reading can understand. The plan may be read by managers who know little about your specialty area.

Project Questions

The first project question asks if it is true that [state the problem] exists and its extent.

The second project question asks what the specific causes of the problem are.

The third project question asks how to solve the problem.

The fourth project question asks how to implement and evaluate the possible solutions and/or how to make them operational.

Objectives and Evaluation

Long-Range Goals

Before presenting the project objectives, remind the reader of the ultimate goals of the project that may not be reached by the time the project is over. Perhaps you might take the problem and reword it so that it focuses on the elimination of the problem.

Project Objectives

Present each project objective in numerical order and give it a brief name. State what you will accomplish for each. You can write the project objectives by taking each project question and rewording it to indicate that it is answered. Each objective must have a due date and success criteria that show how you will prove that it was accomplished. Select and present the relevant enabling objectives under each project objective you will deal with and include due dates and success criteria. A specific plan may have some or all of the following objectives.

Project Objective 1: To Prove the Problem Exists and Its Extent

By [date] I will demonstrate that the problem exists and its extent. My success criteria are that my data will meet or exceed the criteria for proving that there is a problem set in enabling objective 1f, _____ [someone at a peer level who will concentrate on the accuracy of your data and calculations] will check and approve my data results, and _____ [the key management person who becomes *the client*] will be convinced that the problem exists.

The criteria for this objective are written so that you do not have to know beforehand the criteria to prove the problem. There is an enabling objective to design the detailed data collection and to designate what levels the data must reach to prove the problem.

Enabling Objective 1a: To Determine the Plan of Work for the Project

By [date] the agreement describing the scope, objectives, and conditions of this project will be approved in [written or oral] form by _____ [the client].

Enabling Objective 1b: To Identify the Parameters
of the Project (Importance, Relevant Steps,
Operational Definitions, Normal Loads)

By [date], if not already done, I will have identified the importance of the problem
with regard to outcomes or other performance standards, relevant steps related to the
problem and/or operational definitions of relevant variables to be collected, normal
work loads, and the number of observations to be made [choose what applies]. I will
have the approval of _____ [the relevant key management person].

Enabling Objective 1c: To Identify the Causes to Be Studied

By [date], I will have decided whether to add additional causes to the original list
of possible causes. After asking at least [number of] staff what they think the causes
of the problem are and after reviewing the literature, I will be ready with a list of the
causes I will study.

Enabling Objective 1d: To Design Detailed
Data Collection for Proving the Problem and Objective Causes

By [date], I will have designed and field tested the method and data collection
forms. I will have the approval of _____ [the management person with whom you
will work most regularly] and the data collection forms will be successfully field
tested: *all* who will use the forms will be able to work with them, and the needed
data will be able to be collected without problems.

Enabling Objective 1e: To Schedule Data Collection
on Proof of Problem (Approval for Start Date)

By [date], I will be ready to begin data collection. I will have approval from the
people involved or supervising each area of data collection before I begin, and all
who will collect data will be ready and have starting dates or appointments.

Enabling Objective 1f: To Identify the Criteria to Prove the Problem

By [date], I will have determined what levels my data must reach to prove there
is a problem. _____ [key management person, client] will approve.

Project Objective 2: To Identify Causes of the Problem

By [date], I will have identified the causes of the problem. My success criteria are that, for each possible cause I identify as a real cause, my data will meet or exceed the criteria for proving that cause, as set in Enabling Objective 2c. _____ [someone at a peer level who will concentrate on the accuracy of your data and calculations] will check and approve my data results, and _____ [the key management person, client] will be convinced that these are the causes.

The criteria for this objective are written so that you do not have to know beforehand all the causes you will study and what management would set as proof that a cause is real. There are enabling objectives for you to use to select all the causes to study, design the data collection, and designate what levels the data must reach to prove the causes.

Enabling Objective 2a: To Design
Additional Data Collection on Causes

By [date], additional methods and forms will be designed on causes. They will be approved by _____ [a key management person]. The data collection forms will be successfully field tested: *all* who will be using the forms will be able to work with them, and the needed data will be able to be collected without problems.

Survey instruments or questionnaires will have their content approved by an expert; the results of dry-run testing (field testing) will show that the items are comprehensible to the field-test population, who will be similar to the intended subjects; this will include at least three people similar to each job title or subject type to be studied. If knowledge levels are being tested, the test group will include experts and novices, and the test items will be able to discriminate experts from novices; that is, most experts will answer correctly and most novices will answer incorrectly.

Enabling Objective 2b: To Schedule Data Collection for
Causes Not Already Dealt With (Approval for Start Date)

By [date], I will be ready to begin data collection. I will have approval from the people involved or supervising each area of data collection before I begin, and all the people who will collect data or be surveyed will be ready and have starting dates or appointments.

Enabling Objective 2c: To Identify the Criteria to Prove Each Cause

By [date], I will have identified for each cause being studied what the data for each cause must show for it to be an actual cause. _____ [key management person, client] will approve.

Project Objective 3: To Identify Solutions

By [date], I will have solutions to the problem. My success criteria are that my solutions will reflect the causes proved, will fit within management's feasibility limits, and will be approved by _____ [key management person, client] who has the authority to implement the solutions.

Enabling Objective 3a: To Identify Management's Feasibility Limits

By [date], I will have a list of feasibility limits that management will set for any solutions to be accepted. _____ [key person], whom I will interview about the feasibility limits, will approve the accuracy of my list summarizing the feasibility limits.

Enabling Objective 3b: To Get Ideas on Possible Solutions

By [date], I will have ideas about solutions for the proved causes from interviews with at least [number of] staff and a review of the literature [perhaps the sources used to find additional causes].

Enabling Objective 3c: To Get Feedback on Selected Solutions

By [date], I will have selected a set of solutions and will have positive feedback from at least [number of] staff out of [number], whom I will ask to respond to my suggestions.

Project Objective 4: To Implement, Evaluate, and Make Solutions Operational

By [date], the solutions will be part of the regular operations of the institution. My success criteria are that implementation will be complete, evaluation will show that the solutions meet or exceed the criteria set in Enabling Objective 4a, and that [the institutional decision makers] will have adopted the solutions as standard operating procedures. The solutions will appear in manuals, policy documents, staff orientation curricula, staff evaluation protocols, or as appropriate to the nature of the solutions; new standards or indicators will be adopted, and the procedures and monitoring techniques will be in use.

Enabling Objective 4a: To Design an Implementation and Evaluation Plan

By [date], I will have designed a plan to try out the solutions in the department (institution), designed the data collection forms to be used (after an appropriate period of time) to compare the old results with the results after using the solutions, identified the success criteria to prove the success of the solutions, and received approval of these from _____ [by management person, client].

Enabling Objective 4b: To Schedule Implementation and Data Collection

By [date], I will have approval from all relevant supervisors and staff for the dates the new solutions will be in place and for data collection.

Enabling Objective 4c: To Determine Whether the Solutions Are Successful

By [date], it will be determined whether the data from the evaluation have met or exceeded the criteria for proving success set in Enabling Objective 4a. _____ [someone at a peer level who will concentrate on the accuracy of your data and calculations] will check and approve my data results, and _____ [key management person, client] will be convinced.

Enabling Objective 4d: To Identify the Steps to Make the Solutions Operational

By [date], I will have identified what staff, changes, procedures, staff training, manuals, other written documents, and monitoring must be accounted for to make the solutions operational, and I will have made arrangements to accomplish each required step.

Enabling Objective 4e: To Determine the New Standards or Indicators
Required to Monitor Solutions or Participate in a Reference Database

By [date], a decision will be made about how to monitor the new solutions,
including new standards, data collection, and indicators; a decision will also be made
about whether to include the data in a reference database.

Plan of Work

Table 1.1 presents the objectives for the project in order of their due dates. It is a
Plan of Work and Evaluation Design. Column 1 presents the objectives, column 2
shows their expected due dates, and column 3 will show the dates the objectives are
completed. Column 4 presents the success criteria and column 5 will present my
actual results and comments. [Present Table 1.1, as described earlier. This provides
an easy-to-follow timetable for the project and a later means of summarizing your
results.]

Agreement on Ethics and Standards

The client [give titles] agrees to the following standards for ethical conduct of the
project: [Include the list agreed upon].

Appendix 2

<hr/>

Detailed Tables and Practice Exercises

Case 1: Getting Nursing Home Residents Into Physical Therapy in a Timely Fashion[1]

<hr/>

This appendix shows how the data collection instruments for Case 1 were laid out and presents the summary data collected. The figures are excerpted from tables used in the case, shown in truncated form as models. The tables report complete data. Included are exercises offered to enrich the reader's experience through practice with and interpretation of the data and results.

Final List of Possible Causes

<hr/>

Exercise

Before reviewing the list of causes developed by Anna, try your hand at thinking of possible causes yourself.

1. Examine the generic list of causes in Chapter 2 and then see what you would select and what else you can come up with. Ask yourself what might interfere with starting a patient on physical therapy.

Data Collection

Exercise

1. How would you design tables to show the extent of the problem?
2. What would you collect at the same time to account for the possible causes? How?

A codesheet, Figure A2.1, "Model Codesheet for Patient ID Information," listed the 74 residents in the study along the left-hand stub by code numbers 1 through 74. These were the current or new residents. The data in the codesheet were originally arrayed in order by patient ID number. Once the patients' ranks for waiting for physical therapy were calculated, the data were rearranged and presented in ascending order by rank, with rank defined by the number of days wait. This made it possible to visually inspect the data to see associations by rank. Ranks went from 1 (4 days) to 20 (27 days). Waits with the same number of days received the same rank. Figure A2.1 shows the way the table was set up, with the first and last entries and the totals.

Figure A2.2, "Raw Data on Physical Therapy Consults and Orders for Physical Therapy Care," included the key dates by patient code, rank, physician code, and whether there was a PT consult at intake. The columns cover the dates for intake, the X-ray and orthopedist consult orders for fracture patients, the physical therapy request for a consult order, when a nurse was enlisted to ask the physician for the PT consult, the PT consult order, when X rays were taken, the orthopedist consult, the physical therapy request for the physiatrist, when the physical therapy order was received from the physiatrist, the order to start physical therapy, and the total days wait. The first and last two entries and the totals are shown.

Note that for most figures and tables there is a sentence in parentheses below the figure or table that indicates the table number assigned in the original project. This is because summary tables give the source of the original data by table numbers that correspond to numbers assigned in the project.

Figure A2.3, "Additional Raw Data on Physical Therapy Consults and Orders," shows dates for other consults ordered, when they were done, and the number of days the physiatrist was away during a given patient's wait.

Figure A2.4, "Number of Days to Being Put on Physical Therapy," calls for the elapsed days wait to start physical therapy in categories needed to prove the problem. These include waits according to whether the patient had a fracture or not, was continuing or starting physical therapy, and whether the patient arrived from a hospital, was already a resident, or came from home. The completed table showed the total wait and the wait over 3 days for fracture patients and over 7 days for all others. At the bottom were summary data by patients and days and the calculated averages (days divided by patients).

Table A2.1 was designed to summarize all the data needed to prove the problem. It summarizes days of wait, days over the limit, patients, patients

(text continues on p. 331)

Figure A2.1 Model Codesheet for Patient ID Information

Patient ID	Rank (Name Not shown)	Hospital Yes	No	Name	Nursing Home	Own Home	Admit New	Readmission	PT Need Continuation	New	Medical Diagnosis	Special Orders
3	1	x			our					x	CVA/CHF	
59	20		x	COM.				x	x		Fracture (hip)	XR Orthopedics
Total 74	20	56	18		14	4	37	22	21	53		

NOTE: This was Codesheet 2 for the project.

Figure A2.2 Model Table for Raw Data on Physical Therapy Consults and Orders for Physical Therapy Care

Patient ID	Date	Intake MD ID	PT Consult Order? Yes	No	Fracture Date of X-ray Order	Date of Orthopedics Order	PT Stage Date Consult Requested By PT	By RN	Date of PT Consult Order	Rank	Fracture Dates X-Ray Done	Orthopedist Came	PT Activity Dates PT Request for Physician	Physiat. Order Received	PT Start	Net Total Days
3	1/15[a]	5	x				1/15		1/18	1			1/18	1/18	1/19	4
20	3/18	8		x			3/19		3/18	1			3/19	3/21	3/22	4
56	7/13	3	x		7/18	7/18	7/15		8/5	20	7/20	7/23	8/6	8/8	8/9	27
59	7/13	3		x	7/15	7/15	7/15		8/3	20	7/16	7/23	8/6	8/8	8/9	27
Total 74		32		42	14	7		5		20						854

NOTE: This was Table 1.1 for the project.
a. Patient was a resident and physical therapy care was requested. Date is physical therapy request date.

| Patient ID | Intake Date[a] | MD ID | Special Tests, Consults (Not X Rays) Ordered | | | | Dates the Physiatrist Had No Replacement | | |
| | | | At Once | | Order Date | Date Done | Days Between Request for Consult & Consult | | |
			Yes	No			1/1 to 1/17	2/5 to 2/20	7/2 to 7/9
2	1/13	6					2		
7	1/13	7					3		
48	6/23	5	x		6/23	6/28			
4	12/30	4					22		
56	7/13	3		x	7/18	7/23			
59	7/13	3		x	7/15	7/23			
Total 18	xxxx	7	2	8	10	10	29	20	8

Figure A2.3 Model Table for Additional Raw Data on Physical Therapy Consults and Orders

NOTE: This was Table 1.2 for the project.

a. If patient was a resident and physical therapy care was requested, date is physical therapy request date.

Patient ID	Coming From Hospital								Residents				Coming From Home			
	With Fracture				Without Fracture				With Fracture		Without Fracture		With Fracture		Without Fracture	
	Continuing		Starting		Continuing		Starting		Starting		Starting		Starting		Starting	
	Total	>3	Total	>3	Total	>7	Total	>7	Total	>3	Total	>7	Total	>3	Total	>7
27					4	0										
17															7	0
Total patients	5	5	8	8	15	12	28	17	1	1	13	6	0	0	4	1
Total days	73	58	119	95	159	61	331	142	19	16	126	53	0	0	27	3
Average days	14.6	11.6	14.9	11.9	10.6	5.1	11.8	8.4	19.0	16.0	9.7	8.8	–	–	6.8	3.0

Figure A2.4 Model Table: Number of Days to Being Put on Physical Therapy

NOTE: This was Table 1.3 for the project.

Table A2.1	Summary of Patients' Wait for Physical Therapy (Exercise)									

	Days			*Patients*			*Average Days*			
Patient Origin;							*Percentage*			
With or Without		*Over*			*Over*		*Patients*			
Fracture; Starting	*Total*	*Limits*		*Total*	*Limits*		*Over*			
or Continue PT	*Days*	*> 7*	*> 3*	*Patients*	*> 7*	*> 3*	*Limits*	*Total*	*> 7*	*> 3*
From Hospital										
W. fracture, continue	73	—	58	5		5	100.0	14.6	—	11.6
W. fracture, starting	119	—	95	8		8	100.0	14.9	—	11.9
Total Fracture	192	—	153	13		13	100.0	14.8	—	11.8
W/O fracture, cont.	159	61	—	15	12	—	80.0	10.6	5.1	—
W/O fracture, starting	331	142	—	28	17	—	60.7	11.8	8.4	—
Total W/O fracture	490	203	—	43	29	—	67.4	11.4	7.0	—
Residents										
W. fracture, start	19	—	16	1	—	1	100.0	19.0	—	16.0
W/O fracture, starting	126	53	—	13	6	—	46.2	9.7	8.8	—
Coming From Home										
W. fracture starting	0	—	0	0	—	0	—	—	—	—
W/O fracture starting	27	3	—	4	1	—	25.0	6.8	3.0	—

	Days		*Patients*		*Average Days*		
					Percentage		
					Patients		
	Total	*Over 3/7*	*Total*	*Over 3/7*	*Over*		*Over 3/7*
	Days	*Limits*	*Patients*	*Limits*	*Limits*	*Total*	*Limits*
Total hospital	682	?	56	?	75.0	?	8.5
Total residents	?	69	?	7	?	10.4	9.9
Total from home	27	?	4	?	?	6.8	?
Total fracture	?	169	14	14	?	15.1	?
Total without fracture	643	259	?	36	60.0	?	7.2
Grand total	854	?	74	?	67.6	?	8.6

NOTE: This was Table 1.4 for the project.

over the limit, percent of patients over the limit, and average days of wait for every patient category in which Anna was interested. Some of the entries have question marks; these are filled in in Table A2.2.

Exercise

1. Before looking at Table A2.2, try to see if you understand the data and the way they were derived by filling in the blank spaces marked by question marks in Table A2.1. Calculate the missing figures yourself and compare with the data in Table A2.2.

Table A2.2 Summary of Patients' Wait for Physical Therapy

Patient Origin; With or Without Fracture; Starting or Continue PT	Days			Patients			Average Days			
	Total Days	Over Limits >7	>3	Total Patients	Over Limits >7	>3	Percentage Patients Over Limits	Total	>7	>3
From hospital										
W. fracture, continue	73	—	58	5		5	100.0	14.6	—	11.6
W. fracture, starting	119	—	95	8		8	100.0	14.9	—	11.9
Total fracture	192	—	153	13		13	100.0	14.8	—	11.8
W/O fracture, continue	159	61	—	15	12	—	80.0	10.6	5.1	—
W/O fracture, starting	331	142	—	28	17	—	60.7	11.8	8.4	—
Total W/O fracture	490	203	—	43	29	—	67.4	11.4	7.0	—
Residents										
W. fracture, start	19	—	16	1	—	1	100.0	19.0	—	16.0
W/O fracture, starting	126	53	—	13	6	—	46.2	9.7	8.8	—
Coming from home										
W. fracture starting	0	—	0	0	—	0	—	—	—	—
W/O fracture starting	27	3	—	4	1	—	25.0	6.8	3.0	—

	Days		Patients		Average Days		
	Total Days	Over 3/7 Limits	Total Patients	Over 3/7 Limits	Percentage Patients Over Limits	Total	Over 3/7 Limits
Total hospital	682	356	56	42	75.0	12.2	8.5
Total residents	145	69	14	7	50.0	10.4	9.9
Total from home	27	3	4	1	25.0	6.8	3.0
Total fracture	211	169	14	14	100.0	15.1	12.1
Total without fracture	643	259	60	36	60.0	10.7	7.2
Grand total	854	428	74	50	67.6	11.5?	8.6

NOTE: This was Table 1.4 for the project.

Proving the Problem

A table to set out the criteria used to prove the problem and show the results comes next. But Table A2.3 is an exercise table: It presents the criteria Anna and the client agreed on for proof of the problem. The far left column shows the 18 measures, including totals and subtotals by risk factors. The measures are stated as a percentage of patients above the limits and as average days of wait. In the next column are the thresholds above which the problem would be said to exist. The column with "x" marks shows the client's approval of these criteria. The far right column gives the source of the data, Table 1.4 (actually

---

Table A2.3 Criteria for Proof of Problem and Results: Waiting for Physical Therapy (Exercise)

Measure	Point Beyond Which Problem Exists (Percentage, Rate, etc.)	OKed	Actual Results	Source
Number of days from admission (or from request for Physical Therapy, if already resident)				
Fracture	> 3 days	x		
Nonfracture	> 7 days	x		
Percentage of patients with wait longer than limits				
Total patients (74)	> 9 %	x	. %	
Fracture	> 9 %	x	. %	
Nonfracture	> 9 %	x	. %	
Total from hospital	> 9 %	x	. %	
Starting therapy				
Fracture	> 9 %	x	. %	
Nonfracture	> 9 %	x	. %	
Continuing therapy				
Fracture	> 9 %	x	. %	
Nonfracture	> 9 %	x	. %	
Total already residents	> 9 %	x	. %	
Starting therapy				
Fracture	> 9 %	x	. %	
Nonfracture	> 9 %	x	. %	
Total from own homes (All starting therapy and nonfracture)	> 9 %	x	. %	
Average days of wait				Table 1.4
Total patients	> 5 days	x	. days	
Fracture	> 3 days	x	. days	
Nonfracture	> 7 days	x	. days	
From hospital	> 5 days	x	. days	
Already residents	> 5 days	x	. days	
From own home	> 5 days	x	. days	

NOTE: This was Table 2 for the Project.

Table A2.2). The results are missing in the second column from the right. You have enough data to complete the results section of Table A2.3.

Exercise

1. Next to each measure for which there is a criterion, fill in the actual results in the column designated and write whether it is *proved, partly proved,* or *not proved* in the far right column.

2. Write a conclusions section dealing with your interpretation of Table A2.3. Discuss your results and any conclusions you draw or insights you have about the problem. The completed table is presented as Table A2.4.

Table A2.4 Criteria for Proof of Problem and Results: Waiting for Physical Therapy

Measure	Point Beyond Which Problem Exists (Percentage, Rate, etc.)	OKed	Actual Results	Source
Number of days from admission (or from request for Physical Therapy, if already resident)				
Fracture	> 3 days	x		
Nonfracture	> 7 days	x		
Percentage of patients with wait longer than limits				Table 1.4
Total patients (74)	> 9 %	x	67.6 %	Proved
Fracture	> 9 %	x	100.0 %	Proved
Nonfracture	> 9 %	x	60.0 %	Proved
Total from hospital	> 9 %	x	75.0 %	Proved
Starting therapy				
Fracture	> 9 %	x	100.0 %	Proved
Nonfracture	> 9 %	x	60.7 %	Proved
Continuing therapy				
Fracture	> 9 %	x	100.0 %	Proved
Nonfracture	> 9 %	x	80.0 %	Proved
Total already residents	> 9 %	x	50.0 %	Proved
Starting therapy				
Fracture	> 9 %	x	100.0 %	Proved
Nonfracture	> 9 %	x	46.2 %	Proved
Total from own homes (All starting therapy and nonfracture)	> 9 %	x	25.0 %	Proved
Average days of wait				Table 1.4
Total patients	> 5 days	x	11.5 days	Proved
Fracture	> 3 days	x	15.1 days	Proved
Nonfracture	> 7 days	x	10.7 days	Proved
From hospital	> 5 days	x	12.2 days	Proved
Already residents	> 5 days	x	10.4 days	Proved
From own home	> 5 days	x	6.8 days	Proved

NOTE: This was Table 2 for the project.

Proving Causes

Now comes the challenge of verifying the causes of the problem.

Exercise

Before seeing what additional data were collected on causes, try the following exercise.

1. Look at the list of possible causes presented with the case and describe the kind of data you would need for each before looking at the remaining descriptions of what was actually done.

Objective Cause Data

Figures A2.5 and A2.6 model how data were presented to show the elapsed days for each step. The data by patient ID are listed separately in rank order for fracture and nonfracture patients. The code numbers of the patients' general physicians (who wrote the PT consult orders) are also shown. Above the bank of columns for each step, Anna suggested the maximum number of days a patient could ideally be expected to wait for the step to occur. These maxima were set to be realistic as well as ideal but were more stringent for fracture patients than for nonfracture patients. The columns for each step show the actual number of days, whether this was within the listed limit (OK), or whether it was over. If over, the number of days over is given. Since some of the steps overlap in time, the total wait is not always as long as the sum of the days for all the steps. There is a column to show which step had the longest wait of more than 2 days and its percentage of the total wait.

Each table had subtotals for fracture and nonfracture patients and average days of wait. Some of the subtotals were for specific consultations, excluded days the physiatrist was away, or excluded patients whose times were affected by RN assistance in obtaining PT consult orders.

Table A2.5 presents summary data for the steps. For each step, it shows total days, days over the limit, the days over the limit as a percentage of the total days, the step's share of the total days over the limit for the wait from admission to the start of physical therapy, the number of patients for whom the step was the longest step over 2 days, and the latter as a percentage of the total patients.

Figure A2.7 is the model for a worksheet developed for each physician, based on elapsed time by steps and aggregated for each. There were subtotals for each general physician's relevant steps. The subtotals became inputs for later analysis of the physicians' performance (Table A2.6). Negative and zero days of elapsed time were given a value of 1 so as to not wash out of the denominator in percentage calculations. This was not applied to days over the limit.

Table A2.6 was designed to rank the physicians in relation to the waits based on data prepared in the worksheets. The table shows the MD code, the number of patients covered by the physician among the 74 patients of the study, and, in column a, the total days from admission to the physical therapy consult order because this was where the physicians' responsibility ended. Negative and zero days of elapsed time in the original data were given a value of 1 when numbers were added to totals so as to not wash out the denominator in percentage calculations. This was not done for total days over the limit.

Number of Days Between Steps (not necessarily additive) for Fracture Patients

	Maximum Days: 0			Maximum Days: 0			Maximum Days: 1			Maximum Days: 1			Maximum Days: 0			
	Admit Date to Admit Notice & PT Screening			Admit Date to Order for X Ray or Consult[b]			X-ray Order to Date X Rays Taken			MD Consult Order to Date of PT Consult[b]			Admit Date to PT Consult Order			
Patient ID	Number of Days	OK	Over	Number of Days	OK	Over	Number of Days	OK	Over	Number of Days	OK	Over	Number of Days	OK	Over	MD ID
Fracture patients																
50	1		1	0		×	2		1				0	×		7
69	0	×	0	0		×	2		1				0	×		4

Number of Days Between Steps (Are not necessarily additive) for Patients Without Fracture

	Maximum Days: 1			Maximum Days: 0				Maximum Days: 1			Maximum Days: 1			
	Admit Date to Admit Notice & PT Screening			Admit Date to Order for X Ray or Consult[b]			NA	MD Consult Order to Date of PT Consult[b]			Admit Date to PT Consult Order			
Patient ID	Number of Days	OK	Over	Number of Days	OK	Over		Number of Days	OK	Over	Number of Days	OK	Over	MD ID
Nonfracture patients														
3[a]	0	×	0								3	×	2	5
20	1	×	0								0	×	0	8

Figure A2.5 Model Table: Elapsed Time Between Steps, up to Physical Therapy Consult Order

NOTE: This was Table 2.1 for the project.
a. Indicates that patient was a resident and physical therapy was requested. Admit date is physical therapy request date.
b. Consults may be Orthopedic, Neurologic, or for Cardiology.

Number of Days Between Steps (Not necessarily additive)

Maximum Days:	0 PT Consult Order to PT Request for Physiatrist			1 PT Requests Physiatrist to PT Order			1 PT Order to PT Start Date						Longest Wait Over 2 Days	
Patient ID	Number of Days	OK	Over	Number of Days	OK	Over	Number of Days	OK	Over	MD ID	Total From Admission to PT Start	Rank Order, Total Days of Wait[a]	Name	Percentage of Total
Fracture patients														
⌐50	3		3	1	x	0	2		1	7	6	3	CO/PTR	50.0
└69	3		3	2		1	1	x	0	4	6	3	CO/PTR	50.0
Nonfracture patients														
⌐3	0	x	0	0	x	0	1	x	0	5	4	1	AD/PTCO	75.0
└20	1		1	2		1	1	x	0	8	4	1		

Figure A2.6 Model Table: Elapsed Time From Physical Therapy Consult Order to Start of Treatment

NOTE: This was Table 2.2 for the project.

a. Shortest wait equals lowest rank; equal waits are of equal rank. CO/PTR = Consult to PT request; AD/PTCO = Admit to PT consult order.

Table A2.5 Summary Data on Days Over the Limit by Step

					Longest Over 2 Days	
Steps	Total Days	Total Over Limit[a,b]	Percentage Over Limit[a]	Percentage Share of Total Over Limit (428)[b]	Number of Patients[c]	Percentage of 74 Patients
Admit to treatment	854	428	50.1	100.0	65	87.8
Admit to screening	101	57	56.4	13.3	0	0.0
Admit to X-ray order	31	32	103.2	7.5	1	1.4
X-ray order to X ray	26	15	57.7	3.5	0	0.0
Admit to Orthopedics order	31	32	103.2	7.5	1	1.4
Orthopedics consult order to orthopedics consult	49	42	85.7	9.8	0	0.0
Admit to other consult order	9	9	100.0	2.1	0	0.0
Other consult order to consult	18	15	83.3	3.5	2	2.7
Admit to PT consult order	365	328	89.9	85.3	26	35.1
PT consult order to PT Request for physiatrist	185	142	76.8	33.2	34	45.9
Request for physiatrist to PT start order	221	97	43.9	22.7	13	17.6
Start order to treatment	66	9	13.6	2.1	1	1.4

SOURCE: Tables 1.4, 2.1, and 2.2.

NOTE: This was Table 2.3 for the project.

a. The number of days over the limit can exceed the number of days of wait because some waiting days are negative numbers, when one date precedes another.
b. The total days over the limit equals 778, but because many of the steps overlap, the actual days over the limit from admission to the start of treatment is used.
c. Some patients had more than one step of equal length.

Column b is the total days over the limit for the step. Column b/a is the excess wait rate for each physician (column b as a percent of column a). In the bank of columns below, column b/a is ranked in column j. Note that 62.5% for

	From Admission to Order for X-Ray or MD Consult			From Admission to PT Consult Order		
		Number of Days Between Steps		*MD ID: 2*		
				0 Allowed for Fractures, 1 Allowed for Nonfractures		
Patient ID	*0 Allowed (Fractures)*					
	Days	Adjusted	Over Limit	Days	Adjusted[a]	Over Limit
19	11	11	11	11	11	11
13				5	5	4
57				0	1	0
10				7	7	6
70				12	12	11
32				14	14	13
1 Fracture	11	11	11			
6 Total				49	50	45

Figure A2.7 Model Table: Elapsed Time and Days Over the Limit for Steps Related to General Physicians

NOTE: This was Worksheet 1 for the project.

a. Negative and zero days of elapsed time were given a value of 1 so as not to wash out of the denominator in percentage share calculations. This was not applied to days over the limit.

physician 7 is the lowest rate in column b/a; he is rank 1 in column j. Percentage share of patients is shown in column c and ranked in the bank below, column k. The physicians' shares of days over the limit are calculated in column d and are ranked below in column l.

To find disproportionate shares of the excess wait, Anna subtracted each MD's share of total patients (c), from the MD's share of excess days (d). A positive number means a disproportionate share of excess waits. This is shown in column d-c and is ranked below in column m.

A similar analysis was done for days between admission and the X-ray order or other consults (column e through column g – i); this covers the 14 X-ray consults and three other consults, for a total of 17. The ranks appear below in columns n through q.

In the lower bank, the sum of ranks for the two sets of data are given in columns r and s. The sum of ranks j to m and n to q are presented in a single column so the reader can compare MD ranks reflecting all patients with MD ranks for patients with special consults, primarily fracture patients. All 8 ranks are added in column t, on the left, and the total of these rank scores is ranked in the far-left column u, which is the column of interest.

The final rank u is a composite measure of responsibility for the results; the scores in column t show MD 8 with a score of 8. He appeared only for the first set of 4 ranks and has a final rank of 1 in column u. He had no special consults. He was given a final rank of 1, assuming his performance would be similar in the other steps.

Table A2.6 Summary Data on MDs in Relation to Consult and X-Ray Orders

		Days Between Admit and Physical Therapy Consult Order						Days Between Admit and X Ray or Consult Order						
MD ID	No. of Patients	Total Days: Admit to PT Consult Order a*	Total Days Over Limit For the Step b	Rate: Percentage Over Limit b/a*	Percentage Share of 74 Patients c	Percentage Share of Total Days Over Limit (328) d*	Share of Days Over Minus Share of Total Patients d-c	Total Days to Order X Ray and Consults e*	Total Days Over Limit for the Steps f	Rate: Percentage of Days Over Limit f/e*	Percentage Share of Total Days Over Limit (41) g	Number of Patients With Fracture Plus Consults h	Percentage of Patients With Fracture Plus Consults (17) i	Share of Days Over Minus Share of Fracture Patients With Consults g-i
2	6	50	45	90.0	8.1	13.7	5.6	11	11	100.0	26.8	1	5.9	20.9
3	14	110	98	89.1	18.9	29.9	11.0	8	8	100.0	19.5	3	17.6	1.9
4	12	61	50	82.0	16.2	15.2	-1.0	4	3	75.0	7.3	2	11.8	-4.5
5	9	25	17	68.0	12.2	5.2	-7.0	6	0	0.0	0.0	6	35.3	-35.3
6	6	32	26	81.2	8.1	7.9	-0.2	1	0	0.0	0.0	1	5.9	-5.9
7	12	32	20	62.5	16.2	6.1	-10.1	9	8	88.9	19.5	2	11.8	7.7
8	4	16	12	75.0	5.4	3.7	-1.7	–	–	–	–	0	–	–
9	11	69	60	87.0	14.9	18.3	3.4	11	11	100.0	26.8	2	11.8	15.0
Total	74	395	328	77.7	100.0	100.0	xxx	50	41	75.8	99.9	17	100.1	xxx

* Negative and zero days of elapsed time were given a value of 1 so as not to wash out of denominator in percentage calculations. This was not applied to days over the limit.

MD ID	Final Rank of (t) u	Total Ranks: Sum of j to q t	Ranks j to m; n to q		Rank (b/a) j	Rank (c) k	Rank (d) l	Rank (d − c) m	Sum of j to m r	Sum of n to q s	Rank (f/e) n	Rank (g) o	Rank (i) p	Rank (i-g) q
2	6	38	6	6	8	2	5	7	22	16	4	4	1	7
3	8	43	8	5	7	6	8	8	29	14	4	3	3	4
4	5	29	5	3	5	5	6	4	20	9	2	2	2	3
5	2	16	2	2	2	3	2	2	9	7	1	1	4	1
6	3	20	4	1	4	2	4	5	15	5	1	1	1	2
7	4	23	3	4	1	5	3	1	10	13	3	3	2	5
8	1**	8	1	–	3	1	1	3	8	–	–	–	–	–
9	7	39	7	6	6	4	7	6	23	16	4	4	2	6

NOTE: This was Table 2.4 for the project. Rank: Higher number means greater amount of days over limit or rate; equal values get equal ranks.

** Although 8 only appears for the first set of 4 ranks, even if this physician received a rank of 4 ranks, a rank of 8 for the second group, the sum would keep him or her in first place.

341

Subjective Cause Data: Interviews and Questionnaires

The questionnaire presented to the physicians is Figure A2.8. Table A2.7 presents the physicians' responses, but it is set up for another exercise. It arranges the responses to the questionnaire in ascending order by physician rank, with the MD codes in the stub and a bank of possible answers under each summarized question across the top. Physicians in ranks 1 through 4 had the fewest problems; ranks 5 through 8 had the most. The answers were totalled for all eight physicians and for the two groups of ranks. Below the totals are the percentage distributions. The "correct" answers are indicated by asterisks; incorrect answers helped to establish causes.

Exercise

1. Table A2.7 is presented with some percentages missing (indicated by question marks). Try to calculate these yourself to see if you understand how the data were derived. The answers follow in Table A2.8, so you can compare your work.

Criteria to Prove the Causes

Table A2.9 is also set up for an exercise. It shows each of the possible causes and its measure in the first left-hand column. The next column presents the criteria to prove the cause. The column with x's shows management's approval of the criteria. The far-right column shows the tables or other sources the data were drawn from, and here is where the judgment on whether the cause was proved, partly proved, or not proved is entered. To the left is the column with the actual results. The sources in the far-right column refer to the table numbers found beneath the figures and tables.

Exercise

Before looking at the actual results in Table A2.10, try the following exercise:

1. Complete the results section of Table A2.9 for those causes where the results are left blank. In the far-right column, write whether the cause is *proved, partly proved*, or *not proved*. The completed work is in Table A2.10.
2. Write a conclusions section dealing with your interpretation of Table A2.10. Discuss your results and any conclusions you draw or insights you have about the causes. Is there a pattern? Are any interrelated?

Dear Physician:
I am examining the wait of physical therapy patients from the time it is decided they need Physical Therapy (PT) services to when they start. Would you please check the answers below that best express your opinion.

	Agree	*Disagree*	*Don't Know*
1. Fracture patients need to begin physical therapy (PT):			
a. The next day	( )	( )	( )
b. Within 3 days	( )	( )	( )
c. By 7 days	( )	( )	( )
d. By 14 days	( )	( )	( )
2. Nonfracture patients (such as CVA, amputee) need to begin PT:			
a. The next day	( )	( )	( )
b. Within 3 days	( )	( )	( )
c. By 7 days	( )	( )	( )
d. By 14 days	( )	( )	( )
3. At this nursing home residents do not wait too long for PT to begin.	( )	( )	( )
4. It is a usual concern of mine to see that residents start PT early.	( )	( )	( )
5. There is no nursing home policy on how soon PT consults should be written after a resident is admitted.	( )	( )	( )
6. It would be a good idea to order a PT consult ahead of admission when a patient on PT is to be admitted from a hospital.	( )	( )	( )
7. Fracture patients need to have X rays ordered:			
a. Upon admission	( )	( )	( )
b. Within 3 days	( )	( )	( )
c. By 7 days	( )	( )	( )
8. I feel well informed about the steps leading to and following from a PT consult order.	( )	( )	( )
9. If it helps speed things up, I would be in favor of providing the PT department with computerized admission data on patients.	( )	( )	( )
10. How long residents wait to begin PT is not something I am concerned about because it is not a problem.	( )	( )	( )

Figure A2.8 Physician Questionnaire

Solutions

Table A2.11 presents the feasibility limits, the proved causes, and calls for your suggested solutions. This is the opportunity for another exercise.

(text continued on p. 364)

Table A2.7 Responses to Physician Questionnaire (Exercise)

Question 1. When Fracture Patients Need To Begin Physical Therapy

MD ID	a. The Next Day			b. Within 3 Days			c. By 7 Days			d. By 14 Days			Question 4. Concern To Start Early		
	Agree*	Disagree	Don't Know	Agree*	Disagree	Don't Know	Agree	Disagree*	Don't Know	Agree	Disagree*	Don't Know	Agree*	Disagree	Don't Know
8		x		x				x			x		x		
5		x		x				x			x		x		
6		x			x			x		x			x		
7		x		x				x			x		x		
4		x			x		x				x		x		
2		x			x			x			x		x		
9			x	x				x			x		x		
3		x		x			x				x		x		
Total (8)	0	7	1	5	3	0	2	6	0	1	7	0	8	0	0
Ranks 1 to 4 (4)	0	4	0	3	1	0	0	4	0	1	3	0	4	0	0
Ranks 5 to 8 (4)	0	3	1	2	2	0	2	2	0	0	4	0	4	0	0
Percentage of total (8)	0.0	?	12.5	62.5	?	?	0.0	100.0	?	12.5	?	0.0	100.0	?	0.0
Ranks 1 to 4 (4)	0.0	100.0	?	75.0	25.0	?	0.0	100.0	0.0	?	75.0	0.0	?	0.0	?
Ranks 5 to 8 (4)	0.0	75.0	25.0	?	50.0	?	50.0	?	0.0	0.0	?	0.0	100.0	0.0	0.0

* Correct answer.

Question 2. When Nonfracture Patients Need To Begin Physical Therapy

MD ID	a. The Next Day			b. Within 3 Days			c. By 7 Days			d. By 14 Days			Question 10. Concern About Patient Waiting		
	Agree*	Disagree	Don't Know	Agree*	Disagree	Don't Know	Agree*	Disagree	Don't Know	Agree	Disagree*	Don't Know	Agree	Disagree*	Don't Know
8	x			x				x			x			x	
5	x			x				x			x			x	
6	x			x				x			x			x	
7		x			x			x			x			x	
4	x					x		x			x				x
2	x			x			x				x			x	
9		x			x			x			x		x		
3		x			x			x			x		x		
Total															
8	5	3	0	4	3	1	1	7	0	0	8	0	2	5	1
Ranks 1 to 4															
4	3	1	0	3	1	0	0	4	0	0	4	0	0	4	0
Ranks 5 to 8															
4	2	2	0	1	2	1	1	3	0	0	4	0	2	1	1
Percentage of total															
8	62.5	?	?	50.0	?	12.5	?	?	?	0.0	100.0	0.0	25.0	?	12.5
Ranks 1 to 4															
4	75.0	?	?	75.0	?	?	?	100.0	?	0.0	100.0	0.0	0.0	100.0	?
Ranks 5 to 8															
4	?	?	?	25.0	?	25.0	?	75.0	?	0.0	?	?	50.0	25.0	25.0

* Correct answer.

(continued)

TABLE A2.7 Responses to Physician Questionnaire (Exercise) (continued)

MD ID	Q7. When Fracture Patients Need to Have X Rays Ordered — a. At Admission — Agree*	Disagree	Don't Know	b. Within 3 Days — Agree	Disagree*	Don't Know	c. By 7 Days — Agree	Disagree*	Don't Know	Q3. Residents Do Not Wait Too Long — Agree	Disagree*	Don't Know	Q5. No Policy: Write PT Consult Order — Agree*	Disagree	Don't Know
8	x				x			x		x			x		
5	x				x			x		x			x		
6		x			x			x		x			x		
7	x				x			x		x			x		
4			x	x			x			x					x
2	x			x				x				x			x
9		x			x			x		x				x	
3	x				x			x				x	x		
Total															
8	5	2	1	2	6	0	1	7	0	6	0	2	5	1	2
Ranks 1 to 4															
4	3	1	0	0	4	0	0	4	0	4	0	0	4	0	0
Ranks 5 to 8															
4	2	1	1	2	2	0	1	3	0	2	0	2	1	1	2
Percentage of total															
8	62.5	25.0	12.5	25.0	75.0	0.0	12.5	87.5	0.0	75.0	0.0	?	?	?	?
Ranks 1 to 4															
4	75.0	25.0	0.0	0.0	100.0	0.0	0.0	100.0	0.0	?	0.0	0.0	100.0	0.0	0.0
Ranks 5 to 8															
4	?	?	?	?	?	?	75.0	75.0	0.0	50.0	0.0	50.0	25.0	25.0	50.0

* Correct answer.

MD ID	Question 6. Likes Idea of Ordering Consults Ahead			Question 8. Feel Informed About PT Consult Steps			Question 9. Provide PT With Computerized Admit Data		
	Agree	Disagree	Don't Know	Agree	Disagree	Don't Know	Agree	Disagree	Don't Know
8		x				x	x		
5	x			x			x		
6		x			x		x		
7		x			x		x		
4		x		x					x
2	x				x		x		
9	x			x			x		
3	x				x		x		
Total									
8	?	4	0	3	4	1	7	0	1
Ranks 1 to 4									
4	1	3	0	1	2	1	4	0	0
Ranks 5 to 8									
4	3	1	0	2	2	0	3	0	1
Percentage of total									
8	?	50.0	0.0	37.5	?	?	87.5	0.0	?
Ranks 1 to 4									
4	25.0	?	0.0	?	50.0	25.0	?	0.0	0.0
Ranks 5 to 8									
4	73.0	25.0	?	50.0	50.0	0.0	75.0	?	25.0

NOTE: This was Table 2.5 for the project.

347

Table A2.8 Responses to Physician Questionnaire

| | Question 1. When Fracture Patients Need to Begin Physical Therapy | | | | | | | | | | | | Question 4. Concern to Start Early | | |
| | a. The Next Day | | | b. Within 3 Days | | | c. By 7 Days | | | d. By 14 Days | | | | | |
MD ID	Agree*	Disagree	Don't Know	Agree*	Disagree	Don't Know	Agree	Disagree*	Don't Know	Agree	Disagree*	Don't Know	Agree*	Disagree	Don't Know
8		×		×				×			×		×		
5		×		×				×			×		×		
6		×			×			×		×			×		
7		×		×				×			×		×		
4		×			×		×				×		×		
2		×			×			×			×		×		
9			×	×				×			×		×		
3		×		×			×				×		×		
Total															
8	0	7	1	5	3	0	2	6	0	1	7	0	8	0	0
Ranks 1 to 4															
4	0	4	0	3	1	0	0	4	0	1	3	0	4	0	0
Ranks 5 to 8															
4	0	3	1	2	2	0	2	2	0	0	4	0	4	0	0
Percentage of total															
8	0.0	87.5	12.5	62.5	37.5	0.0	25.0	75.0	0.0	12.5	87.5	0.0	100.0	0.0	0.0
Ranks 1 to 4															
4	0.0	100.0	0.0	75.0	25.0	0.0	0.0	100.0	0.0	25.0	75.0	0.0	100.0	0.0	0.0
Ranks 5 to 8															
4	0.0	75.0	25.0	50.0	50.0	0.0	50.0	50.0	0.0	0.0	100.0	0.0	100.0	0.0	0.0

* Correct answer.

Question 2. When Nonfracture Patients Need to Begin Physical Therapy

Question 10. Concern About Patient Waiting

MD ID	a. The Next Day Agree*	Disagree	Don't Know	b. Within 3 Days Agree*	Disagree	Don't Know	c. By 7 Days Agree*	Disagree	Don't Know	d. By 14 Days Agree	Disagree*	Don't Know	Q10 Agree	Disagree*	Don't Know
8		X		X				X			X			X	
5		X		X				X			X			X	
6		X		X				X			X			X	
7	X				X			X			X			X	
4		X		X				X			X				X
2		X				X	X				X			X	
9	X				X			X			X		X		
3	X				X			X			X		X		
Total	3	5	0	4	3	1	1	7	0	0	8	0	2	5	1
Percentage of total	37.5	62.5	0.0	50.0	37.5	12.5	12.5	87.5	0.0	0.0	100.0	0.0	25.0	62.5	12.5
Ranks 1 to 4	1	3	0	3	1	0	0	4	0	0	4	0	0	4	0
Ranks 1 to 4 %	25.0	75.0	0.0	75.0	25.0	0.0	0.0	100.0	0.0	0.0	100.0	0.0	0.0	100.0	0.0
Ranks 5 to 8	2	2	0	1	2	1	1	3	0	0	4	0	2	1	1
Ranks 5 to 8 %	50.0	50.0	0.0	25.0	50.0	25.0	25.0	75.0	0.0	0.0	100.0	0.0	50.0	25.0	25.0

* Correct answer.

(continued)

TABLE A2.8 Responses to Physician Questionnaire (continued)

| | Question 7. When Fracture Patients Need to Have X Rays Ordered | | | | | | | | | Question 3. Residents Do Not Wait Too Long | | | Question 5. No Policy: Write PT Consult Order | | |
| | a. At Admission | | | b. Within 3 Days | | | c. By 7 Days | | | | | | | | |
MD ID	Agree*	Disagree	Don't Know	Agree	Disagree*	Don't Know	Agree	Disagree*	Don't Know	Agree	Disagree*	Don't Know	Agree*	Disagree	Don't Know
8	x				x			x		x			x		
5	x				x			x		x			x		
6		x			x			x		x			x		
7	x				x			x		x			x		
4			x	x			x			x					x
2	x				x			x				x		x	
9		x		x				x		x					x
3	x				x			x				x	x		
Total	5	2	1	2	6	0	1	7	0	6	0	2	5	1	2
Ranks 1 to 4	3	1	0	0	4	0	0	4	0	4	0	0	4	0	0
Ranks 5 to 8	2	1	1	2	2	0	1	3	0	2	0	2	1	1	2
Percentage of total	62.5	25.0	12.5	25.0	75.0	0.0	12.5	87.5	0.0	75.0	0.0	25.0	62.5	12.5	25.0
Ranks 1 to 4	75.0	25.0	0.0	0.0	100.0	0.0	0.0	100.0	0.0	100.0	0.0	0.0	100.0	0.0	0.0
Ranks 5 to 8	50.0	25.0	25.0	50.0	50.0	0.0	25.0	75.0	0.0	50.0	0.0	50.0	25.0	25.0	50.0

* Correct answer.

MD ID	Question 6. Likes Idea of Ordering Consult Ahead			Question 8. Feel Informed About PT Consult Steps			Question 9. Provide PT With Computerized Admit Data		
	Agree	Disagree	Don't Know	Agree	Disagree	Don't Know	Agree	Disagree	Don't Know
8		x				x	x		
5	x			x			x		
6		x			x		x		
7		x			x		x		
4		x		x					x
2	x				x		x		
9	x			x			x		
3	x				x		x		
Total 8	4	4	0	3	4	1	7	0	1
Ranks 1 to 4 4	1	3	0	1	2	1	4	0	0
Ranks 5 to 8 4	3	1	0	2	2	0	3	0	1
Percentage of total 8	50.0	50.0	0.0	37.5	50.0	12.5	87.5	0.0	12.5
Ranks 1 to 4 4	25.0	75.0	0.0	25.0	50.0	25.0	100.0	0.0	0.0
Ranks 5 to 8 4	73.0	25.0	0.0	50.0	50.0	0.0	75.0	0.0	25.0

NOTE: This was Table 2.5 for the project.

Table A2.9 Criteria for Proof of Causes and Results (Exercise)

Cause and Measure	Proof Required to Prove the Cause	OKed	Actual Results		Source

Client Risk Factors
Whether patient has a fracture

Proof Required to Prove the Cause: If fracture pts. have a higher % of patients waiting > 3 days than nonfracture patients waiting > 7 days; and if the average wait is longer for fracture patients

OKed: x

Actual Results:
	Fracture	Nonfracture
Percentage > 3 or 7	. %	. %
Average wait (days)	.	.

Source: Table 1.4

Whether patient came from

Hospital
Own home
Current resident

Proof Required to Prove the Cause: If within fracture and nonfracture groupings, pts. in one of the three categories has a higher % of pts. > limits and if the average wait is longer

OKed: x

Actual Results:
	Fracture Percentage > 3	Nonfracture Percentage > 7
over the limit		
Hospital	. %	. %
Own home	none	. %
Resident	. %	. %
Average wait	(days)	
Hospital	.	
Own home		.
Resident		

Source: Table 1.4

Whether starting or continuing physical therapy

Proof Required to Prove the Cause: As above

OKed: x

Actual Results:
	Fracture Percentage > 3	Nonfracture Percentage > 7
Starting	100.0%	60.7%
Continuing	100.0%	80.0%
Average wait	(days)	
Starting	11.5	
Continuing	11.6	

Source: Table 1.4 / Not proved

352

Diagnosis	Diagnosis as percentage of patients ranked 10 to 20 is more than 10% higher than its percentage of patients ranked 1 to 4 and its percentage of total patients is over 14%	x			

		Ranks 10 to 20		Ranks 1 to 4		Codesheet 2
		No.	%	No.	%	
	Patients	21		26		Proved for Fracture
	CVA	9	43%	12	46%	
	Fracture	6	29%	2	8%	
	Total CVA	30		% of pts:	41%	
	Total Fracture	14		% of pts:	19%	

Whether X rays and consults are needed (days to order and days to have done)	Special order's percentage of days over its limit is > 15% of total wait over the limit for all patients (428 days)	x		

Consult	Percentage days over limit	Percentage share days over limit	Codesheet
X ray	82.5%	11.0%	Table 2.1
Orthopedics	92.5%	17.3%	Table 2.3
Neurology, Cardiology	88.9%	5.6%	Proved for Orthopedic consult

Related to staff

Specific MDs	An MD ranks high in these criteria: 1. Rate of days over limit 2. Disproportionate share of days over limit for PT consult 3. Over limit for special orders 4. One to three MDs stand out	x		

MD ID	Final Rank	Rate of days over limit		Percentage of days over limit minus percentage of patients		Codesheet
		PTCO	Other	PTCO	Other	
8	1	75%	–	–1.7	–	Table 2.4
5	2	68%	0%	–7.0	–35.3	
6	3	81%	0%	–0.2	–5.9	Proved for MDs 2, 3, 9
7	4	62%	89%	–10.1	7.7	
4	5	82%	75%	–1.0	–4.5	
2	6	90%	100%	5.6	20.9	
9	7	87%	100%	3.4	15.0	
3	8	89%	100%	11.0	1.9	

(continued)

Table A2.9 Criteria for Proof of Causes and Results (Exercise) (continued)

Cause and Measure	Proof Required to Prove the Cause	OKed	Actual Results			Source
			Wrong answers			
			Q.1 %	Q.2 %	Q.7 %	
Knowledge that there are consequences of > 3 or 7 days delay	If 60% or more MDs do not answer 2 out of 3 correctly:	×	Total			Table 2.5
Question 1. Answer should be agree, a/b	When fracture patients should begin PT		Ranks 1-4 . %	. %	. %	
Question 2. Answer should be agree, a/b/c	When nonfracture patients should begin		5-8 . %	. %	. %	
Question 7. Answer should be agree, a	When X rays should be ordered and ranks 5 to 8 do worse					
			Disagree/ Don't Know Q.4 %	**Agree/ Don't Know** Q.10 %		
Unconcerned attitude towards the problem	If 60% or more answer Question 4 Disagree or Don't Know (concern for early PT)	×	Total	. %		Table 2.5
Question 4. Answer should be agree	Question 10 Agree/Don't Know (Not concerned; not a problem); and ranks		Ranks 1-4% . %	. %		
Question 10. Answer should be disagree	5 to 8 do worse (2 of 2)		5-8 . %	. %		
			Q.3	**Agree/ Don't Know** Q.3 %		
MDs not aware of problem	If 60% or more answer Agree or Don't Know or ranks 5 to 8 do worse: Residents don't wait too long	×	Total	. %		Table 2.4 Table 2.5
Question 3. Answer should be disagree			Ranks 1-4 . %			
			5-8 . %			

Related to Institution			Percentage over limit	Percentage of days over limit	
Specific steps	If percentage of days over the limit is > 20% and if this is > 15% of total days over limit (428)	x	1. Admit–Screening	56.4	13.3	Table 2.1
1. Time from admit to PT screening			2. Admit–X-ray order	103.2	7.5	Table 2.2
2. Time from admit to X-ray order	(For 2, 3, 4, just fracture patients)		3. X-ray order–X ray	57.7	3.5	Table 2.3
3. Time from X-ray order to visit	(Too few other MD consults to be considered here)		4. Orthopedic consult order–visit	85.7	9.8	Proved for Steps 5, 6, 7
4. Time from Orthopedic consult order to visit			5. *Admit–PTCO*	*89.9*	*85.3*	
5. Time from admit to PT consult order			6. *PTCO–PT request*	*76.8*	*33.2*	
6. Time from PT consult order to PT request for physiatrist			7. *PT request–PTSO*	*43.9*	*22.7*	
7. Time from request for physiatrist to PT start order			8. PTSO–Start	13.6	2.1	
8. Time from PT start order to PT start						

NOTE: Because of overlap, adds to more than 100%.

				Yes	No	
No defined policy related to how long a wait is allowed and when steps should occur	Interview with management finds there is no policy:	x	Policy on:			Interview
	1. When to write PT consult order		1. When consult		x	
	2. When to order X ray		2. When X rays		x	Proved
	3. When physiatrist responds to PT request		3. When physiatrist responds		x	
	4. Maximum wait for physical therapy		4. Maximum allowable waits		x	
	or					

(continued)

Table A2.9 Criteria for Proof of Causes and Results (Exercise) (continued)

Cause and Measure	Proof Required to Prove the Cause	OKed	Actual Results	Source
	If 60% or more answer Agree or Don't Know (no policy for how soon for PT consult order) to Question 5		Question 5. Agree / Don't Know Total ___ %	Table 2.5
The way the work is organized 1. No action prior to admit even if patient comes from a hospital	If verified in interview with management and if PT consult order is a problem or	x	1. PT consult order is a problem. Verified: there is no action prior to admit even if patient comes from a hospital.	Table 2.1 Table 2.2 Table 2.3
2. PT/X-ray/ortho-pedist orders not automatic on admit	If tests or consults are a problem or		2. Orthopedic consult is a problem. Verified X-ray orthopedic orders are not automatic on admit.	Proved for all four
3. Physiatrist acts once per week	If physiatrist visit is a problem or		3. Physiatrist visit is a problem. Verified physiatrist acts on Saturdays only	
4. PT waits for days physiatrist comes to issue request	If physiatrist visit is a problem and PT request is also a problem		4. Physiatrist visit & PT request both problems; verified PT waits until Friday.	
Other 5. Too many steps for patients to pass through	If residents don't have any step > 2 days but are above the limit anyway or	x	5. Percentage with total wait over and no step > 2 days: none	

356

No coverage for physiatrist when away	If more than 2 steps qualify as the longest step > 2 days over limit for > 10% of patients	x	Number of steps longest > 2 days over limit for 10 % or more of patients: 3 steps	Table 2.3 Proved
	If calculating the step without days psychiatrist was away makes the step less a problem by 1 day or more	x	Average days: Including days away / Excluding days away. Time from PT request to physiatrist order: 3.0 / 2.3. Total wait: 11.5 / 10.9	Table 2.2 Not proved
Physical Therapy does not have timely access to admission information (this affects step between admit notice and screen date).	If verified in interview with management and > 10% of residents wait more than 1 day for this step	x	Residents wait > 1 day: 28 of 74 residents is 37.8%. Verified: PT does not have timely access to admit information and this delays decision to screen	Interview Table 2.1 Proved
Lack of communication about the steps (MDs do not know what the steps are) Question 8. Answer would be Disagree or Don't Know	If 60% or more answer Disagree or Don't Know (don't know the steps) and ranks 5 to 8 do worse than 1 to 4	x	Question 8 Disagree/Don't Know. Total . % Ranks 1-4 . % 5-8 . %	Table 2.5

Table A2.10 Criteria for Proof of Causes and Results

Cause and Measure	Proof Required to Prove the Cause	OKed	Actual Results		Source
Client Risk Factors Whether patient has a fracture	If fracture pts. have a higher % of patients waiting 3 days than nonfracture patients waiting > 7 days; and if the average wait is longer for fracture patients	x	<u>Fracture</u> Percentage > 3 or 7 100.0% Average wait (days) 15.1	<u>Nonfracture</u> 60.0% 10.7	Table 1.4 Proved
Whether patient came from Hospital Own home Current Resident is	If within fracture and nonfracture groupings, pts. in one of the three categories has a higher % of pts. > limits and if the average wait is longer	x	Fracture Percentage <u>> 3</u> Percentage over the limit Hospital 100.0% Own home none Resident 100.0% Average wait Hospital Own home Resident	Nonfracture Percentage <u>> 7</u> 67.4% 25.0% 46.2% <u>(days)</u> 12.2 6.8 10.4	Table 1.4 Proved for Hospital (nonfracture)
Whether starting or continuing physical therapy	As above	x	Fracture Percentage <u>> 3</u> Starting 100.0% Continuing 100.0% Average wait Starting Continuing	Nonfracture Percentage <u>> 7</u> 60.7% 80.0% <u>(days)</u> 11.5 11.6	Table 1.4 Not proved

| Diagnosis | Diagnosis as percentage of patients ranked 10-20 is more than 10% higher than its percentage of patients ranked 1-4 and its percentage of total patients over 14% | x |

	Ranks 10 to 20		Ranks 1 to 4		
	No.	%	No.	%	
Patients	21		26		
CVA	9	43%	12	46%	
Fracture	6	29%	2	8%	
Total CVA:	30		% of pts:	41%	
Total Fracture:	14		% of pts:	19%	

Proved for Fracture

| Whether X rays and consults are needed (days to order and days to have done) | x |

Consult	Percentage days over limit	Percentage share days over limit
X ray	82.5%	11.0%
Orthopedics	92.5%	17.3%
Neurology, Cardiology	88.9%	5.6

Table 2.1
Table 2.3
Proved for Orthopedic consult

Related to staff

Specific MDs — An MD ranks high in these criteria:

1. Rate of days over limit
2. Disproportionate share of days over limit for PT consult
3. Or over limit for special orders
4. One to three MDs stand out

x

MD ID	Final Rank	Rate of days over limit		Percentage of days over limit minus percentage of patients	
		PTCO	Other	PTCO	Other
8	1	75%	–	-1.7	–
5	2	68%	0%	-7.0	-35.3
6	3	81%	0%	-0.2	-5.9
7	4	62%	89%	-10.1	7.7
4	5	82%	75%	-1.0	-4.5
2	6	90%	100%	5.6	20.9
9	7	87%	100%	3.4	15.0
3	8	89%	100%	11.0	1.9

Table 2.4
Proved for MDs 2, 3, 9

(continued)

Table A2.10 Criteria for Proof of Causes and Results (continued)

Cause and Measure	Proof Required to Prove the Cause	OKed	Actual Results				Source

Group 1

Cause and Measure	Proof Required to Prove the Cause	OKed		Wrong answers			Source
				Q.1 37.5%	Q.2 0.0%	Q.7 37.5%	
Knowledge that there are consequences of > 3/7 days delay	If 60% or more MDs do not answer 2 out of 3 correctly:	x	Total				Table 2.5
Question 1. Answer should be agree, a/b	When fracture patients should begin PT		Ranks				Not proved
Question 2. Answer should be agree, a/b/c	When nonfracture patients should begin		1-4	25.0%	0.0%	25.0%	
Question 7. Answer should be agree, a	When X rays should be ordered and ranks 5 to 8 do worse		5-8	50.0%	0.0%	50.0%	

Group 2

Cause and Measure	Proof Required to Prove the Cause	OKed		Disagree/ Don't Know	Agree/ Don't Know	Source
				Q.4 0.0%	Q.10 37.5%	
Unconcerned attitude toward the problem	If 60% or more answer Question 4 Disagree/Don't Know (concern for early PT)	x	Total			Table 2.5
Question 4. Answer should be agree	Question 10. Agree/Don't Know (Not concerned; not a problem), and ranks 5 to 8 do worse (2 of 2)		Ranks			Not proved
Question 10. Answer should be disagree			1-4	0.0%	0.0%	
			5-8	0.0%	75.0%	

Group 3

Cause and Measure	Proof Required to Prove the Cause	OKed		Agree/ Don't Know	Source
				Q.3	
MDs not aware of problem	If 60% or more answer Agree or Don't Know or ranks 5 to 8 do worse: Residents don't wait too long	x	Total	100.0%	Table 2.4
Question 3. Answer should be disagree			Ranks		Table 2.5
			1-4	100.0%	Proved for all
			5-8	100.0%	

Related to Institution

Specific steps

1. Time from admit to PT screening
2. Time from admit to X-ray order
3. Time from X-ray order to X ray
4. Time from Orthopedic consult order to visit
5. Time from admit to PT consult order
6. Time from PT consult order to PT request for physiatrist
7. Time from request for physiatrist to PT start order
8. Time from PT start order to PT start

If the percentage of days over the limit is > 20% and if this is > 15% of total days over the limit (428)   x

(For 2, 3, 4, just fracture patients)

(Too few other MD consults to be considered here)

	Percentage over limit	Percentage of days over limit	
1. Admit–Screening	56.4	13.3	Table 2.1
2. Admit–X-ray order	103.2	7.5	Table 2.2
3. X-ray order–X ray	57.7	3.5	Table 2.3
4. Orthopedic consult–visit	85.7	9.8	Proved for
5. *Admit–PTCO*	89.9	85.3	Steps 5, 6, 7
6. *PTCO–PT request*	76.8	33.2	
7. *PT request–PTSO*	43.9	22.7	
8. PTSO–Start	13.6	2.1	

NOTE: Because of overlap, adds to more than 100%.

No defined policy related to how long a wait is allowed and when steps should occur   x

Interview with management finds there is no policy:
1. When to write PT consult order
2. When to order X ray
3. When physiatrist responds to PT request
4. Maximum wait for physical therapy

or

Policy on:	Yes	No	
1. When consult		x	Interview
2. When X rays		x	
3. When physiatrist responds		x	Proved
4. Maximum allowable waits		x	

(continued)

Table A2.10 Criteria for Proof of Causes and Results (continued)

Cause and Measure	Proof Required to Prove the Cause	OKed	Actual Results	Source
	If 60% or more answer Agree or Don't Know (no policy for how soon for PT consult order) to Question 5		Question 5. Agree/ Don't Know / Total = 87.5%	Table 2.5
The way the work is organized 1. No action prior to admit even if patient comes from a hospital	If verified in interview with management and if PT consult order is a problem or	x	1. PT consult order is a problem. Verified: there is no action prior to admit even if patient comes from a hospital	Table 2.1 Table 2.2 Table 2.3
2. PT/X-ray/ortho-pedist orders not automatic on admit	If tests/consults are a problem or		2. Orthopedic consult is a problem. Verified: X-ray orthopedic orders are not automatic on admit.	Proved for all four
3. Physiatrist acts once per week	If physiatrist visit is a problem or		3. Physiatrist visit is a problem. Verified: physiatrist acts on Saturdays only	
4. Patient waits for days physiatrist comes to issue request	If physiatrist visit is a problem and PT request is also a problem		4. Physiatrist visit and PT request both problems. Verified: PT waits until Friday.	
Other 5. Too many steps for patients to pass through	If residents don't have any step > 2 days but are above the limit anyway or	x	5. Percentage with total wait over limit and no step > 2 days: none	

362

Issue	If criterion		Data / Results	Source / Status
	If more than 2 steps qualify as the longest step > 2 days over limit for > 10% of patients		Number of longest steps > 2 days over limit for 10% or more of patients: 3 steps	Table 2.3 Proved
No coverage for physiatrist when away	If calculating the step without days physiatrist was away makes the step less a problem by 1 day or more	x	Average days: Including days away / Excluding days away — Time from PT request to physiatrist order: 3.0 / 2.3; Total Wait: 11.5 / 10.9	Table 2.2 Not proved
Physical Therapy does not have timely access to admission information (This affects step between admit notice and screening date)	If verified in interview with management and > 10% of residents wait more than 1 day for this step	x	Residents wait > 1 day: 28 of 74 residents is 37.8%. Verified: PT does not have timely access to admit information, and this delays decision to screen	Interview Table 2.1 Proved
Lack of communication about the steps (MDs do not know what the steps are) Question 8. Answer would be Disagree or Don't Know	If 60% or more answer Disagree or Don't Know (don't know the steps) and ranks 5 to 8 do worse than 1 to 4	x	Question 8. Disagree/Don't Know — Total 62.5%; Ranks 1-4 75.0%; 5-8 50.0%	Table 2.5 Partly proved

Table A2.11 Causes, Constraints, and Solutions (Exercise)

Feasibility Limits:	1. No increase in nonmedical professional staff. 2. Additional documentation by MDs to be limited. 3. Additional costs not to exceed $1,000.

Causes Proved	*Solutions*
Physical Therapy does not have timely admission information	
Fracture patients PT, X-ray, & orthopedic consult orders not automatic at admission Response to X-ray order and order for orthopedist consult	
Patients coming from hospital	
Step covering PT consult order	
Step covering PT request for physiatrist Step covering physiatrist Physiatrist acts once per week	
Too many steps for patient to pass through	
No defined policy on wait for PT and individual steps	
Specific MDs MDs not aware of problem Lack of communication about the steps	

Exercise

Before looking at the actual proposals in Table A2.12, try the following exercise:

1. Fill in your own solutions on Table A2.11.
2. Write about your solution(s), explaining why you think they are relevant, feasible, and effective. The actual solutions are in Table A2.12.

Table A2.12 Causes, Constraints, and Solutions

Feasibility Limits: 1. No increase in nonmedical professional staff.
2. Additional documentation by MDs to be limited.
3. Additional costs not to exceed $1,000.

Causes Proved	*Solutions*
Physical Therapy does not have timely admission information	Set policy: Admission office will notify PT the same day a patient is adtted via an admission card. PT access to computerized admissions data will be suggested as part of ongoing expansion planning.
Fracture patients PT, X-ray, & orthopedic consult orders not automatic at admission Response to X-ray order and order for orthopedist consult	Set policy: New admissions or current residents with fracture must receive orders for X rays, orthopedic consult, and physical therapy consult upon admission or injury. X-ray and orthopedist orders and consults shall be answered promptly.
Patients coming from hospital Step covering PT consult order	Set policy: all new admissions and readmissions receiving physical therapy prior to admission must receive a PT consult order upon admission. All new admissions and readssions with recent diagnosis of fracture, CVA, amputation, and dementia must receive a PT consult order upon admission.
Step covering PT request for physiatrist Step covering physiatrist Physiatrist acts once per week	Physical therapy must screen the patient within one day of admission and notify physiatrist of a PT consult order the same day as the screening. The physiatrist shall be on call for acute fractures, will visit residents at once, shall answer PT consults 3 times per week, and may prescribe a weight-bearing status for a fracture and place the resident on program while waiting for an orthopedic consult to be answered.
Too many steps for patient to pass through	Steps reduced from 8 to 6: 1. PT consult, X-ray, and orthopedist consult orders automatic for fractures/PT candidates as appropriate 2. PT screens patient and requests physiatrist on admission 3. X-ray is taken for fracture patients 4. Physiatrist evaluates and orders PT program 5. Orthopedist answers consult order 6. PT program begins day after PT order is given
No defined policy on wait for PT and individual steps	Write policy: PT program begins within 3 days of admission for fracture patients and within 7 days of admission for patients without fractures. For steps, see above.
Specific MDs MDs not aware of problem Lack of communication about the steps	Each MD shall receive a copy of the new policy. MDs shall be made aware of problem or policy at a facility medical board meeting at which this report will be presented

Exercise

1. How do you think management responded to the suggestions in Table A2.12? Why?

2. Assuming that all the solutions proposed by Anna were accepted, answer the following questions:

   a. What changes in operations are being proposed?

   b. If there are any, state for each change the staff who will be involved.

   c. Which administrators have to be involved?

   d. Will anyone have resistance to the changes? Why? What would you do about it?

   e. Anything to be newly designed?

   f. If so, who will design it and who must approve?

   g. In what order should the changes be introduced?

   h. Describe what will now be different for each staff member involved.

   i. What meetings will be needed? When?

   j. Will any staff training be needed? If so, designed by whom? Given by whom? To whom? When?

   k. Will the changes affect the interface with any other departments? How? How will this be introduced?

   l. For each change, what could go wrong? How would you handle it?

   m. How long a period should elapse before the solution is evaluated?

   n. What data need to be collected to evaluate the solutions? When? For how long? Do you need new forms? New tables?

   o. What will be the success criteria to evaluate the solutions?

   p. What indicators would you recommend be adopted to monitor the solutions?

Note

1. Yvette L. Santana was the internal consultant for this project.

Background Reading
Related to the Cases

Case 1

Bobath, B. (1990). *Adult hemiplegia: Evaluation and treatment*. Oxford, England: Heinemann Medical.

Carey, R. G., Seibert, J. H., & Posavac, E. J. (1988, May). Who makes the most progress in inpatient rehabilitation? An analysis of functional gain. *Archives of Physical Medicine and Rehabilitation, 69*, 337-343.

Carr, J. H. & Shepard, R. B. (Eds.). (1987). *Movement science: Foundations for physical therapy in rehabilitation*. Gaithersburg, MD: Aspen.

Davies, P. M. (1985). *Steps to follow: A guide to treatment of adult hemiplegia*. New York: Springer-Verlag.

Dodds, T. A., Martin, D. P., Stolov, W. C., & Deyo, R. A. (1993, May). A validation of the functional independence measurement and its performance among rehabilitation inpatients. *Archives of Physical Medicine and Rehabilitation, 74*, 531-536.

Di Domenico, R. L. & Ziegler, W. Z. (1989). *Practical rehabilitation techniques for geriatric aides*. Gaithersbur, MD: Aspen.

Donatelli, R. & Owens-Burkhardt, H. (1981, Fall). Effects of immobilization on the extensibility of periarticular connective tissue. *Journal of Orthopedic and Sports Physical Therapy, 3*, 67-72.

Donnan, G. A. (1991, November). Early intervention in acute stroke. *Australian Family Physician, 20*, 1575-1580.

Foy, S. S. & Mitchell, M. M. (1990). Factors contributing to learned helplessness in the institutionalized aged: A literature review. *Physical and Occupational Therapy in Geriatrics, 9*, 1-23.

Hayes, S. H. & Carroll, S. R. (1986, May). Early intervention care in the acute stroke patient. *Archives of Physical Medicine and Rehabilitation, 67*, 319-321.

Kauffman, T. (1986, January-February). Skeletal muscle and the aging process: Implications for physical therapy. *Clinical Management in Physical Therapy, 6*, 18-21.

Kottke, F. J. (1966, June). The effects of limitation of activity upon the human body. *Journal of American Medical Association, 196*, 825-830.

Kottke, F. J. & Lehman, J. F. (Eds.). (1990). *Krusen's handbook of physical medicine and rehabilitation* (4th ed.). Philadelphia, PA: W. B. Saunders.

Lewis, C. B. (1989). *Improving mobility in older persons: A manual for geriatric specialists.* Gaithersburg, MD: Aspen.

Molloy, D. W., Beerschoten, D. A., Borrie, M. J., Crilly, R. G., & Cape, R. D. (1988, January). Acute effects of exercise on neuropsychological function in elderly subjects. *Journal of American Geriatric Society, 36,* 29-33.

O'Neil, M. B., Woodard, M., Susa, V., Hunter, L., Mulrow, C. D., Gerety, M. B., & Tuley, M. (1992, August). Physical therapy assessment and treatment protocol for nursing home residents. *Physical Therapy, 72,* 596-604.

O'Sullivan, S. B. & Schmitz, T. J. (1981). *Physical rehabilitation: Assessment and treatment* (2nd ed.). Philadelphia, PA: F. A. Davis.

Payton, O. D. & Poland, J. L. (1983, January). Aging process: Implications for clinical practice. *Physical Therapy, 63,* 41-48.

Petchers, M. K., Roy, A. W., & Brickner, A. (1987, December). A post-hospital nursing home rehabilitation program. *The Gerontologist, 27,* 752-755.

Rapoport, J. & Judd-Van Eerd, M. (1989, January). Impact of physical therapy weekend coverage on length of stay in an acute care community hospital. *Physical Therapy, 69,* 32-37.

Richards, C. L., Malouin, F, Wood-Dauphinee, S., Williams, J. I., Bouchard, J. P., & Brunet, D. (1993, June). Task-specific physical therapy optimization of gait recovery in acute stroke patients. *Archives of Physical Medicine and Rehabilitation, 74,* 612-620.

Somers, F. P. (1991, July). Long term care and federal policy. *American Journal of Occupational Therapy, 45,* 628-635.

Stewart, D. L. & Abeln, S. H. (Eds.). (1993). Documenting functional outcomes in physical therapy. St. Louis, MO: C. V. Mosby.

Thompson, R. F., Crist, D. M., Marsh, M., & Rosenthal, M. (1988, February). Effects of physical exercise for elderly patients with physical impairments. *Journal of the American Geriatric Society, 36,* 130-135.

Umphred, D. A. (Ed.). (1990). *Neurological rehabilitation* (2nd ed.). St. Louis, MO: C. V. Mosby.

Case 2

German, K., Nuwahid, F., Matthews, P., & Stephenson, T. (1993, February). Dangers of long waiting times for outpatient appointments at a urology clinic. *British Medical Journal, 306,* 429.

Hancock, W. M. & Isken, M. W. (1992, November). Patient scheduling methodologies. *Journal of Social Health Systems, 3,* 83-94.

Schneider, G. (1992, June). A new approach to staying on time. *Journal of Clinical Orthodontics, 26,* 344-346.

Shanks, J. (1993, January 2). Asking patients about their treatment. *British Medical Journal, 306,* 65.

Swage, T. & Mudd, D. (1993, March 6). Waiting times for outpatient appointments. *British Medical Journal, 306,* 657.

Case 3

Bozzo, P. (1991). *Implementing quality assurance*. Chicago: American Society of Clinical Pathologists.

Clevenger, R. R. (1985, May). A protocol for verifying critical values. *Medical Laboratory Observer, 17*, 72-74, 76.

Jahn, M. (1993, September). Stats too high, yet labs cope: Turnaround time, Part 2. *Medical Laboratory Observer, 25*, 33-38.

Kaufman, H. W. & Collins, C. (1994, August). Notifying clients of life threatening results. *Medical Laboratory Observer, 26*, 44-45.

Kost, G. J. (1990, February 2). Critical limits for urgent clinician notification at US medical centers. *Journal of the American Medical Association, 263*, 704-707.

Kost, G. J. (1993, March). Using critical limits to improve patient outcomes. *Medical Laboratory Observer, 25*, 22-27.

Lundberg, G. D. (1990, February 2). Critical (panic) value notification: An established laboratory practice policy. *Journal of the American Medical Association, 263*, 709.

Martin, B. G. & Kurec, A. S. (1989). Staffing and scheduling of laboratory personnel. In J. R. Synder & D. A. Senhauser (Eds.), *Administration and supervision in laboratory medicine* (pp. 199-217). Philadelphia, PA: J. B. Lippincott.

Mass, D. (1989). Motivation-managerial assumptions and effects. In J. R. Synder & D. A. Senhauser (Eds.), *Administration and supervision in laboratory medicine* (pp. 66-72). Philadelphia, PA: J. B. Lippincott.

Peterson, P. & Emancipator, K. (1994, September 14). *Critical values: No need to panic* (teleconference). New York: American Society of Clinical Pathologists.

Steindel, S. J. (1994, March). Critical values: When they're reported, how they're used. *CAP Today, 8*, 22-26.

Case 4

Butler, D. J., Turkal, N. W., & Seidl, J. J. (1992, January-February). Amputation: Preoperative psychological preparation. *Journal of the American Board of Family Practice, 5*, 69-73.

Carey, R. G., Seibert, J. H., & Posavac, E. J. (1988, May). Who makes the most progress in inpatient rehabilitation? An analysis of functional gain. *Archives of Physical Medicine and Rehabilitation, 69*, 337-343.

Chan, K. M. & Tan, E. S. (1990, November). Use of lower limb prosthesis among elderly amputees. *Annals of the Academy of Medicine, Singapore, 6*, 811-816.

Daly, R. & Flynn, R. J. (1985). A brief consumer satisfaction scale for use in in-patient rehabilitation programs. *International Journal of Rehabilitation Research, 8*, 335-338.

Gerhards, F., Florin, I., & Knapp, T. (1984). The impact of medical reeducational and psychological variables on rehabilitation outcomes in amputees. *International Journal of Rehabilitation Research, 7*, 379-388.

Goldberg, R. T. (1984, January). New trends in the rehabilitation of lower extremity amputees. *Journal of Rehabilitation Literature, 45*, 2-11.

Kerstein, M. D., Zimmer, H., Dugdale, F. E., & Lerner, E. (1974, October). Amputations of the lower extremity: A study of 194 cases. *Archives of Physical Medicine and Rehabilitation, 55,* 454-459.

Klein, D. & Campbell, A. (1995, June-July). The CQI pathway: Botsford General Hospital utilized Continuous Quality Improvement to decrease the length of stay for amputee patients. *Rehab Management, 8,* 89-90, 92, 94-95. [This article appeared after the Case 4 study was completed. It is interesting because it used the CQI root-cause (fishbone diagram) approach to finding causes. The causes found were essentially the same as in Case 4 but did not include *as many* and missed several that may have been equally relevant, given the Case 4 results.]

Torres, M. M. & Esquenazi, A. (1991, May). Bilateral lower limb amputee rehabilitation. A retrospective review. *Western Journal of Medicine, 5,* 583-586.

Case 5

Cooper, P. & Butterbaugh, D. (1993, Spring). Health service development for physician/medical records: A 1980s model, a 1990s application and refinement. *Health Care Management Review, 18,* 7-14.

Davidhizar, R. & Policinski, H. (1994, March). Getting along with the difficult physician. *Health Care Supervisor, 3,* 11-16.

Friedman, B. A. (1985, November). A streamlined system for test requisitions. *Medical Laboratory Observer, 17,* 74-78.

Larson, E. B., Donell, S., & Scott, D. H. (1984, November). Inadequate medical order writing and delivery. *Quality Review Bulletin, 10,* 353-355.

Case 6

Brashear, H. R. & Raney, R. B. (1986). *Handbook of orthopaedic surgery* (10th ed.). St. Louis, MO: C. V. Mosby.

Buckwald, E., Rusk, H. A., Deaver, G. G., & Covalt, D. A. (1952). *Physical rehabilitation for daily living.* New York: McGraw Hill.

Chabas, D. & Scheiber, M. (1986, December). Suprascapular neuropathy related to use of crutches. *American Journal of Physical Medicine, 5,* 298-300.

Cozen, L. (1984, January). Walking aids: Select the right one, teach its use, and avoid damage elsewhere. *Consultant, 24,* 268-273, 276.

Lawton, E. B. (1963). *Activities of daily living for physical rehabilitation.* New York: McGraw Hill.

Palmer, M. L. & Toms, J. E. (1980). *Manual for functional training* (3rd ed.). Philadelphia, PA: F. A. Davis.

Case 7

Corbett, J. V. (1987). *Laboratory tests and diagnostic procedures with nursing diagnoses* (2nd ed.). Norwalk, CT: Appleton & Lange.

Devgun, M. S. (1989). Delay in centrifugation and measurement of serum constituents in normal subjects. *Clinical Physiology and Biochemistry, 34,* 189-197.

Garza, D. & Becan-McBride, K. (1989). *Phlebotomy handbook* (2nd ed.). Norwalk, CT: Appleton & Lange.

Greenson, J. K., Farber, S. J., & Dubin, S. B. (1989, February). The effects of hemolysis on creatine kinase determination. *Archives of Pathology Laboratory Medicine, 113,* 184-185.

Lynch, M. J. & Raphael, S. S. (1983). *Lynch's medical laboratory technology* (4th ed.). Philadelphia, PA: W. B. Saunders.

O'Bannan, R. H. (1988, November). The effects of improper specimen handling on lab tests. *Medical Laboratory Observer, 11,* 42-47.

Pai, S. H., Marie, & Cyr-Manthey, M. (1991, June). Effects of hemolysis on chemistry tests. *Laboratory Medicine, 22,* 408-410.

Walters, N. J., Estridge, B. H., & Reynolds, A. P. (1996). *Basic medical laboratory techniques* (3rd ed.). Albany, NY: Delmar.

Zilva, J. F., Pennall, P. R., & Mayne, P. D. (1988). *Clinical chemistry in diagnosis and treatment* (5th ed.). Chicago, IL: Year Book Medical.

Case 8

Allan, E. L. & Barker, K. N. (1990, March). Fundamentals of medication error research. *American Journal of Hospital Pharmacy, 47,* 555-571.

Barker, K. N. & Pearson, R. E. (1992). Medication distribution systems. In T. R. Brown (Ed.), *Handbook of institutional pharmacy practice* (pp. 325-361). Bethesda, MD: Society of Health-System Pharmacists.

Becker, M. D., Johnson, M. H., & Longe, L. R. (1978, April). Errors remaining in unit dose carts after checking by pharmacists versus pharmacy technicians. *American Journal of Hospital Pharmacy, 35,* 432-434.

Buchanan, T. L., Barker, K. N, Gibson, J. T., Jiang, B. C., & Pearson, R. E. (1991, October). Illumination and errors in dispensing. *American Journal of Hospital Pharmacy, 48,* 2137-2145.

McGhan, W. F., Smith, W. E., & Adams, D. W. (1983, April). A randomized trial comparing pharmacists and technicians as dispensers of prescriptions for ambulatory patients. *Medical Care, 21,* 445-453.

Means, B. J., Derewicz, H. J., & Lamy, P. P. (1975, February). Medication errors in a multidose and a computer-based unit dose drug distribution system. *American Journal of Hospital Pharmacy, 32,* 186-191.

Taylor, J. & Gaucher, M. (1986, February). Medication selection errors made by pharmacy technicians in filling unit dose orders. *Canadian Journal of Hospital Pharmacy, 39,* 9-12.

Case 9

Lewis, H. W. (1990). *Technological risk*. New York: W. W. Norton.

Lofgren, D. J. (1989). *Dangerous premises: An insider's view of OSHA enforcement*. Ithaca, NY: New York School of Industrial and Labor Relations Press.

Moeller, D. W. (1992). *Environmental health*. Cambridge, MA: Harvard University Press.

New York State Department of Labor. (1987). *Toxic substances information, training, and education* (Part 820, §§ 820.1-820.7). Albany, NY: New York State Department of Labor.

Puckett, S. B. & Emery, A. R. (1988). *Managing AIDS in the workplace*. Reading, MA: Addision-Wesley.

White, L. (1983). *Human debris: The injured worker in America*. New York, NY: Seaview/Putnam.

Case 10

Austin, E. K. (1981). *Guidelines for the development of continuing education offerings for nurses*. New YorK: Appleton-Century-Crofts.

Chu, L. K. & Chu, G. S. (1991, February). Feedback and efficiency: A staff development model. *Nursing Management, 22*, 28-31.

Hedlund, N. L. (1991, April). How can I, as a nurse manager, help staff nurses function? *Journal of Nursing Quality Assurance, 3*, 75-77.

Jacobsma, B. (1991, February). A balancing act: Continuing education for staff nurses. *Journal of Psychosocial Nursing and Mental Health Services, 29*, 15-21.

Katz, J. M. (1991, January). Quality monitoring and evaluation in staff development. *Journal of Nursing Staff Development, 7*, 15-20.

Puetz, B. E. (1987). *Contemporary strategies for continuing education in nursing*. Gaithersburg, MD: Aspen.

Tobin, H. E., Yoder-Wise, P. S., & Hull, P. K. (1979). *The process of staff development: Components for change* (2nd ed.). St. Louis, MO: C. V. Mosby.

Case 11

Badzek, L. A. (1992, June). What you need to know about advance directives. *Nursing '92, 22*, 58-59.

Davidson, K. W., Hackler, C., Caradine, D. R., & McCord, R. S. (1989, November). Physicians' attitudes on advance directives. *Journal of the American Medical Association, 262*, 2415-2419.

Emanuel, L. L., Barry, M. J., Stoeckle, J. D., Ettelson, L. M., & Emanuel, E. J. (1991, March 28). Advance directives for medical care: A case for greater use. *New England Journal of Medicine, 324*, 889-895.

LaPuma, J., Orentlicher, D., & Moss, R. I. (1991, July 17). Advance directives on admission: Clinical implications and analysis of the Patient Self Determination Act of 1990. *Journal of the American Medical Association, 266,* 402-405.

Tolmie, M. E. (1992, May). Discuss advance directives. *Nursing 1992, 22,* 8.

Case 12

Austin, S. M., Balas, E. A., Mitchell, J. A., & Ewigman, B. G. (1994). Effect of physician reminders on preventive care: Meta-analysis of randomized clinical trials. *Proceedings of the Annual Symposium of Computer Applications in Medical Care,* 121-124 (Program in Health Services Management, U. of Missouri-Columbia. Grant No.: HS 07268 HS AHCPR).

Banks, N. J. & Palmer, R. H. (1990. July-August). Clinical reminders in ambulatory care. *HMO Practice, 4,* 131-136.

Berger, D., Braverman, A., Sohn, C. K., & Morrow, M. (1989, April 1). Patient compliance with aggressive multimodal therapy in locally advanced breast cancer. *Cancer, 61,* 1453-1456.

Coffey, R. J., Harrison, B. J., Bedrosian, D. S., Mueller, M. M., & Steele, A. M. (1991). Computerized clinic scheduling system at the University of Michigan Medical Center. *Journal of Society for Health Systems, 2,* 81-89.

Curran, J. S. & Halpert, R. D. (1989, Winter). Patient no-shows—A costly problem. *Radiology Management, 1,* 20-23.

Davidson, R. A., Fletcher, S. W., Retchins, S., & Duh, S. (1984, November). A nurse-initiated reminder system for the periodic health examination. Implementation and evaluation. *Archives of Internal Medicine, 11,* 2167-2170.

Frame, P. S., Zimmer, J. G., Werth, P. L., & Martens, W. B. (1991, September-October). Description of a computerized health maintenance tracking system for primary care practice. *American Journal of Preventive Medicine, 7,* 311-318.

Garr, D. R., Ornstein, S. M., Jenkins, R. G., & Zemp, L. D. (1993, January-February). The effect of routine use of computer-generated preventive reminders in a clinical practice. *American Journal of Preventive Medicine, 9,* 55-61.

Garrett, T. J., Ashford, A., Savage, D. G., & Garret, T. J. (1986, August 1). Oncology clinic attendance at an inner city hospital. *Cancer, 58,* 793-795.

Gruzd, D. C., Shear, C. L., & Rodney, W. M. (1986, July-August). Determinants of no-show appointment behavior: The utility of multivariate analysis. *Family Medicine, 18,* 217-220.

Hoagland, A. C., Morrow, G. R., Bennett, J. M., & Carnrike, C. L. (1983, April). Oncologists' views of cancer patient noncompliance. *American Journal of Clinical Oncology, 6,* 239-244.

Kinne, D. W. (1991). The surgical management of primary breast cancer. *Ca—Cancer Journal for Clinicians, 41,* 71-84.

Manfredi, C., Lacey, L., & Warnecke, R. (1990, January). Results of an intervention to improve compliance with referrals for evaluation of suspected malignancies at neighborhood public health centers. *American Journal of Public Health, 80,* 85-87.

Moran, W. D., Nelson, K, Wofford, J. L., & Velez, R. (1992, September-October). Computer-generated mailed reminders for influenza immunization: A clinical trial. *Journal of General Internal Medicine, 7*, 535-537.

Moser, S. E. (1994, September). Effectiveness of postcard appointment reminders. *Family Practice Research Journal, 14*, 281-288.

Quattlebaum, T. G., Darden, P. M., & Sperry, J. B. (1991, October). Effectiveness of computer-generated appointment reminders. *Pediatrics, 88*, 801-805.

Case 13

Health Care Financing Administration. (1988). *483-Interpretive guidelines: Intermediate care facilities for the mentally retarded.* New York: United States Department of Health and Human Services.

Health Care Financing Administration. (1991-1992). *Statement of deficiencies and plan of corrections.* New York: United States Department of Health and Human Services.

New York State Commission on Quality Care for the Mentally Disabled. (1990-1991). Annual report.

Case 14

Cummins, R. O., Chesemore, K., & White, R. D. (1990, August 22). Defibrillator failures. Causes of problems and recommendations for improvement. Defibrillator Working Group. *Journal of the American Medical Association, 264*, 1019-1025.

Dickinson, E. (1991, May). Who's in charge? *Emergency, 23*, 30-59.

Gibbs, W., Eisenberg, M., & Damon, S. K. (1990, March). Dangers of defibrillation: Injuries to emergency personnel during patient resuscitation. *American Journal of Emergency Medicine, 8*, 101-104.

Lightfoot, S. (1992, February). First responder defibrillation. *Emergency, 24*, 33-35.

Lipton, H. (1990, March). A call gone bad. *Emergency, 22*, 16-17.

Mercer, S. (1993, February). Automated external defibrillation. *Emergency, 25*, 36-39.

Rod, R. (1991, May). Stand back for P.D. *Emergency, 23*, 43-45.

White, R. D. (1993, February). Maintenance of defibrillators in a state of readiness. *Annals of Emergency Medicine, 22*, 302-306.

White, R. D. & Chesemore, K. F. (1992, April). Charge! FDA recommendations for maintaining defibrillator readiness. *Journal of Emergency Medical Services, 17*, 70-72, 82.

Index